Algorithms for Intelligen

MW00574838

Series Editors

Jagdish Chand Bansal, Department of Mathematics, South Asian University, New Delhi, Delhi, India

Kusum Deep, Department of Mathematics, Indian Institute of Technology Roorkee, Roorkee, Uttarakhand, India

Atulya K. Nagar, School of Mathematics, Computer Science and Engineering, Liverpool Hope University, Liverpool, UK

This book series publishes research on the analysis and development of algorithms for intelligent systems with their applications to various real world problems. It covers research related to autonomous agents, multi-agent systems, behavioral modeling, reinforcement learning, game theory, mechanism design, machine learning, meta-heuristic search, optimization, planning and scheduling, artificial neural networks, evolutionary computation, swarm intelligence and other algorithms for intelligent systems.

The book series includes recent advancements, modification and applications of the artificial neural networks, evolutionary computation, swarm intelligence, artificial immune systems, fuzzy system, autonomous and multi agent systems, machine learning and other intelligent systems related areas. The material will be beneficial for the graduate students, post-graduate students as well as the researchers who want a broader view of advances in algorithms for intelligent systems. The contents will also be useful to the researchers from other fields who have no knowledge of the power of intelligent systems, e.g. the researchers in the field of bioinformatics, biochemists, mechanical and chemical engineers, economists, musicians and medical practitioners.

The series publishes monographs, edited volumes, advanced textbooks and selected proceedings.

More information about this series at http://www.springer.com/series/16171

Praveen Kumar Khosla · Mamta Mittal ·
Dolly Sharma · Lalit Mohan Goyal
Editors

Predictive and Preventive Measures for Covid-19 Pandemic

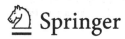 Springer

Editors
Praveen Kumar Khosla
Centre for Development of Advanced
Computing (C-DAC),
Ministry of Electronics & IT
Mohali, Punjab, India

Mamta Mittal
Department of Computer Science
and Engineering
G. B. Pant Government Engineering College
New Delhi, India

Dolly Sharma
Department of Computer Science
and Engineering
Amity University
Noida, Uttar Pradesh, India

Lalit Mohan Goyal
Department of Computer Engineering
J. C. Bose University of Science
and Technology
Faridabad, India

ISSN 2524-7565   ISSN 2524-7573   (electronic)
Algorithms for Intelligent Systems
ISBN 978-981-33-4235-4   ISBN 978-981-33-4236-1   (eBook)
https://doi.org/10.1007/978-981-33-4236-1

This Springer imprint is published by the registered company Springer Nature Singapore Pte Ltd.
The registered company address is: 152 Beach Road, #21-01/04 Gateway East, Singapore 189721,
Singapore

Preface

COVID-19 is as of now one of the most hazardous diseases around the globe. The spread is such that it has crossed every single geological limit. As COVID-19 spreads over the world, information about the infected people, messages on preventive measures and updates on cures are of most extreme significance. The need of the hour is to focus on quick and precise detection, extraction of graphical features, clinical analysis, develop medicates/drugs quicker, anticipate the spread of the ailment, foresee the next pandemic and so forth. The necessity is to investigate the help of new advancements like artificial intelligence (AI), big data, computer vision and machine learning to battle against the new novel coronavirus. This pandemic has set off an extraordinary interest for advanced well-being innovation like digital health technology solutions and releasing information to prevail upon this pandemic. Prevention from this disease is possible only if its propagation can be restricted. Thus, this book focuses on the predictive and preventive measures to be taken during this pandemic. It has been organized into 17 chapters.

Chapter 1 "Mitigate the Impact of Covid-19: Telehealth" discusses that COVID-19 pandemic has accelerated the adoption of telemedicine solutions which obviate the need of in-person consultation. This elucidates the top-line telemedicine solutions prevalent in India and USA which can be embraced by the readers. Under the leadership of leading author of this chapter, a team rolled out two variants of telemedicine solutions for use by national populace. One facilitates doctor-to-doctor consultations and the other patient-to-doctor consultations. Both solutions put together have logged more than 10,00,000 consultations as of December, 2020. More than 30,000 doctors have been onboarded at national level. In a short span of its rollout, it has emerged as the largest solution although several Indian organizations are active in this domain for the last two decades. Its mandated use of Web app, mobile app, cloud services and video conference services is capable of handling more than 25000 hits/sec. Its uniqueness lies in forwarding the consultation to the next higher hope if higher level of specialization needs to be referred. The design and implementation of Indian National Telemedicine Solution is a perfect case for adoption by fast-spreading community of telemedicine providers and aspirants. It makes it amply clear that teleconsultation is much more than just the two-way audio–video chat.

Chapter 2 "Epidemic Models in Prediction of COVID-19" discusses the role of COVID-19 data assessment and reviewed epidemic models. The impact of self-quarantine and isolation in control of COVID-19 among individuals to have a better contribution toward the well-being of nationalities has presented. They further discussed that, researchers are focusing on developing epidemic models to forecast risk severity by the use of country-wise data and since no approved vaccination or immediate medicine to cure of COVID-19 other than controlling virus spread by isolation, testing, and contact tracing is possible.

Chapter 3 "SIQRS Epidemic Modelling and Stability Analysis of COVID-19" presents the spread of COVID-19 infectious immigrants with effect of quarantine which is investigated using SIQRS epidemic model. The rate of natural death in COVID-19 is embedded in this model. The mathematical equations are solved using Runge–Kutta fourth-order method carried by the numerical simulation and graphical interpretation using MATLAB software. Authors have discussed the stability analysis of infection-free and endemic equilibrium with the help of basic reproduction number. It has also observed that the endemic infective class size decreases in quarantine class, which also leads to disease extinction.

Chapter 4 "Mental Health Analysis of Students in Major Cities of India During COVID-19" analyzes psychological stress due to COVID-19 pandemic through user-generated content on Twitter for major cities of India. In this study, the lexica relating to depression has been used for identifying depressing tweets. The depressing content has been analyzed for major cities of India. The results show that there exists a relational pattern between the number of coronavirus cases, number of recovered cases and the total number of depressing tweets. A sentiment analysis of the tweets has been carried out to determine the severity of psychological stress level among general public. Further, the results have been compared for four major cities of India, viz. Rajasthan, Delhi, Mumbai and Bangalore. Finally, a demographic categorization has been made based on the sentiment analysis results.

Chapter 5 "Analyzing the Impact on Online Teaching Learning Process on Education System During New Corona Regime Using Fuzzy Logic Techniques" studies the impact of lockdown on the teaching–learning process, with the objective to assess the quality of online classes and challenges associated with them. The study is based on responses from students of diverse academic backgrounds of education institutions of Punjab region. Responses related to online teaching have been collected, processed and analyzed on various parameters, using fuzzy logic techniques for studying the impact of online teaching–learning process on the education system during corona regime.

Chapter 6 "Healthcare 4.0 in Future Capacity Building for Pandemic Control" explains the status of telemedicine in different countries, technologies that can further improve the status, and how it has emerged as a priceless boon for COVID and non-COVID patients. There is a paradigm shift in healthcare services since the spread of this pandemic. It is no doubt true that telemedicine has emerged as the essential technology in these times as it minimizes the point of contact between patients and doctors. Though it is not yet adopted widely, still it has a vast potential and has grown exponentially since the spread of the disease. It has undoubtedly replaced the conventional method of providing medical services. Moreover, tele-medicine has bridged several gaps in the healthcare sector including the shortage of doctors, access to rural areas and others and can bring about a revolution in the health sector.

Chapter 7 "Preventive Behavior Against COVID 19: Role of Psychological Factors" focuses on the psychological factors influencing preventive behavior against COVID 19. Personal protective practices such as hand hygiene, use of face mask and social distancing are being suggested by the health officials as preventive behavior against COVID 19. Since these preventive measures are largely behavioral, psychological factors need to be considered in context to the preventive behavior against COVID-19. Significant association of preventive behavior with psychological factors like perceived susceptibility, severity, risk and fear of a disease has been reported. Adherence of the general public to the recommendations of the health officials helps in mitigating and management of COVID-19.

Chapter 8 "Impact of the COVID-19 on Consumer Behavior Towards Organic Food in India" includes the social and economic behavior of consumers in food sector during COVID-19, how consumer will behave after pandemic attack of corona in organic food sector, and what is the future of organic food market in India after COVID-19. Due to unavailability of vaccine against coronavirus, the people recognize immunity as ammunition against coronavirus. So, now, they understand the value of nutritive food which can increase their immune system and prevent from coronavirus. There is a huge opportunity in the Indian market to motivate the consumer to buy more and more organic food; it is time to shift from conventional food to organic food. The data has been observed by ASSOCHEM Indian organic food market which is going to be raised by 40,000 million to approximately 1,20,000 million in 2020 after COVID-19.

Chapter 9 "Socioeconomic Impacts and Opportunities of COVID-19 for Nepal" aims to examine the socioeconomic and health impacts of COVID-19. It is based on secondary data, a review of budget statements, policy intervention and documents related to COVID-19 and its consequences. This also rings true in Nepal, where reports are increasingly coming that the poor became more vulnerable to the COVID-19. The disruption of transportation and human movement as a part of containing COVID-19 has troubled socioeconomic activities and resulted in a health crisis in Nepal. Nevertheless, this chapter further argues that the crisis of COVID-19 will eventually lead to an opportunity in terms of reforms in the socioeconomic and health sectors in Nepal.

Chapter 10 "Strategic Decision in Long and Short Run for Cross-Country Commodity Market in the Post-COVID 19 Era" accepts the price association and dependencies for agricultural products which is one of the biggest challenges mainly when there is an outbreak of COVID-19. As per this issue, the present research considers few selected food crops, i.e., corn, wheat, rice and soy for three different countries, i.e., USA, India and China, to identify price movements and price associations in the short and long run. This outcome is beneficial mainly to the farmers in price fixation and decision on trading at the national or international platform; this is also useful for the investors to invest in agro-sectors in post-COVID-19 eras rather than investing in an unpredictable stock market or indices.

Chapter 11 "Prediction of Novel Coronavirus (nCOVID-19) Propagation Based on SEIR, ARIMA and Prophet Model" develops mathematical and prediction models of a new coronavirus (nCoVid19). The forecasting system and mathematical modeling of real-world dataset have been a challenge. They have presented the modeling based on SEIR by formulating the fractional equation for real-time data and also modeled how the infection decreases if people maintain social distancing. The predictions are done by ARIMA and Prophet models in order to analyze the spread of virus. The proposed novel methodology yields better results and establishes the importance of social distancing.

Chapter 12 "Innovative Strategies to Understand and Control COVID-19 Disease" presents that SARS-CoV-2 is closely related to the bat coronavirus RaTG13. A mutation in the spike S-protein is under the scrutiny for its possible role in an increased degree of contagiousness over earlier coronaviruses. Pathogenicity of SARS-CoV-2 is being understood with every growing number of COVID-19 patients and accumulated clinical data. The scientific and medical world has accelerated the pace of research in search of effective vaccines; as of now, there are 321 vaccine candidates, 32 of which are under trials. Besides a worldwide medical and health emergency, COVID-19 has hit the economies and societies very hard. Hence, there is an urgent need for developing innovative approaches for proper utilization of technologies to control infections, reduce pathogenicity, treat the patients and develop post-COVID-19 care.

Chapter 13 "An Investigation on COVID 19 Using Big Data Analytics and Artificial Intelligence" presents that big data and data analytics are quite helpful techniques to predict and to find the recovery and mortality rate in many hospitals of many countries. Thus, authors have compared three different data analytic models—logistic regression, Kaplan–Meier analysis and SIR models—used for prediction of COVID-19 using myocardial injury dataset and concluded with a favorable result on the SIR model. The challenges so far faced by big data and data analytics add a recommendation for other countries to get involved with big data and data analytics on COVID-19.

Chapter 14 "Rise of Online Teaching and Learning Processes During COVID-19 Pandemic" raises, discusses and presents potential solutions to different affairs of the online teaching and learning process and presents a comparative analysis of Internet-based educational/teaching platforms being employed by educational practitioners all around the world during the global COVID-19 crises. It also analyzes a brief survey on Indian teachers about their experiences, expectations and suggestions on online teaching and learning practices.

Chapter 15 "Robotic Technology for Pandemic Situation" imparts the knowledge that the automatic robots can be employed to maintain the protocol of social distancing that helps to break the chain of virus transmission. To make the medical staff's work easy and to minimize the exposure and direct contact to the deadly virus, a feasible idea would be to employ robots that are fully automated in its functioning and are competent in performance. They can be used for different purposes like cleaning the floors and automatic cleaning of toilets. They can also be employed to visit patients at regular intervals of time to provide food, medicines, checking temperature, etc., and help the frontline workers in this pandemic situation.

Chapter 16 "Face Mask Detection Using AI" discusses the artificial intelligence and its subsets, namely machine learning, deep learning and deep learning frameworks followed by a simple implementation for face mask detection system. This system enables to identify who is without a required face mask. These systems work with the existing surveillance systems along with innovative neural network algorithms to check whether a person has worn a face mask or not. Thus, this system can be very helpful in taking preventive measures and can be considered as COVID tracking tools for safety.

Chapter 17 "Machine Learning Tools to Predict the Impact of Quarantine" presents various machine learning models that are being explored by the researchers to develop tools to help in quantifying the effects of considering quarantine as a measure in several parts of the world. Neural network-based model, big data dashboards and crowd counting algorithms using CNN are being developed by various countries to monitor the impact of virus in various regions. This chapter attempts to provide a thorough investigation and insights into various machine learning tools and technologies which could help in measuring the effects of quarantine and isolation strategies adopted. The learning from the case studies can benefit the researchers to focus on building more effective tools around these concepts.

The editors are very thankful to all the members of Springer (India) Private Limited, especially Prof. J. C. Bansal and Aninda Bose for the given opportunity to edit this book.

Mohali, India	Praveen Kumar Khosla
New Delhi, India	Mamta Mittal
Noida, India	Dolly Sharma
Faridabad, India	Lalit Mohan Goyal

Contents

Editors and Contributors

About the Editors

Dr. Praveen Kumar Khosla received M.Tech. in Electronics & Communication from National Institute of Technology, Kurukshetra. He was awarded University Medal for being a topper. He passed Ph.D. in Electronics & Communication from Thapar University. He has recently passed a course in Advance Artificial Intelligence in Cyber Security from Carnegie Melon University, USA. He joined DRDO as Scientist B in 1986. He rose to become Scientist G in 2014. In the intervening period, he was Founder of Embedded Systems Division of TBRL. The embedded products developed under his leadership have been successfully inducted into on-board systems such as missiles and aircraft. In 2018, he took over C-DAC, Mohali, as Executive Director. At C-DAC, he is working in the field of cyber security, healthcare technologies, e-governance, agri-electronics and artificial intelligence. Cyber threat management system and national tele-consultation systems, which were developed under his leadership, have been successfully delivered to national level agencies. He is instrumental in bringing a turnaround in C-DAC Mohali in 2019–2020. He has published in several national and international journals, written book chapters and guided Ph.D. students. His relentless efforts have enabled scientists to unravel the previously unforeseen and latent issues in defence systems. His work in IT systems has benefited millions of people. He is receipient of Digital India Award 2020 in category "Innovation in Pandemic" from President of India.

Dr. Mamta Mittal graduated in Computer Science & Engineering from Kurukshetra University Kurukshetra in 2001 and received Master's degree (Honors) in Computer Science & Engineering from YMCA, Faridabad. She has completed her Ph.D. from Thapar University Patiala in Computer Science and Engineering. She has been teaching from the last 16 years with emphasis on data mining, machine learning, soft computing and data structure. She is a lifetime member of CSI. She has published and communicated number of research papers in SCI, SCIE, Scopus indexed journals and attended many workshops, FDPs and seminars. She has filed two patents; one is on human surveillance system and another on wireless copter for explosive handling and diffusing. Presently, she is working at G.B. PANT Government Engineering College, Okhla, New Delhi (under Government of NCT Delhi), and supervising Ph.D. candidates of GGSIPU (Guru Gobind Singh Indraprastha University), Dwarka, New Delhi. She is Main Editor of the book entitled "Data Intensive Computing Application for Big Data" published by IOS press, Netherland, and another book entitled "Big Data Processing Using Spark in cloud" by Springer. She is Managing Editor of International Journal of Sensors, Wireless Communications and Control published by Bentham Science. She is working on DST approved Project "Development of IoT based hybrid navigation module for mid-sized autonomous vehicles." She is Reviewer of many reputed journals, has chaired number of conferences and has delivered invited talks.

Dr. Dolly Sharma graduated in Computer Science & Engineering from Kurukshetra University in 2004 and received Masters in Information Technology with honors from Panjab University, Chandigarh, in 2007. She was the second University topper. She has completed Ph.D. in Computer Science and Engineering from Punjab Engineering College, Chandigarh. She is currently working as Associate Professor in Amity University, Noida. She has a rich teaching experience of around 13 years. Her area of interests includes bioinformatics, grid computing and data mining. She has published a number of research papers and book chapters indexed in Scopus and SCI. She has contributed as Reviewer in important conferences and journals. She has chaired international conferences and delivered invited talks. She is a lifetime member of ISTE and AIENG.

Dr. Lalit Mohan Goyal has completed Ph.D. from Jamia Millia Islamia, New Delhi, in Computer Engineering, M.Tech. (Honors) in Information Technology from Guru Gobind Singh Indraprastha University, New Delhi, and B.Tech. (Honors) in Computer Engineering from Kurukshetra University, Kurukshetra. He has 16 years of teaching experience in the area of theory of computation, parallel and random algorithms, distributed data mining & cloud computing. He has completed a project sponsored by Indian Council of Medical Research, Delhi. He has published many research papers in SCI indexed & Scopus indexed journals, and conferences. Two patents filed by him are also now published online. He is Reviewer of many reputed journals & conferences. He has given many invited talks in FDP and conferences. Presently, he is working at J. C. Bose Univ. of Sc. & Tech. YMCA Faridabad in the Department of Computer Engineering.

Contributors

Ajay Agarwal Department of Computer Science and Engineering, Dehradun Institute of Technology (DIT University Dehradun), Dehradun, India

Ashi Agarwal National Institute of Technology Raipur, Raipur, India

Basant Agarwal Department of Computer Science and Engineering, Indian Institute of Information Technology Kota (MNIT Campus Jaipur), Jaipur, India

Francesco Amenta Telemedicine and Tele Pharmacy Center, School of Medicinal and Health Products Sciences, University of Camerino, Camerino, Italy; Research Department, International Radio Medical Center (C.I.R.M.), Rome, Italy

J. Ashwinth Department of Information Technology, MIT Campus, Anna University, Chennai, India

Gopi Battineni Telemedicine and Tele Pharmacy Center, School of Medicinal and Health Products Sciences, University of Camerino, Camerino, Italy

Jangyadatta Behera Department of Mathematics, S.K.C.G. (Autonomous) College, Paralakhemundi, Odisha, India

Kashish Chachra DS Web Tech (Australia), Ambala Cantt, India

Anamika Chaturvedi UP Institute of Design, Noida, India

Deepak Chaudhary Tribhuvan University, Kathmandu, Nepal

Nalini Chintalapudi Telemedicine and Tele Pharmacy Center, School of Medicinal and Health Products Sciences, University of Camerino, Camerino, Italy

Rajeev Kumar Dang UIET, Panjab University SSG Regional Centre, Hoshiarpur, Punjab, India

Binayak Dihudi Department of Mathematics, KIST, Jatni, Bhubaneswar, Odisha, India

Lalit Mohan Goyal Department of CE, J. C. Bose University of Science and Technology, YMCA, Faridabad, India

Priyanka Harjule Department of Mathematics, Indian Institute of Information Technology Kota (MNIT Campus Jaipur), Jaipur, India

M. Irfan Qureshi Proteomics and Bioinformatics Lab, Department of Biotechnology, Jamia Millia Islamia, Delhi, India

S. Karthika Department of Information Technology, MIT Campus, Anna University, Chennai, India

Amandeep Kaur Computer Science and Engineering, Punjab Engineering College (Deemed to be University), Chandigarh, India

Praveen Kumar Khosla Centre for Developement of Advance Computing (C-DAC), Ministry of Electronics & IT, Mohali, Punjab, India

Arya Kumar Faculty of MBA, College of IT and Management Education, Biju Patnaik University of Technology, Bhubaneswar, India

Koushal Kumar Sikh National College, Guru Nanak Dev University, Qadian, Punjab, India

Jagmohan Mago Department of Computer Science and Applications, Apeejay College of Fine Arts, Jalandhar, Punjab, India

Neeru Mago DCSA, Panjab University SSG Regional Centre, Hoshiarpur, Punjab, India

Sonia Mago Department of Physics, Swami Sant Dass Public School, Jalandhar, Punjab, India

Kabita Maharjan Tribhuvan University, Kathmandu, Nepal

G. Maria Jones Department of Computer Science and Engineering, Saveetha Engineering College, Chennai, India

X. Mercilin Raajini Department of ECE, Prince Shri Venkateshwara Padmavathy Engineering College, Chennai, India

Mamta Mittal Department of CSE, G. B. Pant Government Engineering College, Okhla, New Delhi, India

Neerja Mittal Computational Instrumentation, CSIR-CSIO, Chandigarh, India

Tarini Charan Panda Department of Mathematics, Ravenshaw University, Cuttack, Odisha, India

Bhagwati Prasad Pande Department of Computer Applications, LSM Govt. PG College, Pithoragarh, Uttarakhand, India

Saini Pooja Department of Computer Science and Engineering, Ambala College of Engineering and Applied Research, Ambala, Haryana, India

D. Poornima Department of EEE, Sri Ramakrishna Institute of Technology, Coimbatore, Tamil Nadu, India

Saini Preeti Chitkara University, Rajpura, Punjab, India

Sadia Qamar Proteomics and Bioinformatics Lab, Department of Biotechnology, Jamia Millia Islamia, Delhi, India

Mujibur Rahman Galgotias University, Greater Noida, India

G. Rajesh Department of Information Technology, MIT Campus, Anna University, Chennai, India

Yerra Shankar Rao Department of Mathematics, GIET Ghangapatana, Bhubaneswar, Odisha, India

Md Rashid Chand Galgotias University, Greater Noida, India

Aswin Kumar Rauta Department of Mathematics, S.K.C.G. (Autonomous) College, Paralakhemundi, Odisha, India

S. Sangeetha Department of EEE, Sri Ramakrishna Institute of Technology, Coimbatore, Tamil Nadu, India

Mahendra Sapkota Tribhuvan University, Kathmandu, Nepal

R. Shanmugapriya Department of Information Technology, MIT Campus, Anna University, Chennai, India

Richa Singh Department of Psychology, Vasanta College for Women, Varanasi, India

Amna Syeda Proteomics and Bioinformatics Lab, Department of Biotechnology, Jamia Millia Islamia, Delhi, India

Anurag Upadhyay Department of Psychology, Udai Pratap Autonomus College, Varanasi, India

Jagjot Singh Wadali Centre for Development of Advanced Computing, Mohali, India

S. Godfrey Winster Department of Computer Science and Engineering, SRM Institute of Science and Technology, Kattankulathur, Chengalpattu, India

Chapter 1
Mitigate the Impact of Covid-19: Telehealth

Praveen Kumar Khosla, Mamta Mittal, Lalit Mohan Goyal, and Kashish Chachra

1 Introduction

It is an unprecedented trying time while Covid-19 pandemic spreads its tentacles across the globe. Figure 1 shows the current strength of humans affected by Covid-19 [1]. Precincts of even premier medical institutes are breeding ground of hospital infection, more so Covid-19 infections. Often, a patient falls prey to Covid-19 infection during usual visit to the outdoor patient department (OPD). As a response to the threat of infection, Governments have ordered closure of most of the OPDs across the countries, leaving non-Covid patients in the lurch.

In such scenarios, it is imperative to provide treatment to the patients even when the doctor and the patient are distant apart, thereby making in-person visits redundant. In this regard, rapid developments in Republic of India are more brought out as an example, while similar situation exists in most other countries. Tele-consultation seems to be the obvious answer. However, in pre-Covid-19 era, it has not been so popular. It was touted as an attempt to provide consultation to rural masses or support in nation disasters. The major impediment has been the state guidelines which had either prohibited it or allowed only doctor to doctor consultations. With the result, the doctors have remained apprehensive of tele-consultations.

P. K. Khosla (✉)
Centre for Developement of Advance Computing (C-DAC), Ministry of Electronics & IT, A-34, Industrial Area, Mohali, Punjab, India
e-mail: drpkhosla@gmail.com

M. Mittal
Department of CSE, G. B. Pant Government Engineering College, Okhla, New Delhi, India

L. M. Goyal
Department of CE, J. C. Bose University of Science and Technology, YMCA, Faridabad, India

K. Chachra
DS Web Tech (Australia), Ambala Cantt, India

© The Author(s), under exclusive license to Springer Nature Singapore Pte Ltd. 2021
P. K. Khosla et al. (eds.), *Predictive and Preventive Measures for Covid-19 Pandemic*,
Algorithms for Intelligent Systems, https://doi.org/10.1007/978-981-33-4236-1_1

1

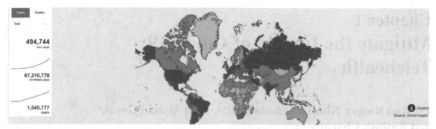

Globally, as of 5:13pm CET, 8 December 2020, there have been 67,210,778 confirmed cases of COVID-19, including 1,540,777 deaths, reported to WHO.

Fig. 1 Global spread of Covid (*Source* WHO)

1.1 Healthcare Infrastructure in India

Public healthcare providers are responsible for offering Primary Healthcare system in India. As shown in Fig. 2, secondary and tertiary health care are provided by Govt Medical Colleges or Community Healthcare Centres and Civil Hospitals in the districts.

While the secondary and tertiary health care are provided by both public and private healthcare providers. During and post-Covid-19, it has emerged that out patient department (OPD) services will be availed by the patients from the confines and comfort of their house through telemedicine solutions as shown in Fig. 3. Health and Wellness Centres (HWCs) constituting primary care will still remain relevant. The patients who need preliminary tests for vital parameters or do not have access

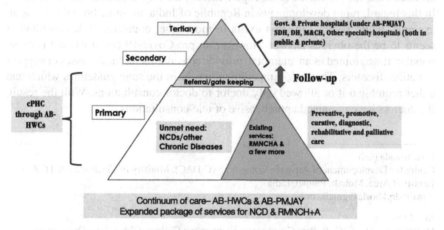

AB-HWCs Ayushman Bharat- Health & Wellness Centres; *AB-PMJAY* Ayushman Bharat- Pradhan Mantri Jan Arogya Yojana; *cPHC* Comprehensive Primary Health Care; *DH* District hospitals; *NCD* Non-communicable diseases; *M&CH* Mother and Child Health; *RMNCH+A* Reproductive Maternal, Newborn, Child and Adolescent Health; *SDH* Social determinants of health

Fig. 2 Hierarchy of healthcare systems in India

Fig. 3 Telehealth solution to OPD

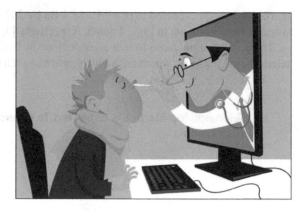

to Laptop/desktop or smartphone can visit HWC where a paramedic renders the necessary help. Patients having smartphone but not tech savy shall also visit HWCs. The doctors would either treat them by themselves or refer the patient to secondary or tertiary hospital.

The Governments have worked at accelerated pace to release the telemedicine guidelines [2, 3]. It is pertinent to mention that the development in India is typically also representative of development in other countries. The leading author leads development of Indian National Telemedicine solution a system which completed more than 10,000 consultations in second month of its roll-out. In India, the guidelines were issued on 25 March 2020, and gazette notification was released on 14 May 2020. Some of the salient of such recent guidelines have been

- to do away with state guidelines which prohibited tele-consultations
- client centric
- any registered medical practitioner can practice
- any mode of communication such as audio, video, social media can be followed
- patient and the doctor, both need to identify each other
- either party can discontinue the consultation
- the jurisdiction is any state of India.

  However, these guidelines do not cover

- Management/ownership of data
- HW, SW, building and maintenance
- Remote surgery prohibited
- Artificial intelligence-based solutions can support doctors but cannot advise patients.

Based on such guidelines, an ecosystem is getting evolved wherein exponential growth of telemedicine solutions is expected. In USA, President Trump has reported 11,000 consultation/ week in pre-Covid era which increased to 650,000 consultations/week post-Covid era. The forecast of the expected trend in the telemedicine market in India is expected to reach US$5.4 Bn by 2025 with a CAGR of 31% and world at large is shown in Figs. 4 and 5, respectively [4, 5].

There is 700% increase in tele-consultations in India. Table 1 lists the leading telemedicine solutions which are actively providing telemedicine services. Leading

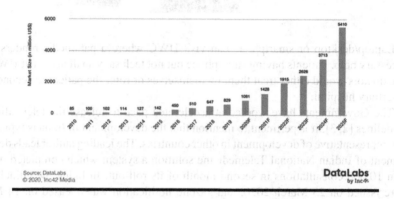

Fig. 4 Forecast of telemedicine market in India

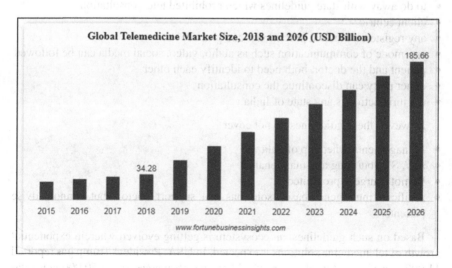

Fig. 5 Forecast of global telemedicine market

Table 1 Prominent telemedicine solutions in practice

Source of information	[3]	[6]	[4]	[5]
1	SteadyMD.com	Analog Eclipse	Practo	eSanjeevaniOPD.in
2	MDLIVE	Arka Technologies	Doc Prime	Swasth
3	Sherpaa	ConcertCare	M Fine	StepOne
4	LiveHealth Online	Express Clinics	Call Health	Tata Biridgital
5	PlushCare	Kushala	Lybrate	Tech Mahindra
6	DoctorOnDemand	Neurosynaptic Communications		
7	BetterHelp.com	Rijuven India		
8	First Opinion	TeleVital India		
9	Teladoc	Vidmed Tele Health		
10	AmericanWell			

Coloumn [3], [6], [4] and [5] mention names of products which render telemedicine services

eSanjeevaniOPD.in has been developed under the leadership of leading author of this chapter.

1.2   Telehealth

It covers all aspects of education of healthcare providers in non-clinical settings as well as tele-consultations to patients and referral to higher specialised doctors. That can be in clinical settings. It is broader term than telemedicine.

1.3   Telemedicine

Telemedicine is a method by which a doctor can examine, investigate, monitor and treat patient in distant place using two-way audio and/or video consultations in clinical settings. Telemedicine is part of telehealth. m-Health and e-Health are other two terms used frequently which need to be understood. m-Health is the use of mobile devices such as a mobile phone or tablet to support the practice of health care. e-Health is the healthcare practice supported by electronic processes and broader than m-Health.

1.4   Why Telehealth Has Come of Age Now

- **Enough Internet bandwidth available now**—2 Mbps Internet bandwidths are all that are required to conduct tele-consult including two-way audio video chat, sharing demographics and generating e-prescription. Several earlier implementations banked on VSAT satellite communications.
- **440 million Smartphone users in India and 3.5 billion in world** [7]—All these users can access telemedicine facilities using mobile apps in their phones.
- **Covid-19**—In-person consultation can spread infection to healthcare professionals and the fellow patients. Telemedicine is natural alternative to in-person visit.
- **Patient to doctor consultation is legal now**—The newer guidelines are more forthcoming and meeting the need of hour.
- **Adoption of technology by doctor and patient**—There is a push of social distancing which motivates the two stake holders to embrace telehealth services.
- **Cost of VC is reducing**—Cost of peer-to-peer consultation from People Link is prohibitive. A perpetual licence doctor–patient video conference is Rs. 250,000/-. Now that the utilisation of video conference will shoot up, the prices are expected to fall drastically.
- **Younger generation is tech savy**—Younger generation of doctors and patients is tech savy and is familiar with use of Web app and mobile app. They quickly learn telemedicine solutions and begin to use it.

2   Telemedicine Solution eSanjeevaniOPD

No telemedicine program can be created overnight [8], but building on previous doctor to doctor consultation solution, team lead by leading author has built the doctor to patient system in a short span of 19 days thereby meeting the challenges posed by onset of Covid-19. With the funding of Ministry of Health and Family Welfare (MoHFW), Government of India, a telemedicine solution was developed by C-DAC. eSanjeevaniOPD version 1.0 has been designed to be an extremely simple and easy-to-use telemedicine system that requires minimal effort from the user [9]. The system logged more than 223,000 consultations on 8 Sep 2020.

2.1   Overview of Architecture

The major sub-systems of the telemedicine system are cloud services, the Web app for doctor, mobile app/Web app for patient, the video conferencing solution and consoles for administrative functions. Figure 6 depicts these sub-systems. The process flow for realisation of eSanjeevaniOPD telemedicine solution is described in Fig. 7. A

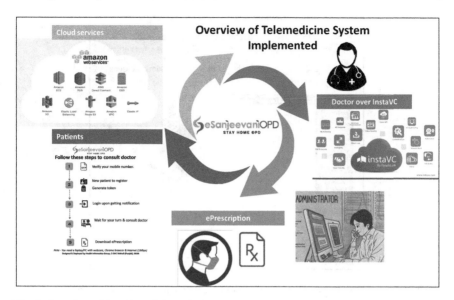

Fig. 6   Overview of the telemedicine solution

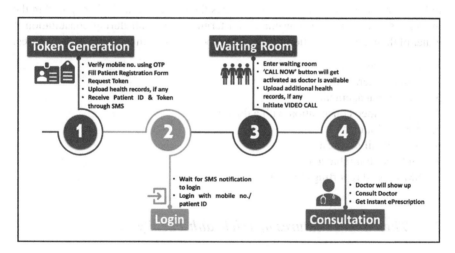

Fig. 7   Process flow for realisation of eSanjeevani telemedicine solution

patient fills up a form for registration after his mobile phone no is verified using a SMS. In case patient wishes to seek an appointment, he generates a token number.

The patient is notified through an SMS when his turn matures and is prompted to login using the token number. Doctor's availability is displayed through a "Call Now" button. When patient presses this button, the doctor on the far end accepts the consultation. Thereafter, two-way audio video consultation starts. At the end of consultation, physician generates an e-prescription and explains the medicines

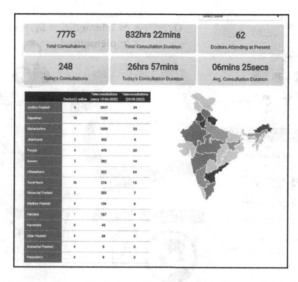

Fig. 8 Figure depicts the geographical spread of the solution implementation in India

to be taken. Thereafter, physician terminates the consultation. As is required in the guidelines, the patient or consultant can terminate the call during consultation if either of them are not satisfied. The whole process passes through following phases:

1. Patient registration
2. Token generation
3. Queue management
4. Audio–video consultation with a doctor
5. e-prescription
6. SMS/email notifications
7. Fully configurable admn
8. SMS-based reporting (Fig. 8).

2.2 The Salient Features of Telehealth Facility

Telehealth facility has number of salient features which are quite helpful in such pandemic time as well as future point of view.

- Cloud-based online OPD system
- Real-time patient to doctor video consultations
- Supports fully managed token-based queuing service
- Archives records and consultations for follow-up reviews
- Short learning and adoption curve
- Further customisations as per need possible
- Provision of text chat in case two video chats fail

- Modelled on EHR guidelines of MoHFW, GoI and SNOMED CT-based e-prescription enabled
- Rapid deployment—web app and mobile app
- Efficient SMS notifications and alerts
- Based on first-in-first out service delivery.

Two-way audio video consultation is captured in Fig. 9, and number of consultations carried out each day is shown in Fig. 10.

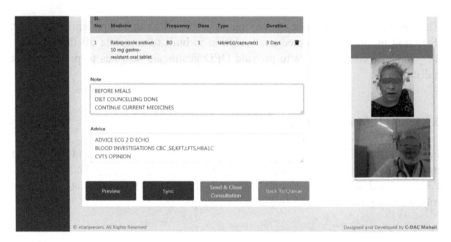

Fig. 9 Tele-consultation in progress between doctor and patient in the solution under discussion

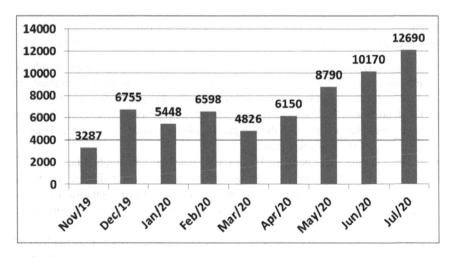

Fig. 10 Tele-consultation per month of eSanjeevani (HWC)

3 Detailed Architecture of Telehealth Model

The architecture of telehealth model has shown in Fig. 11. It has the following components.

3.1 Presentation Layer

This layer presents the application to the end-users who can be a patient or a doctor. TeleOPD mobile app telemedicine solution is built to integrate all the COVID-19 pandemic circumstances to provide OPD healthcare services to patients from a distance.

3.1.1 OTP-Based Authentication

Patient can avail OPD services by registering through mobile number and verification using OTP. After patient successfully registered on TeleOPD app, he/she will get PatientID and Token No. through SMS on mobile no. OTP authentication is more robust and secure than the static username and passwords.

3.2 Application Layer

Application layer contains the app logic through which patient/doctor can enter the system to avail the OPD services or offer the services to patients remotely.

- Through API controller, the patient will login with their registered mobile no and token no. (already generated through OTP authentication), and eSanjeevani engine provides patient queue no. and entry patient in the waiting queue room.
- Token no. is valid only for current day when patient generated the token. If patient forgets his token number, he/she can get the token no. with their registered mobile no. through OTP authentication.
- Patient can cancel the generated token with their registered mobile no.
- ASP.NET SignalR provides real-time code push from server-side content to the connected clients simultaneously, it helps to provide real-time signalling to control the availability of doctor–patient status (maintaining patient waiting queue status, available online doctor, doctor already in-call, etc.).
- Through SignalR ability, API service layer provides services to make video call between patient and doctor. The Patient will get the online available doctor status and request to doctor for consultation just by clicking on the call now button. While on the doctor end, the doctor will get VC call notification to initiate the

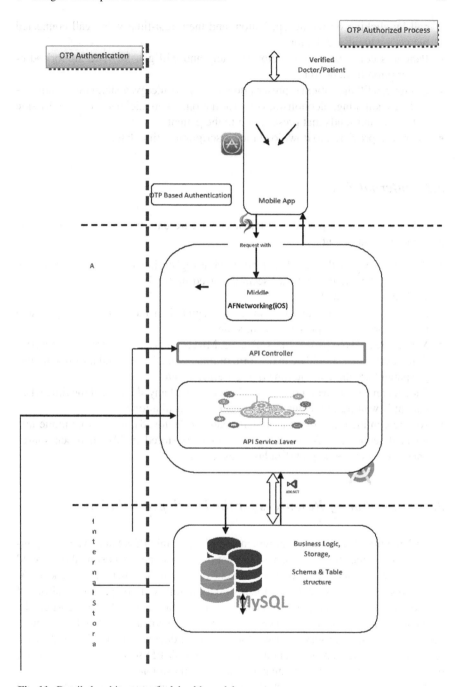

Fig. 11 Detailed architecture of telehealth model

call by clicking on the accept button, and then, real-time video call connected between patient and doctor.

- Patient is consulting with doctor remotely and will get the valid authorised e-prescription from doctor.
- Doctor can fill the patient e-prescription diagnosis (allergy, general information—diabetes, smoking, alcoholism, BP information, Rx medicines, etc.) side by side in the VC and sends that prescription to the patient.
- There is a provision to download the prescription at time later.

3.3 Internal Storage

The data access layer provides efficient and secure data transactions meeting the application requirements.

- Patient can upload their medical records while registering or generating new token, all the medical documents are securely saved in the database for the references while consulting with doctor.
- SNOMED CT and RxNorm listing is integrated in the app for allergies and medications in the e-prescription module.
- Medical records of patient like CT scans, MRI reports, X-rays, previous prescription reports, etc., should be in the form of images, pdf's, etc., and max documents per patient are three at the time of registering token.
- Patient can also upload more medical documents if any skipped, at the time when patient is waiting in the queue room for their consultation turn.
- All the confidential information data (patient/ doctor ids, token no, mobile no., medical records, etc.) of doctor and patient is stored in MySql (open source database) with the help of data layer resources.

3.4 Allocation of Resources for the Developed Solution

Table 2 mentions the hosting requirement for eSanjeevaniOPD/eSanjeevaniAB application and provides figures which a new user may expect before hosting it on a cloud service. It was tested for 25,000 concurrent users, that is, experiencing 25k hits/s. These concurrent users can be doctors, patients, administrators, persons desirous of only the registration and persons trying to become familiar with the Website. The application server hosts the main eSanjeevani engine with about 100 MB of deployable code. The staging server is used for training of doctors, onboarding of doctors, running code under development and the like. SNOMED server caters to database of allergies, drugs, provisional diagnosis and immunisation.

A schema of 50 MB incremental/month emerged after optimal design of database in MySQL. Database server supported the schema. For an average of 250 consultations/day, a storage of 2.5 GB incremental/month was estimated to be adequate.

Table 2 Hosting requirements for eSanjeevani telemedicine solution

a	Application server	VM (LINUX)—2 Cores, 4 vCPUs, 3.1 GHz, 32 GB RAM
b	Staging server	(LINUX)—1 Core, 2 vCPUs, 2.5 GHz, 16 GB RAM
c	SNOMED server	VM (LINUX), Apache Tomcat—2 Cores, 4 vCPUs, 3.1 GHz, 32 GB RAM
d	Database server	VM/RDS-Managed Service (MySQL)—4 Cores, 8 vCPUs, 3.1 GHz, 64 GB RAM
e	Storage	5 TB SSD
f	architecture	Scalable/CDN architecture, as per real time/LIVE load matrix
g	Bandwidth	Minimum 10 Mbps

The architecture reported here is scalable. The dashboard shows CPU usage. An alert is generated if the value exceeds 90%. Additional cluster gets allotted without allowing application to crash. The cloud services of Amazon Web Services (AWS) were considered for hosting as they offered the services free of cost during Covid time. Description of eSanjeevani AWS Cloud Architecture: the users of eSanjeevani telemedicine system are physicians, paramedics, master trainers and patients. The solution has been hosted on AWS servers. There are separate application and database servers allocated. As shown in Fig. 12, a remote user or remote admin can login into the eSanjeevani through Internet gateway in AWS server. Remote

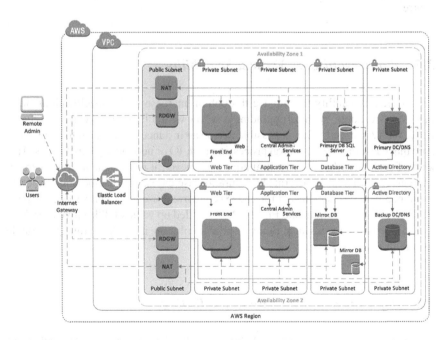

Fig. 12 Hosting of eSanjeevani solution on cloud services of AWS

desktop gateway (RD gateway) grants eSanjeevani users or admin on public networks access to Windows desktops and applications hosted in AWS cloud services. The RD gateway component uses secure sockets layer (SSL) to encrypt the communications channel between clients and the server. The elastic load balancer automatically distributes incoming application traffic across multiple targets, such as Amazon EC2 instances, containers, IP addresses and Lambda functions.

The eSanjeevani AWS server can handle the varying load of application traffic in a single availability zone or across multiple availability zones. The NAT gateway provides eSanjeevani users or admin, available AWS managed service which makes it easy to connect to the Internet from instances within a private subnet in an Amazon Virtual Private Cloud (Amazon VPC). A private subnet sets that route to a NAT instance. Private subnet instances need a private IP and Internet traffic is routed through the NAT in the public subnet.

Simultaneously, remote desktop gateway starts accessing the Web tier, application tier and the database tier so that user and admin in a client–server can access eSanjeevani application can access a Web application that has the frontend, the backend and the database. The data submitted in eSanjeevani application by doctors and patients is stored in database tier simultaneously through RDP gateway. The eSanjeevani AWS model has two availability zones, and it is a logical data centre in a region available for use by any AWS customer. Each zone in a region has redundant and separate power, networking and connectivity to reduce the likelihood of two zones failing simultaneously. A common misconception is that a single zone equals a single data centre.

3.5   eSanjeevani Uses Vertical Scalability

The vertical scalability takes place through an increase in the specifications of an individual resource, such as upgrading a server with a larger hard drive or a faster CPU. With Amazon EC2, it is possible to stop an instance and resize it to an instance type that has more RAM, central processing unit, IO or networking capabilities. This kind of scalability has its own limitations. However, it is convenient to implement and can be sufficient in several short duration use cases. The telemedicine solution explained here has been tested for 25,000 concurrent users/s. Figure 13 shows peak of 27.5k active users/min, and Fig. 14 shows scaled up value of 37k active users/min experienced three weeks later. Being a scalable solution, it is able to adjust to variable load requirements.

3.6   Importance of Cross Platform Testing

In implementing such a solution, Web app, Android native app and iOS native app are used. The iOS uses "Objective C", but Android programming uses Java. Both

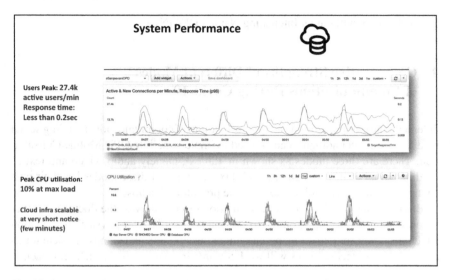

Fig. 13 System performance observed from dashboard in early days of deployment

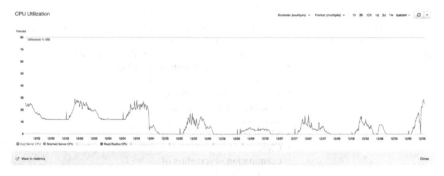

Fig. 14 Active connections increase to 37,000 three weeks later and still processing successfully

of these being built on separate platforms and require extra fixes to be made in the application to recognise strings arriving from another language platforms. Therefore, cross platform testing, especially, from Android to iOS gains paramount importance, as uninterrupted service during Covid-19 is more important.

3.7   Interoperability

Mobile app is interoperable with all the e-Health applications at C-DAC. It also complies with international standards such as

1.   Digital Imaging and Communications in Medicine (DICOM) [10]

2. Technology without an Interesting Name (TWAIN).

4 Comparative Strengths of Different Modes of Communications During Covid-19

Telemedicine guidelines allow use of any medium of communication including social media. Several technologies can be used to implement Tele OPD Mobile Consultation. There are three modes as shown in Table 3, namely audio, video and text as used in textual chat, messaging, email, fax, etc. Each of these modes has their own strengths, weaknesses and contexts, while providing diagnosis.

Broadly, though telemedicine consultation offers safety to the doctor and other fellow patients from contagious conditions, it is no replace for physical examination which may look for palpation, percussion or auscultation and entails physical touch and feel. Newer technologies will work towards improvements in such drawback.

Table 3 Comparison of different modes of communication

Mode	Strengths	Limitations
Video, tele OPD mobile APP video on platforms such as chat	• Similar to an in-person consultation, soft real-time discussion • Convenient to identification patient • Doctor and patient can see each other, and care giver can assist • Visual cues can be observed • Close examination/observation of patient is feasible	• Requires 2 Mbps internet connectivity • Privacy of patient is a challenge
Audio phone, VOIP, apps and the like	• It is fast and operable • Easy accessibility • Suitable for urgent requirements • Does not require separate infrastructure • Privacy can be ensured • Real-time discussion	• Non-verbal observation can be missed • Physical examination is not feasible • Difficult to identify the patient
Text-based, verbal chat-based, tele OPD mobile solution with mobile apps and SMS	• Easy to operate • Documentation and identification may be inherently available • Suitable when two-way audio video chat fails	• Examination of patient is most difficult • Specialisations such as psychiatry require building positive report with the patient. In this case, it is not possible

In the implemented solution, all the three modes have been used. If video chat fails due to poor Internet connectivity, text chat comes in handy.

5 Conclusion

Driven by Covid-19, the telehealth solutions will be ubiquitous. They will be embraced by masses and adopted by all sections. Newer solutions catering to needs of different specialisations of medicine will be rapidly developed and would remain in demand. Such solutions will play crucial role in slowing down the spread of Covid-19 pandemic. In future, a stage would come when physician will look for vital parameters of patients. Many points of need devices will have to be developed to aid doctors in decision support. It could be for measurement of respiration, fundus parameters, dermatology studies, blood glucose levels and the like. These points of need devices will not only be used by patients but also by paramedics in Health and Wellness Centres. US $5.5 billion Indian market by 2025 offers ample opportunity in the domain of telemedicine.

Acknowledgements The work reported here is a team effort. We acknowledge the efforts of Dr. S. P. Sood, Sh. Rajesh Kaushish and team of C-DAC in carrying out this work.

References

1. https://covid19.who.int/. Accessed on 20 May 2020
2. Ohannessian R, Duong TA, Odone A (2020) Global telemedicine implementation and integration within health systems to fight the COVID-19 pandemic: a call to action. JMIR Public Health Surveill 6(2):e18810
3. Smith WR et al (2020) Implementation guide for rapid integration of an outpatient telemedicine program during the COVID-19 pandemic. J Am Coll Surg 231(2):216–222.e2
4. https://telemedicine.cioreviewindia.com/vendors/2019/0. Accessed on 23 May 2020
5. https://www.aarogyasetumitr.in. Accessed on 23 May 2020
6. https://onlinemedicalcare.org/best-online-doctor-medical-services/. Accessed on 23 May 2020
7. https://www.statista.com/statistics/330695/number-of-smartphone-users-worldwide/. Accessed on 24 May 2020
8. Hagge D, Knopf A, Hofauer B (2020) Telemedicine in the fight against SARS-COV-2-opportunities and possible applications in otorhinolaryngology: narrative review. HNO. https://doi.org/10.1007/s00106-020-00864-7
9. Hollander JE, Carr BG (2020) Virtually perfect? Telemedicine for COVID-19. N Engl J Med 382(18):1679–1681
10. Wadali JS, Sood SP, Kaushish R, Syed-Abdul S, Khosla PK, Bhatia M (2020) Evaluation of free, open-source, web-based DICOM viewers for the Indian national telemedicine service (eSanjeevani). J Digit Imaging 1–15
11. https://inc42.com/datalab/telemedicine-market-opportunity-in-indian-healthtech/. Accessed on 23 May 2020

Chapter 2
Epidemic Models in Prediction of COVID-19

Gopi Battineni, Nalini Chintalapudi, and Francesco Amenta

1 Introduction

After an origination of the novel pandemic known as COVID-19 in early days of 2020, this illness has spread across the world and more than 180 countries are suffering by this deadly disease. Researchers confirmed that COVID-19 was a kind of transmission disease that developed by severe acute respiratory syndrome-coronavirus-2 (i.e., SARS-CoV-2) [1] and contains the little protein spikes of novel coronavirus and SARS which presented in Fig. 1. This virus easily transmitted between human to human either by having physical contact with infected person or by tiny droplets released from a person during conversation, sneeze, or cough. The risk of COVID-19 is high for the people who had respiratory diseases like asthma or breathing issues and comparatively moderate for everyone.

The basic reproduction number (R0) is a factor that defines the transmission speed of epidemic occurrence and is largely highlighted in the medical literature [3]. The World Health Organization (WHO) and other established researches are estimating that this value is between 1.4 and 3.8 in the areas that are affected in the first diffusion phase. For instance, in Wuhan, where this pandemic initiated the R0 was evaluated to 2.2 (95% CI, 1.4–3.9). In Italy, this value extending from 2.76 to 3.25 (95% CI, 0.7–19) [4]. Preventive measures can be powerful in a decrease in infection transmission in the overall population and characterized mass gatherings. So far, the transmission rate has not been fully measured. However, it has the capacity of easy spreading in current society without imposition of preventive measures.

G. Battineni (✉) · N. Chintalapudi · F. Amenta
Telemedicine and Tele Pharmacy Center, School of Medicinal and Health Products Sciences, University of Camerino, Camerino 62032, Italy
e-mail: gopi.battineni@unicam.it

F. Amenta
Research Department, International Radio Medical Center (C.I.R.M.), Rome 00144, Italy

© The Author(s), under exclusive license to Springer Nature Singapore Pte Ltd. 2021
P. K. Khosla et al. (eds.), *Predictive and Preventive Measures for Covid-19 Pandemic*,
Algorithms for Intelligent Systems, https://doi.org/10.1007/978-981-33-4236-1_2

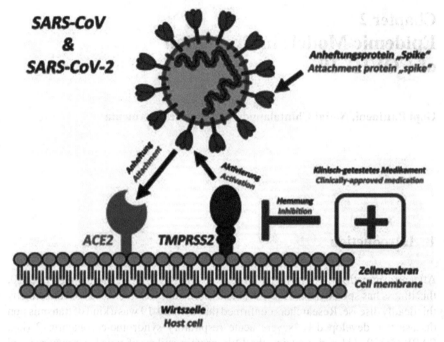

Fig. 1 Protein 'spike' representation of SARS-CoV and SARS-CoV-2 [2]

Some computing models highlighted the influence of maintaining social distance in order to control the COVID-19 spread either by use of parameters that influences early information of SARS coronavirus epidemiological study [5], or not implemented on a worldwide scale [6]. However, there is a wide scope of potential uses with epidemic modeling techniques such as mathematical, time series, machine learning (ML), and deep learning models are covering clinical and cultural issues developed by the COVID-19 pandemic. For the moment, some of them only produce enough information to show operational effects.

ML-based advances are considered as vital approaches in prediction of early spread of COVID-19. Researchers are utilizing ML algorithms to examine the infection, test potential medicines, patient evolution, investigate the public medical effects, and so on. From a genome structural point of view, ML and deep learning can identify the virus structure, evaluated existing medications that again can be used for disease treatment [7]. Moreover, it suggests new compounds that might be promising for medication advancement, distinguishes potential vaccine outcomes, improves find, and better get infection infectivity and seriousness. From a clinical point of view, deep learning model can aid COVID-19 analysis from medical imaging, give elective approaches to follow disease spread with non-intrusive devices, and forecast the patient outcomes depend on multi-data inputs including electronic health records (i.e., EHR).

At the same time, it is important to design an epidemic model by mathematical equations which can also effectively calculate the COVID-19 transmission rates and to propose distinct mitigation measures. Whenever a novel pandemic-like COVID-19 occurs, immediate drug finding is somehow difficult to identify. Because of its widespread nature, the number of infected cases had to be predicted to control pandemic [8]. Most studies used SEIR mathematical models to predict the spread of disease. These models are also called compartmental models and each compartment represents groups of people namely susceptible, exposed, infectious, and recovered. In addition to them, Ivorra et al. [9] mentioned other groups such as hospitalized but ready to die (H_D), infected but undetected (I_U), home quarantined (H_R), recovered without identification (R_U), and recovered after detection (R_D) are included to basic SEIR parameters.

In the worldwide effort to slow down the COVID-19 spread, many countries have been followed home quarantine and social distancing to prevent the effects of the pandemic. Most of the COVID-19 prediction studies involved mainly three types of epidemic modes such as time series, mathematical, machine learning, and deep learning models. This chapter aims to present the available mathematical, predictive, and ML models for the best usages of COVID-19 pandemic modeling. The remaining sections will review the different modeling strategies that include statistical, time series, differential equations based, machine learning, and predictive modeling approaches.

2 Time Series Models

Time series modeling is a measure of outcomes over a consistent time. A model with series data has many time types and represents various stochastic processes. The modeling can vary in three different integrated processes such as autoregressive (AR), integrated (I), and moving average (MA), and these three models are entirely dependent on previous data sets. The combination of the above three-class models can develop an autoregressive moving average (ARMA) [10], and autoregressive integrated moving average (ARIMA) models [11]. In this section, authors provide a glimpse of the intervention of these time series models to forecast the COVID-19.

2.1 ARMA Modeling

ARMA modeling is formed by integrating AR(p) with MA(q) models.

- AR(p) models explain mean reversion and momentum effects usually observed in weather forecasting.
- MA(q) models capture the shock effects that are detected in white noise terms. These shock effects would cause because of unexpected events.

Most often this modeling refers to ARMA (p, q) where is p is polynomial of autoregressive function and q is a polynomial of moving average function [10]. The time series equation of ARMA modeling is presented as

$$X(t) = c + e(t) + \sum_{i=1}^{p} aXt - i + \sum_{i=1}^{q} bXt - i \tag{1}$$

where, c: constant, $e(t)$: error term, a: autoregressive model parameter, and b: moving average model parameter.

For $p = 1$ and $q = 1$, the model equation presented as

$$X(t) = e(t) + ax(t - 1) + be(t - 1) + e(t) \tag{2}$$

2.2 ARIMA Modeling

An amplified version of the ARMA model is ARIMA which successfully managed predictions of stock forecasting, sports, weather, etc. [11]. Basically, ARIMA model consists of three key parameters such as p, d, and q. Here, p is an autoregressive parameter, d is a difference between integrated components (i.e., $I(d)$), and q is error value (i.e., a fundamental value of former error rates e_t).

Based on these parameters, the ARIMA time series modeling equation can written as

$$X(t) = c + e(t) + Ø1y\,dt - 1 + Ø2y\,dt$$
$$- 2 + \cdots + Øny\,dt - n + \theta 1et - 1 + \theta q\ et - q + et \tag{3}$$

The log polynomial function of ARIMA model can presented as

$$Ø(L)(1 - L)d\,yt = \theta(L)et \tag{4}$$

For multiple log polynomials, the presentation is

$$\left[1 - \sum_{i=1}^{p} Øi\,Li \right](1 - L)d\,yt = [1 + \theta j\,Lj]et \tag{5}$$

Several studies are available regarding the involvement of AR, MA, ARMA, and ARIMA models in COVID-19 forecasting and suggestions on preventive measures. For instance, Chintalapudi et al. [4] implemented these models to forecast the Italy COVID-19 situation after having a continuous lockdown of two months. By this, author did prediction of infected cases with an accuracy of 93.75% and recovered cases with an accuracy of 84.4%. Outcomes suggested that by conducting 60-day lockdown measures and self-isolation can control disease transmission rate by 66%.

Saleh et al. [12] used the above prediction models to predict the current pandemic spread in Saudi Arabia and proposed public health policies. The authors involved all four models such as AR, MA, ARMA, and ARIMA to identify the best fit model. Above all, ARIMA outperformed the other three models. Qiuying et al. [13] adopted ARIMA models to check epidemic Italy by comparing Hubei, China. The time series ARIMA models were employed to calculate the newly infected cases and deaths and predict 10-day COVID-19 situation of Italy and produce a theoretic base for other studies.

Muhammad [14] published a study on a more rational approach with coupling Kalman filter with the ARIMA models to do accurate forecasting of the COVID-19 outbreak prevalence, registered, and recovered cases and deaths in Pakistan. The model predicted the values with a 95% confidence interval. Moreover, Zeynep [15] used these models to calculate COVID-19 prevalence of three worst-affected nations such as Spain, Italy, and France. ARIMA (1, 2, 0), ARIMA (0, 2, 1), and ARIMA (0, 2, 1) models are well suited to do epidemic forecasting for Spain, Italy, and France. By implementing these models, it can be possible to recommend more policies and precautionary measures to the local public for controlling the disease.

Khan et al. [16] also adopted ARIMA models to calculate COVID-19 cases in India. The developed model forecasted the cases of 50 days. The ARIMA (1, 1, 0) model was best suited and the highest R^2 value was calculated as 0.95.

3 Epidemic Models with Mathematics

This section presents the different mathematical models available to predict the COVID-19 and cumulative number of infected individuals over the days.

3.1 SEIR Compartmental Model

Many infectious diseases have a latent phase such as the period between the people is infected but not yet infectious and this delay is called the incubation period. The WHO confirmed the incubation for SARS-CoV-2 is at least fourteen days [17]. This delay between getting an infection and becoming contagious adds another state called exposed state E and keeps infected individuals moving from S to E and from E to I compartments before transfer into the infectious state. The recovered (R) population depends upon the sickness length.

The SEIR epidemic model simulates the time variations of an epidemic phenomenon and helps to have a mathematical understanding of infectious disease spreading. It presents relationships among people with disease contraction, present

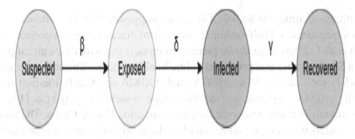

Fig. 2 Compartmental SEIR model

infected, and those who have been recovered or of death at a given time in a population. SEIR model works on both mutual and dynamic connection of four different compartments such as S, E, I, R. Susceptible population (S) is potentially subjected to infection. The compartmental SEIR model is presented in Fig. 2.

In SEIR models, virus spread follows the transition state orders like $S \rightarrow E \rightarrow I \rightarrow R$. When susceptible individuals having contact with virus then change to exposed state. Thereafter, it follows an infectious state and ultimately recovers dead. With including a new transition state (susceptible to exposure), the infection probability rate is the same as before (i.e., all susceptible can be exposed immediately). Each suspected person can be exposed with β (beta) rate of new cases per day, and γ (gamma) represents recovery rates. The new transition probability E to I is one as every exposed individual turn into infected, and the population E and the rate have new parameter δ (delta). These parameters can vary among suspects and infectious comportments since it depends on people's interaction. If the person has been contacted with COVID-19 infected person transmission rate is defined $\frac{dS}{dt} \leq 0$, and if infected person is recovered or dead is defined as $\frac{dR}{dt} \geq 0$.

If N is an overall population in a county or region, the SEIR compartmental equation with regular time interval t can be written as

$$N = S(t) + E(t) + I(t) + R(t) \tag{6}$$

and parameters.

β is probability number infections caused by single infected person (i.e., $\beta = \frac{D}{S}$; $0 < \beta < 1$), δ is the rate of exposed individuals turns into infectious cases, and γ is recovery rate of infected patients (i.e., $\gamma = 1/D$; where D is the number of days is required to spread disease by an infected person).

The transmission rates of each compartment in SEIR model can be derived as

$$\frac{dS}{dt} = -\beta . I \frac{S(t)}{N(t)}$$

$$\frac{dE}{dt} = \beta . I . \frac{S(t)}{N(t)} - \delta E$$

$$\frac{\mathrm{d}I}{\mathrm{d}t} = \delta.E - \gamma I$$

$$\frac{\mathrm{d}R}{\mathrm{d}t} = \gamma I$$

The 'R' function to be dependent on the input of initial values of S, R, E, and I concerning time (t) in days.

Many studies have attempted these models to understand COVID-19 dynamics. Shaobo et al. [18] provided a comprehensive view of COVID-19 dynamics by adopting SEIR compartment models. Authors design SEIR compartmental models by including some general prevention strategies like hospitals, quarantine centers, and exterior inputs. The model has verified the epidemic in Hubei, China and by introducing the stochastic and seasonal parameter infections, chaos with nonlinear dynamics was found. Moreover, Jose et al. [19] also implemented these models to evaluate the infected cases and casualties in Northern Italy. Results highlighted that social distancing, isolation activities, and diffusion knowledge helps in the under-standing of COVID-19 dynamics and it is also necessary to maximize the process to the lockdown effectiveness.

3.2 Models with Control Information

The models with mitigation data are pivotal to the policymakers to procure medical supplies, designate human resources and emergency clinic beds, and guarantee the manageability of the health systems all through the highpoint and epidemic dura-tion. Global researchers have played out various scientific displaying and numerical investigations on COVID-19 outbreak initiation [20].

In SEIR models, the individuals are moved to start with one compartment then onto the next. The conversion rate of 'S' compartment to 'I' compartment is referred as β, 'E' compartment number of people are calculated as βIS. Once βIS individuals are moving from S to E, the numbers are expelled from S and added to E. An isolated or quarantine (Q) compartments can be added to demonstrate the impacts of quarantine were presented in Fig. 3.

A portion (q) of peoples is transferred from I to Q in the quarantine and it is expected that the rest of the people from 'I' compartment can recover with rate γ, or dead with rate di. The individuals that recovered from the 'Q' compartment are excluded from the rate (qt) or died with rate dq.

Let us assume N is infected population then infection rate

$$r(N) = r0 - kN \tag{7}$$

where $r0$: basic reproduction number and k is infection reverse constant that indicates the results of preventive measures. The COVID-19 modeling with the differential equation is presented as

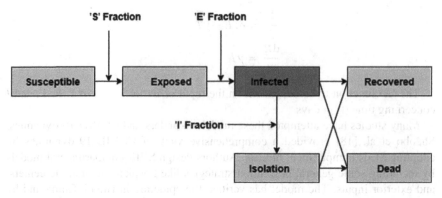

Fig. 3 SEIR model with isolation measures

$$\frac{dN}{dt} = roN\left(1 - \frac{N}{N_{max}}\right) \tag{8}$$

In the above Eq. (8), the first-term $r0N$ presents the natural trend of infection during epidemics when no intervention of control measures, and second term $\frac{-roN_2}{N_{max}}$ presents the afterward effects of preventive measures. The number of the total infected population is measured with the equation mentioned below.

$$N(t) = \frac{N_{max}}{1 + \left(\frac{N_{max}}{N_0} - 1\right)e - ro(t - t_0)} \tag{9}$$

3.3 Spatial Models

Apart from the SEIR models, what is basic is that generally little spatial units, which can act free or express from different regions, are the best way to deal with demonstrating pandemic spread, as it permits conditions inside small areas to be the worst effective modeling. This empowers models likewise to be appropriate at small spatial places like sub-national scales, with the goal that lockdown measures or procedures could be applied all the more explicitly to a territory, for example, urban communities, neighborhoods, or little areas to perceive how powerful they may be [21]. Hasraddin [22] conducted research on the spreading speed and impacts of COVID-19. They reported COVID-19 spreading with the spatial units, and concluded these spatial models, it is possible to examine the connection between affirmed instances of COVID-19, passing thereof, and recuperated cases because of treatment.

For instance, in a small spatial area, 'i' the differential modeling equations of suspected and infected people at time t is mentioned below [23]

$$\frac{\mathrm{d}Sp,i(t)}{\mathrm{d}t} = -\beta i \frac{Sp,iIp,i(t)}{Sp,i(t) + Ip,i(t)} \frac{\mathrm{d}Ip,i(t)}{\mathrm{d}t} \qquad (10)$$

where βi is daily transmission parameter.

The daily discrete equations of the above differential equation were presented as

$$Sp,i(t+1) = Sp,i(t) - \min(P(t), Sp,i(t)) \qquad (11)$$

$$Ip,i(t+1) = Ip,i(t) - \min(P(t), Sp,i(t)) \qquad (12)$$

here $p(t)$ is the poison distribution.

3.4 Spatio-temporal Models

Spatio-temporal information investigation is a rising study region because of the turn of events and utilization of novel computational methods taking into account the examination of huge spatio-temporal databases. Spatio-temporal models emerge when data is gathered across time just as space and has at least of single spatial and single temporal property. In addition to this, Benjamin et al. [24] proposed a between countries' disease spread (BeCoDis) model which developed based on spatio-temporal epidemic information in the research of disease spreading inside and between the countries. Experimental results of BeCoDis models involve outbreak characteristics, epidemic strength, and virus speeding. While estimating the temporal effects on COVID-19 spreading, many studies were attempted to consider only metrological attributes that limit the reliability of the outcome.

Briz-Redon et al. [25] conducted spatio-temporal analysis to explore the daily temperature effects on total COVID-19 registered cases in Spain provinces. In this study, authors considered nonmetro logical factors like age population, density of population in a region, number of travelers, and number of companies that were considered for the analysis. Experimental results did not find any evidence of a reduction of COVID-19 cases at minimum, maximum, and mean temperatures.

3.5 Markov Chain Models

A Markov chain model describes the possible sequential events that each event probability can depend on the state of previous events. There are two types of models such as continuous-time Markov chain (CTMC) model and discrete-time Markov chain (DTMC) models. These models are used in business, share markets, employer planning, and many others. But the prediction results generated by these models are more efficient. Therefore, researchers are adopting these models to predict COVID-19 based on the secondary data available from WHO sites.

Jean Roch et al. [26] adopted these models to identify possible infected cases in Germany which report sick by COVID-19. The developed framework builds on the CTMC model of four states called healthy without infection, sickness, healthy after infection but no symptoms, and dead. The quantitative equation proposed matches the total number of infected persons with the latest observation and ends with infected persons following from sickness probabilities and infection rates.

If N denotes the total population and the initial state is 1 for all people

$$\text{i.e., } S_k(0) = 1; \; k = 1, 2, 3, \ldots, N$$

The probability for random contacts with healthy without infection and sickness individuals will be

$$Pc = \frac{N2(t) + \eta N4(t)}{N1(t) + N2(t) + N4(t)} \tag{13}$$

Here, four states $s = 1, 2, 3, 4$ were considered and $Ns(t)$ is the projected people at particular states at time t and some transition probabilities are resulted as

$$\beta 12 = \beta 14 = \frac{1 - r}{r} \beta 12 \tag{14}$$

r: recovery rate

$$\beta 14 = n_{\text{rec}}^{-1} \tag{15}$$

n_{rec}: number of recovery days

The exponential distribution representation of the particular state that an individual gets sick in day and week is given as

$$Pd(t) = 1 - e^{-\int_t^{t+1} \beta 12(s) ds} \tag{16}$$

$$Pw(t) = 1 - e^{-\int_t^{t+1} \beta 12(s) ds} \tag{17}$$

4 Machine Learning and Deep Learning Models

Artificial intelligence (AI) studies reinforced their proficiency in developing mathematical models to investigate the pandemic spreading by the use of country-wise data. This section presents the machine learning and deep learning models simultaneously that were used to forecast the COVID-19.

4.1   Fb-Prophet Model

Fb-Prophet is a machine learning-based time series forecasting model with nonlinear trends caused by daily, weekly, yearly, and holiday seasonal effects [27]. It is well suited with time series data with several seasons of historical data and strong seasonal effects. It is a fully automatic model with limited manual involvement. Researchers most often used either time series models like ARMA, ARIMA, or SEIR models in epidemic predictions. However, these models have some limitations. In the SEIR model, assumptions are made as each suspect individual has an equal chance of getting contact with another person, and the transmission rate remains the same throughout the epidemic duration. Besides, this model considered having similar transmission rates for both quarantine and non-quarantine populations. On the other hand, time series models deal with one or more values per time step. In time series forecasting models, parameter tuning is mandatory for projections of better accuracy. In automated ARIMA, the input parameters like autoregressive and moving average components are hard to adjust and make better model tuning. However, the Fb-Prophet model does not require the interpolation of missing data; also adds holidays and seasonality in model improvement instead of obtaining better forecasting.

In Fb-Prophet model, a complex time series model with three model components namely non-periodic time series changes (i.e., $g(t)$), seasonal (i.e., $s(t)$), and holiday (i.e., $h(t)$) effects. The combinational equation of three components defined in Eq. 1.

$$y(t) = g(t) + s(t) + h(t) + e_t \qquad (18)$$

where e_t: error term.

To forecast effects caused by seasonal changes, Fb-Prophet model depends on the Fourier series, and seasonal changes characteristic $s(t)$ are measured by the following equation

$$s(t) = \sum_{n=1}^{N} \left(\text{ancos}\left(\frac{2\pi nt}{T}\right) + \text{bnsin}\left(\frac{2\pi nt}{T}\right) \right) \qquad (19)$$

Parameters $a_1, b_1 \ldots a_n, b_n$ has been evaluated by N (where $n = 1\ldots N$) to do seasonal modeling, and T is the time period (i.e., 7 for weekly data and 365.25 for yearly data).

Based on the above equations, some researchers have attempted these models to forecast the pandemic growth. For example, Wang et al. [28] coordinate the most refreshed COVID-19 epidemiological information into the logistic model to fit the top of the epidemic pattern, and afterward, feed the top an incentive into Fb-Prophet model, to evaluate the epidemic trend and foresee the pattern of the pandemic. It is also reported that the Fb-prophet model was used to predict the daily cases registered in Bangladesh [29].

4.2 MIT Machine Learning Model to Predict Quarantine Outcome

A research team from MIT has developed a machine learning model which determines COVID-19 spread. A neural network system was developed to understand control changes caused by preventive measures like quarantine and self-isolation [30]. The study anticipated that the confirmed cases from both Italy and the USA can start to level off by one week from now, however, it depends upon social distancing measures. Simultaneously, it also predicts that if the USA starts to lift the country lockdown, the outcome could be beyond the imagination for the country.

Most of the existing literature is associated with virus prediction by SEIR models. Whereas these models were explored by adding trained models of neural networks. Finally, the developed model successfully identified infected people who were in quarantine. They also mentioned that the developed model shows that quarantine measures are beneficial to decrease virus reproduction number from > 1 to < 1. The learning model 'quarantine control strength function' relates to where we can flatten the curve and be able to observe fewer contaminations.

The developed model autonomously evaluates the data of COVID-19 and integrates two fields including ML and basic epidemiology. COVID-19 data from January to early March was included to train the model, and its forecasts for April were ongoing with the facts, demonstrating the model to be equipped for making clear predictions. The investigation has been carried out in four main hitting regions like Wuhan, South Korea, Italy, and the USA. It analyzed the impacts of quarantine and isolation measures in each country and virus prevention. Figure 4 presents the model outcome of learning patterns in COVID-19 spread.

The developed model highlights by imposing serious quarantine measures in countries like South Korea enables infection control. In places that were slower to actualize government mediations, similar to Italy and the USA, the effective reproduction number of COVID-19 remains more than one that represents a constant rise of infection in these nations. The ML model presents that with the quarantine measures followed by both Italy and the USA leveling the curve at the end of April. In the words of Professor George, 'the developed model has been successful in calculating the R0 value and making sure that governments should continue the preventive measures until the pandemic completely vanishes from the world' [30].

4.3 Deep Learning Models for COVID-19

Deep learning models can make quick decisions in COVID-19 disease diagnosis by involving medical images that are extracted from sources like magnetic resonance imaging (MRI) or computed tomography (CT) [31]. The COVID-19 quantification has been observed by CT scanning with individual characteristics that differ from other pneumonia called influenza-A viral (IAV) pneumonia. Authors

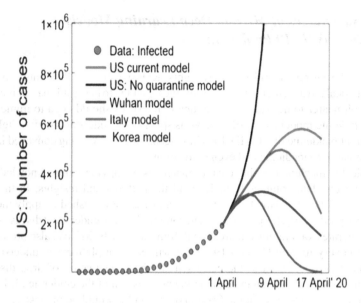

Fig. 4 Model patterns outcome of COVID-19 (*Source* MIT model)

present a screening model to differentiate the pneumonia caused by COVID-19 from IAV pneumonia and well-being individuals over CT images. The preliminary outcomes reported that 86.7% of accuracy was achieved in means of total scans. In this way, deep learning models are effective in early screening of corona virus-infected patients and proposing an additional diagnostic method of frontline medical doctors. Another study conducted an autonomous COVID-19 quantification for chest images by adopting deep learning models [32]. Results mentioned that chest CT combined deep learning software will be the best choice of COVID-19 diagnosis.

Another deep learning model in the diagnosis of COVID-19 by the smartphone embedded sensors were reported [33]. The common symptoms associated with COVID-19 such as headache, nausea, breathing issues, and high body temperature that are classified by the recurrent neural networks (RNN) and convolutional neural networks (CNN) algorithms. Wearable devices such as smartwatches and cameras were used for data collection. A finger sensor was utilized to measure patient temperature. To identify fatigue, camera images, and inertial sensors were used. Based on all these data, COVID-19 severity score was calculated and diagnosed the disease.

The deep learning models integrated with the social media-based natural language process (NLP) help to understand opinions on automatic extraction of COVID-19 [34]. The RNN algorithms were adopted to conduct sentimental analysis on COVID-19 comments. Results highlighted the necessity of understanding public opinion revolving around COVID-19 issues that will guide to related decision making.

4.4 Advantages of ML and Deep Learning Models in COVID-19 Prediction

Because the current world seriously fights against COVID-19, a single piece of technological advancement and resourcefulness tackled to battle this pandemic brings us one bit nearer to defeating it. The healthcare industries should need to immediately adopt epidemic models to predict the virus spread and understand how to fight with the current pandemic of COVID-19. These technologies are being conveyed in areas from research to medicine and even cultivation.

Basically, machine learning enables machines in copying human knowledge and analyzing big data volumes to understand the patterns and insights. In the battle against COVID-19, hospitals and medical industries have rushed to apply their ML expertise, particularly, to speed up patient communication, understand disease spread, and accelerate examination and treatment. Simultaneously, ML can also promote the drug discovery to treat COVID-19, and it will create a platform in understanding the patient body reaction to the coronavirus. The investigation of drug discovery using machine learning can understand the progression of the epidemic [35]. At the same time, COVID-19 is not the first pandemic and it would be the last. As of this, we should have an explicit understanding of ML techniques in the management of pandemics like coronavirus. Hundreds of studies are established across the world to define collective efforts data analysis and propose preventive measures. Therefore, here are some examples of ML works that are helping us to overcome this disease.

ML has already proved that it has the capability of predicting the risks of many diseases. Especially, when medical risk arrives, machine learning is highly interested in three ways such as

Infection risk: Determines COVID-19 risk for specific individuals or groups.

Severity: Understands the risk of a specific group or individual to develop serious COVID-19 symptoms, which requires immediate hospitalization or intensive care.

Risk outcomes: Defines is there any risk with a particular treatment and how likely they are ready to get mortality.

Even machine learning has the potentiality of predicting three risks mentioned, yet it is still a young discipline for COVID-19. More literature and experiments on machine learning have to be developed to have promising results. Besides, we can look at how ML is used in other related areas and understand the risk prediction of COVID-19.

Chatbots are making a mark in the field of medical organizations. Medical chatbots can conduct head-to-head conversations with patients and evaluate each patient's requests. Using a chatbot, the consumers not only get quick and easy access to information but also an interactive platform that is more engaging and personal. The chatbots involved with ML models can help to provide personal medical care and provide information on coronavirus disease at home without being physically available to the hospital [36].

5 Conclusions

There is a large need of implementing epidemic models in the detection and prevention of COVID-19. In this chapter, the authors presented the epidemic models description including mathematical equations and COVID-19 transmission prediction. The authors discussed the different epidemic models including time series, mathematical, machine learning, and deep learning types.

References

1. Andersen KG, Rambaut A, Lipkin WI, Holmes EC, Garry RF (2020) The proximal origin of SARS-CoV-2. Nat Med. https://doi.org/10.1038/s41591-020-0820-9
2. Mousavizadeh L, Ghasemi S (2020) Genotype and phenotype of COVID-19: their roles in pathogenesis. J Microbiol Immunol Infect. https://doi.org/10.1016/j.jmii.2020.03.022
3. Chintalapudi N, Battineni G, Sagaro GG, Amenta F (2020) COVID-19 outbreak reproduction number estimations and forecasting in Marche, Italy. Int J Infect Dis. https://doi.org/10.1016/j.ijid.2020.05.029
4. Chintalapudi N, Battineni G, Amenta F (2020) COVID-19 virus outbreak forecasting of registered and recovered cases after sixty day lockdown in Italy: a data driven model approach. J Microbiol Immunol Infect. https://doi.org/10.1016/j.jmii.2020.04.004
5. Eubank S, Eckstrand I, Lewis B, Venkatramanan S, Marathe M, Barrett CL (2020) Commentary on Ferguson et al 'Impact of non-pharmaceutical Interventions (NPIs) to reduce COVID-19 mortality and healthcare demand. Bull Math Biol. https://doi.org/10.1007/s11538-020-00726-x
6. Usher K, Bhullar N, Durkin J, Gyamfi N, Jackson D (2020) Family violence and COVID-19: increased vulnerability and reduced options for support. Int J Ment Health Nurs. https://doi.org/10.1111/inm.12735
7. Mohamadou Y, Halidou A, Kapen PT (2020) A review of mathematical modeling, artificial intelligence and datasets used in the study, prediction and management of COVID-19. Appl Intell. https://doi.org/10.1007/s10489-020-01770-9
8. Ndaïrou F, Area I, Nieto JJ, Torres DFM (2020) Mathematical modeling of COVID-19 transmission dynamics with a case study of Wuhan. Chaos Solitons Fractals. https://doi.org/10.1016/j.chaos.2020.109846
9. Ivorra B, Ferrández MR, Vela-Pérez M, Ramos AM (2020) Mathematical modeling of the spread of the coronavirus disease 2019 (COVID-19) taking into account the undetected infections. The case of China. Commun Nonlinear Sci Numer Simul. https://doi.org/10.1016/j.cnsns.2020.105303
10. Xiong Y, Yeung DY (2004) Time series clustering with ARMA mixtures. Pattern Recognit. https://doi.org/10.1016/j.patcog.2003.12.018
11. Kalpakis K, Gada D, Puttagunta V (2001) Distance measures for effective clustering of ARIMA time-series. https://doi.org/10.1109/icdm.2001.989529
12. Alzahrani SI, Aljamaan IA, Al-Fakih EA (2020) Forecasting the spread of the COVID-19 pandemic in Saudi Arabia using ARIMA prediction model under current public health interventions. J Infect Public Health. https://doi.org/10.1016/j.jiph.2020.06.001
13. Yang Q, Wang J, Ma H, Wang X (2020) Research on COVID-19 based on ARIMA modelΔ—taking Hubei, China as an example to see the epidemic in Italy. J Infect Public Health. https://doi.org/10.1016/j.jiph.2020.06.019
14. Aslam M (2020) Using the kalman filter with Arima for the COVID-19 pandemic dataset of Pakistan. Data Br. https://doi.org/10.1016/j.dib.2020.105854
15. Ceylan Z (2020) Estimation of COVID-19 prevalence in Italy, Spain, and France. Sci Total Environ. https://doi.org/10.1016/j.scitotenv.2020.138817

16. Khan FM, Gupta R (2020) ARIMA and NAR based prediction model for time series analysis of COVID-19 cases in India. J Saf Sci Resil. https://doi.org/10.1016/j.jnlssr.2020.06.007
17. Lauer SA et al (2020) The incubation period of coronavirus disease 2019 (COVID-19) From publicly reported confirmed cases: estimation and application. Ann Intern Med. https://doi.org/10.7326/M20-0504
18. He S, Peng Y, Sun K (2020) SEIR modeling of the COVID-19 and its dynamics. Nonlinear Dyn. https://doi.org/10.1007/s11071-020-05743-y
19. Carcione JM, Santos JE, Bagaini C, Ba J (2020) A Simulation of a COVID-19 epidemic based on a deterministic SEIR model. Front Public Heal. https://doi.org/10.3389/fpubh.2020.00230
20. Wu JT et al (2020) Estimating clinical severity of COVID-19 from the transmission dynamics in Wuhan, China. Nat Med. https://doi.org/10.1038/s41591-020-0822-7
21. O'Sullivan D, Gahegan M, Exeter DJ, Adams B (2020) Spatially explicit models for exploring COVID-19 lockdown strategies. Trans GIS. https://doi.org/10.1111/tgis.12660
22. Guliyev H (2020) Determining the spatial effects of COVID-19 using the spatial panel data model. Spat Stat. https://doi.org/10.1016/j.spasta.2020.100443
23. Ivorra B, Martínez-López B, Sánchez-Vizcaíno JM, Ramos ÁM (2014) Mathematical formulation and validation of the Be-FAST model for classical swine fever virus spread between and within farms. Ann Oper Res. https://doi.org/10.1007/s10479-012-1257-4
24. Ivorra B, Ngom D, Ramos ÁM (2015) Be-CoDiS: A mathematical model to predict the risk of human diseases spread between countries—validation and application to the 2014–2015 ebola virus disease epidemic. Bull Math Biol. https://doi.org/10.1007/s11538-015-0100-x
25. Briz-Redón Á, Serrano-Aroca Á (2020) A spatio-temporal analysis for exploring the effect of temperature on COVID-19 early evolution in Spain. Sci Total Environ. https://doi.org/10.1016/j.scitotenv.2020.138811
26. Donsimoni JR, Glawion R, Plachter B, Wälde K (2020) Projecting the Spread of COVID-19 for Germany. Wirtschaftsdienst. https://doi.org/10.1007/s10273-020-2631-5
27. Yenidogan I, Cayir A, Kozan O, Dag T, Arslan C (2018) Bitcoin forecasting using ARIMA and PROPHET. https://doi.org/10.1109/ubmk.2018.8566476
28. Wang P, Zheng X, Li J, Zhu B (2020) Prediction of epidemic trends in COVID-19 with logistic model and machine learning technics. Chaos Solitons Fractals. https://doi.org/10.1016/j.chaos.2020.110058
29. Mahmud S (2020) Bangladesh COVID-19 daily cases time series analysis using facebook prophet model. SSRN Electron J. https://doi.org/10.2139/ssrn.3660368
30. Dandekar R, Barbastathis G (2020) Quantifying the effect of quarantine control in Covid-19 infectious spread using machine learning. medRxiv, p. 2020.04.03.20052084, Apr. 2020 https://doi.org/10.1101/2020.04.03.20052084
31. Xu X et al (2020) A deep learning system to screen novel coronavirus disease 2019 Pneumonia. Engineering https://doi.org/10.1016/j.eng.2020.04.010
32. Tao Zhang H et al (2020) Automated detection and quantification of COVID-19 pneumonia: CT imaging analysis by a deep learning-based software. Eur J Nucl Med Mol Imaging. https://doi.org/10.1007/s00259-020-04953-1
33. Maghdid HS, Ghafoor KZ, Sadiq AS, Curran K, Rawat DB, Rabie K (2020) A novel AI-enabled framework to diagnose coronavirus COVID 19 using smartphone embedded sensors: design study. Accessed 22 Aug 2020. [Online]. Available: http://arxiv.org/abs/2003.07434
34. Jelodar H, Wang Y, Orji R, Huang H (2020) Deep sentiment classification and topic discovery on novel coronavirus or COVID-19 online discussions: NLP using LSTM recurrent neural network approach. IEEE J Biomed Heal Inf. https://doi.org/10.1109/jbhi.2020.3001216
35. Vamathevan J et al (2019) Applications of machine learning in drug discovery and development. Nat Rev Drug Discov. https://doi.org/10.1038/s41573-019-0024-5
36. Battineni G, Chintalapudi N, Amenta F (2020) AI chatbot design during an epidemic like the novel coronavirus. Healthcare. https://doi.org/10.3390/healthcare8020154

Chapter 3
SIQRS Epidemic Modelling and Stability Analysis of COVID-19

Aswin Kumar Rauta, Yerra Shankar Rao, Jangyadatta Behera, Binayak Dihudi, and Tarini Charan Panda

Nomenclature

S Susceptible class
I Infected class
Q Quarantine class
R Removed class
R_o Basic reproduction number
α Transmission rate per day from S to I
β Transmission rate per day from I to Q
γ Transmission rate per day from Q to R
σ Recovered rate per day from R to S
μ Rate of infected immigrant to infected class
θ Natural death rate
η COVID-19 death rate

A. K. Rauta · J. Behera
Department of Mathematics, S.K.C.G. (Autonomous) College, Paralakhemundi, Odisha 761200, India
e-mail: aswinmath2003@gmail.com

J. Behera
e-mail: jangyabhr09@gmail.com

Y. S. Rao (✉)
Department of Mathematics, GIET Ghangapatana, Bhubaneswar, Odisha 752054, India
e-mail: sankar.math1@gmail.com

B. Dihudi
Department of Mathematics, KIST, Jatni, Bhubaneswar, Odisha 752050, India
e-mail: bdihudi@gmail.com

T. C. Panda
Department of Mathematics, Ravenshaw University, Cuttack, Odisha 753003, India
e-mail: tc_panda@yahoo.com

© The Author(s), under exclusive license to Springer Nature Singapore Pte Ltd. 2021
P. K. Khosla et al. (eds.), *Predictive and Preventive Measures for Covid-19 Pandemic*,
Algorithms for Intelligent Systems, https://doi.org/10.1007/978-981-33-4236-1_3

1 Introduction

In the current situation, the world is facing pandemic COVID-19 infection with an increasing number of deaths. In the European countries, it spreads from asymptomatic to symptomatic of severe pneumonia followed by mild respiratory infection, cough, cold, sneezing, fever, sour throat and fatigue. On 9 January 2020, China reported to WHO about this respiratory disease which was first detected from Hubei in Wuhan city of China in December 2019. Initially, the novel coronavirus was associated with severe acute respiratory illness and pneumonia. This symptomatic disease with an unknown virus is called a novel coronavirus disease 2019, i.e. COVID-19. Till now no research laboratory and pharmaceutical company discover any vaccine or medicine to cure and suppress this dreadful disease. Hence on 30 January 2020, WHO declared this disease as a public health emergency of international concern. As the basic reproduction number lies in between 2 and 3, so on 11 March 2020 WHO declared this disease as a global pandemic. Normally for the patients suffering from the disease COVID-19, the incubation period is from 5 to 6 days rather than within two weeks from the first day of infection. Many researchers reveal that the incubation period must be of 14 days. In first 1–2 days, the virus is detected in the respiratory tract before the symptoms develop, in moderate case it will prolong for 7–12 days and in case of acute it often remains 14 days. In onset symptomatic virus like viral RNA is identified from the 5th day and in moderate cases, it may remain for four to five weeks.

Therefore, in order to deal with the hypothesis regarding biological and sociological devices which control the transmission of disease and mitigation, etc., the mathematical modelling and its descriptive analysis would be helpful in estimating the transmission dynamics, severity, mitigation measure and the controlling impact of the disease. Many researchers have studied the disease by taking different models and suggested different control measures like social distancing and quarantine of infected individuals. To investigate any new disease, it is essential to understand the background of the infective disease, its mathematical models, stability analysis and effective parameter values. Thus, we have reviewed the following few works of literature related to infections in epidemiology to develop this model.

Al-Sheikh et al. [1] have presented a paper that established the stability of HIV/AIDS with respect to the screening of unaware disease. The paper explains the different aspects of AIDS which is helpful for understanding the modelling of COVID-19. Horst [2] has derived stability analysis for the endemic equilibrium with the help of semi-positive definite operator and Lyapunov theory. The stability analysis presented in this paper can be used to study the stability analysis of current pandemic COVID-19. Ma et al. [3] have investigated the SIR model and explained the global stability using the comparison principle. This model can be used for extending it to SIQRS model and to check the stability behaviours. Erdem et al. [4] have analysed the SIQR influenza model with imperfect quarantine and found the oscillatory behaviour of the model which is alike with the stability behaviours of COVID-19 in some countries like South Korea and China. Lan et al. [5] have investigated the stochastic persistence of diseases using SIQR epidemic model and suggested to use Markov semi-group theory to establish the existence of unique stable stationary distribution. Cao et al. [6] studied the epidemic of susceptible, infectious, quarantine and recovered nodes. The study established that the infective disease eliminates comparatively large white noise. By using the delay parameter in Xia et al. [7] have discussed the SEIQ epidemic model and established the local stability of the model. In Lu et al. [8] have formulated the basic biological models like SIQR, SIR in which they interpreted that food is related to the disease using predator–prey and nonlinear dynamics. They have established Lyapunov function for the existence of periodic stationary point. Mohmood et al. [9] have studied the SIVS model using standard incidence rate and established the global stability based on geometric approaches. Bin et al. [10] have constructed SLIDS compartments based on cellular automata theory that explains the spread of pandemic influenza A (H1N1). They have analysed the different groups like sex ratio, population density, age, etc., with the global stability and local stability, but the study did not demonstrate the individual and their neighbour randomness. Cakir et al. [11] have modelled the COVID-19 by using a simple differential equation and suggested that the infection rate can be reduced using social distancing. Nag [12] has considered the SIS model having both infected and non-infected immigrants and the death rate due to COVID 19 without stability analysis. Kucharski et al. [13] have interpreted the SEIR model with the help of basic reproduction number. They have narrated how the disease declined gradually in Wuhan town of China. Dey et al. [14] have elaborated the data analysis approaches of COVID 19 and concluded that the early detection, management and containment of the spot are only preventive measures of the disease. Nian et al. [15] have examined the dynamic model of COVID-19 and found that containment and effective isolation of the population are essential measures to control COVID-19. Singh et al. [16] have investigated the spread of COVID-19 in India based on age structure and suggested that the lockdown of 21 days is insufficient for India. A complete 49 days or periodic lockdown of 21 + 28 + 18 days with 5 days relaxation of social distancing is necessary to control COVID-19.

The above literature survey concerning different infectious disease motivates many ideas, tools, techniques and methods to explore in research dimension in the development of the study of COVID-19 for control, interpretation and simulation of the data numerically. Some researchers have considered many parameters but did not present the stability analysis. Many authors have presented stability analysis by considering only limited parameters. The papers publications consequently related to COVID-19 have ignored many aspects like infected immigrants, normal death rate, the death rate due to other diseases and quarantine node, etc. So, after a retrospective analysis of many papers, we have considered the SIQRS model with the rate of infected immigrants in infected compartment and rate of natural death in susceptible class and death due to COVID-19 in removed class. The novelty of this paper is the consideration of the infected rate of immigrants directly in the infected compartment with quarantine effect. Also here the authors have derived analytically the stability analysis for locally and globally at infection-free and endemic equilibrium points. Again these results are illustrated in numerically simulations and graphically. So, this research paper is new and original in the area of mathematical modelling of COVID-19.

2 Mathematical Model

Let's consider that the whole number of the individuals is divided into four number of sub-individuals such as Susceptible $S(t)$, Infected $I(t)$, Quarantined $Q(t)$ and Recovered $R(t)$. These individuals change from time to time. Since the whole individuals $N(t)$ are very large so it is divided into different compartments and the size varies continuously from compartment to compartment. The population has constant size N and is sufficiently large so that the size of each compartment is considered as a continuous variable. The number of individuals who may catch the COVID-19 but presently are not affected is considered as a Susceptible class (S). The number of individuals who are currently being infected with COVID-19 carry the disease to a susceptible population; these populations are known as Infective class (I). The Quarantine class (Q) consists of the number of individuals who are either in isolation or under treatment. The Removal Class (R) consists of the number of individuals who are recovered from quarantine and with susceptible-infective populations after treatment of COVID-19. Here, the transformation between the individuals are from Susceptible class to Infective class, then Infective class to Quarantine class and Quarantine class to Removed class, finally back to Susceptible class upon recovery since the COVID-19 has no immunity against it on recovery. So this model is known as the SIQRS model which is diagrammatically shown in Fig. 1.

Now we can take the time range to be very less like one second, so according to the classical epidemic model termed as a Kermack–McKendrick epidemic model, the rate of change of every population of this model is presented by a nonlinear system of ordinary equation

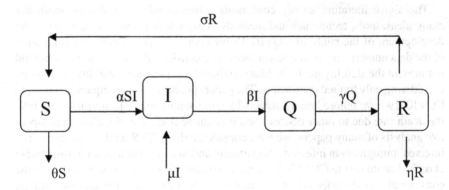

Fig. 1 Compartmental diagram of the model

$$\frac{dS}{dt} = \sigma R - (\theta S + \alpha\, SI)$$

$$\frac{dI}{dt} = \alpha SI + (\mu - \beta)I$$

$$\frac{dQ}{dt} = \beta I - \gamma Q$$

$$\frac{dR}{dt} = \gamma Q - (\eta + \sigma)R \tag{1}$$

In general, this system of the differential equations does not have any closed form. However, by taking different initial values and parameters we have deduced a solution to the above system of equations numerically using Runge–Kutta method for fourth order with the help of mathematical software named as MATLAB.

Basic Assumptions

Since the disease occurs relatively quickly, so the model does not include the birth rate. In this model, the total size of the population is considered as one unit with no latency case. The population is assumed as homogeneously mixing, i.e. the population is well mixed. Here we have assumed that each population is susceptible to borne the diseases, the infection caused due to interaction among the direct and indirect infected populations. Again here it has been taken into consideration that all the populations are uniformly susceptible, with the absence of co-infections and many pathogen infections. Due to the absence of proper vaccination/ medicines, we can use the quarantine/isolation class. Here we can assume from the above system of Eq. (1), all the populations are positive/nonnegative due to the negative solution have no importance in epidemiology. We can take the total population to be a fixed number which is equal to $N = 1$ unit of time, i.e. by adding all the populations. We have built our SIQRS model based on the assumption $N = S + I + Q + R$. The system (1) is closed, positive invariant set $\Omega = \{S(t) + I(t) + Q(t) + R(t) = N(t) : S(t) \geq 0, I(t) \geq 0, Q(t) \geq 0, R(t) \geq 0\}$.

Equilibrium Points and Stability Analysis

In this section, we discuss two equilibrium states
    i..e (1) Infection-free equilibrium state and
    (2) Endemic equilibrium state.
    To obtain the point of equilibriums for the disease-free state, the system of Eq. (1) can be written in a steady-state form as:

$$\sigma R - (\theta S + \alpha\, SI) = 0$$

$$\alpha SI + (\mu - \beta)I = 0$$

$$\beta I - \gamma Q = 0$$

$$\gamma Q - (\eta + \sigma)R = 0 \tag{2}$$

We can found for the infection-free equilibrium point as $\Omega_0 = \{S = 1, I = Q = R = 0\}$

For the Endemic Equilibrium point as $\Omega^* = \{S^*, I^*, Q^*, R^*\}$.

By workout the Eq. (2) altogether, we have

$$S^* = \frac{\beta - \mu}{\alpha}$$

$$I^* = \frac{-\theta}{\alpha}$$

$$Q^* = \frac{-\beta\theta}{\gamma\alpha}$$

$$R^* = \frac{-\beta\theta}{\alpha(\eta + \sigma)}$$

Local Stability Analysis

Theorem 1

When the system of Eq. (2) is asymptotically local stable at the infection-free equilibrium in the given region Ω_0 if $R_0 < 1$, otherwise it is unstable and goes to endemic equilibrium.

Proof Linearization of the system of an Eq. (2) for the infection-free equilibrium $\Omega_0 = \{S(t) = 1, I(t) = 0, Q(t) = 0.R(t) = 0\}$, the Jacobian matrix of (2) is

$$J_{INF} = \begin{pmatrix} -\theta & -\alpha & 0 & \sigma \\ 0 & \alpha + \mu - \beta & 0 & 0 \\ 0 & \beta & -\gamma & 0 \\ 0 & 0 & 0 & -(\eta + \sigma) \end{pmatrix}$$

The characteristic equation is

$$\begin{vmatrix} -\theta - \lambda & -\alpha & 0 & \sigma \\ 0 & (\alpha + \mu - \beta) - \lambda & 0 & 0 \\ 0 & \beta & -\gamma - \lambda & 0 \\ 0 & 0 & 0 & -(\eta + \sigma) - \lambda \end{vmatrix} = 0$$

All the eigenvalues, $\lambda_1 = -\theta, \lambda_2 = -\gamma, \lambda_3 = -(\eta + \sigma), \lambda_4 = \alpha + \mu - \beta$ have negative real parts. For $\lambda_4 = (\alpha + \mu) < \beta, \Rightarrow \lambda_4 = \frac{(\alpha + \mu)}{\beta} < 1,$

i.e. $R_0 = \lambda_4 = \frac{(\alpha + \mu)}{\beta} < 1$

Hence according to the stability criteria for Routh–Hurwitz theorem, the system (2) is asymptotically local stable at infection-free equilibrium Ω_0 if $R_0 < 1$ and when $R_0 > 1$, it is unstable.

Now, for the (EE) endemic equilibrium $\Omega^* = \{S^*, I^*, Q^*, R^*\}$, when $R_0 > 1$, the variation matrix (2) is

$$J_{EE} = \begin{pmatrix} \alpha I^* & \alpha S^* + \mu - \beta & 0 & 0 \\ -\theta - \alpha I^* & -\alpha S^* & 0 & \sigma \\ 0 & \beta & -\gamma & 0 \\ 0 & 0 & 0 & -(\eta + \sigma) \end{pmatrix}$$

Putting the values of S^*, I^* in the above variation matrix, we have

$$J_{EE} = \begin{pmatrix} \alpha\left(-\frac{\theta}{\alpha}\right) & \alpha\left(\frac{\beta-\mu}{\alpha}\right) + \mu - \beta & 0 & 0 \\ -\theta - \alpha\left(-\frac{\theta}{\alpha}\right) & -\alpha\left(\frac{\beta-\mu}{\alpha}\right) & 0 & \sigma \\ 0 & \beta & -\gamma & 0 \\ 0 & 0 & 0 & -(\eta + \sigma) \end{pmatrix}$$

$$J_{EE} = \begin{pmatrix} -\theta & 0 & 0 & 0 \\ 0 & -(\beta - \mu) & 0 & \sigma \\ 0 & \beta & -\gamma & 0 \\ 0 & 0 & 0 & -(\eta + \sigma) \end{pmatrix}$$

The auxiliary roots are

$$\lambda_1 = -\theta$$
$$\lambda_2 = -\gamma$$
$$\lambda_3 = -(\eta + \sigma)$$
$$\lambda_4 = -(\beta - \mu) = \beta(R_0 - 1 - \alpha)$$

Again by Routh–Hurwitz criteria of stability, the system (2) for endemic equilibrium Ω^* is locally asymptotic stable when $R_0 > 1$.

Global Stability Analysis

Theorem 2
When $R_0 > 1$, the endemic equilibrium is globally stable in the region Ω^*.

Proof For proving the global stability in the region Ω^* we are following the Dulac's condition for multiplies $D = 1/I$, in the SI plane of the positive quadrant, so we are using the first two equations of the system (1) are free from Q. Therefore in the positive quadrant of SI plane, we can take two functions F_1 and F_2 such that

$$F_1 = -\theta S - \alpha \, SI$$
$$F_2 = \alpha \, SI - (\mu + \beta)I$$

$$\text{Then} \quad \begin{aligned} DF_1 &= \tfrac{-\theta S}{I} - \alpha S \\ DF_2 &= \alpha S - (\mu + \beta) \end{aligned}$$

$$\therefore \text{We have,} \quad \begin{aligned} &\tfrac{\partial}{\partial S}(DF_1) + \tfrac{\partial}{\partial I}(DF_2) \\ &= \tfrac{\partial}{\partial S}\left(\tfrac{-\theta S}{I} - \alpha S\right) + \tfrac{\partial}{\partial I}(\alpha S - (\mu + \beta)) \\ &= \tfrac{-\theta}{I} - \alpha < 0 \end{aligned}$$

Thus, there is no limit cycle, i.e. periodic solution does not exist in the given region Ω. So as per Poincare–Bendixson theorem, each solution begins in the SI plane of positive quadrants $I(t) > 0$ with time 't' approaching to infinity as S tends to S^* and I tends to I^*. In this case, the closed form of third and fourth equations of the system (1) shows Q tends to Q^* and R tends to R^*. Hence, the system is globally stable in the region in case of endemic equilibrium points of the region Ω^*.

3 Numerical Simulation and Discussion of the Results

In this paper, the nonlinear differential equations are solved using the Runge–Kutta fourth-order method. We are taking the time interval for 200 days with its initial values of the different compartments/ class as: susceptible populations $S(0) = 0.9$, Infected populations $I(0) = 0.1$, Quarantined populations $Q(0) = 0$ and Removed population $R(0 = 0)$. The numerical simulation and graphical representation are done using MATLAB software. By using the Jacobian matrix form, we obtained the basic reproduction number of the given model. These numbers determine the stability of the model. It is found that if the basic reproduction number is more than one the system of the model is unstable and starts to an epidemic. Similarly, if this number is less than one the system is stable. Also by applying the Dulac's principle, we derived the global stability of the model at the endemic equilibrium points. Again by applying the time series and phase portraits, we can illustrate that the proposed model becomes stable in both locally and globally in the given region. The simulated results agree with the mathematical stability of both equilibrium points which are shown in Figs. 2, 3, 4, 5 and 6.

It has been seen from Figs. 2, 3, 4, 5 and 6 that for increasing values of basic reproduction number, the presence of infective immigrants in the system increases the total population initially. But as time goes on more susceptible individuals get infected with the disease and then develops into COVID-19. As time increases, the infective population also increases, which leads to infection of many susceptible individuals due to the absence of control strategies or improper control strategies and the rapid inflow of infected immigrants. They eventually die thereby reducing the total population in the long run. Therefore, the infected classes, quarantine class and recovered class of COVID-19 all initially increase but later reduce to zero. Approximately in 120 days (no epidemic), the infected individuals eventually decrease to zero and in 180 days (epidemic) the infected individuals reach their steady state of 0.0–0.1. For

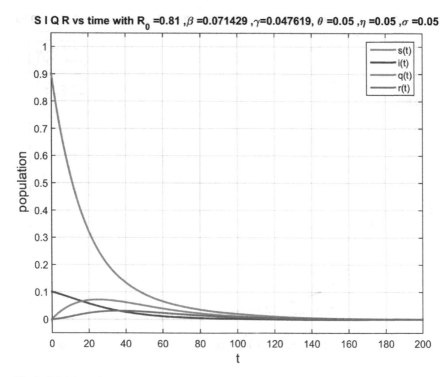

Fig. 2 S I Q R vs time with R_0=0.81

the case of non-epidemic and epidemic, the initial conditions for all the populations of this system are locally stable. The susceptible and infected individuals change with respect to time and decrease until they reach at zero. That is the whole populations get infected with the COVID-19 disease and transferred into the recovered phase.

Figure 7 illustrates that when the basic reproduction number $R_0 < 1$, then the virus wiped out as an infective replaces itself with less than single person. Since, everyone is under susceptible when the disease has disappeared, so the susceptible fraction eventually approaches to one.

Similarly, Fig. 8 explains that the initial infective fraction $I(0)$ is small when the basic reproduction number $R_0 > 1$. If the initial susceptible fraction $S(0)$ is large then S decreases and I increases to a peak value and after it decreases which becomes an epidemic in nature. However, when the infective fraction decreases to a low level, then the susceptible fraction increases slowly due to the recovery of new susceptible.

From Figs. 9 and 10, it is observed that the rate of recovered individuals is increased followed by hospital quarantine. Also, it exhibits that some infected individuals are present in the population. As shown in the Fig. 9, it is clear that the rate of recovered individuals is inversely proportional to susceptible individuals. It shows that due to improper health measures in the hospital the recovered population reduces. Under control, the susceptible population decreases slowly and remains constant in

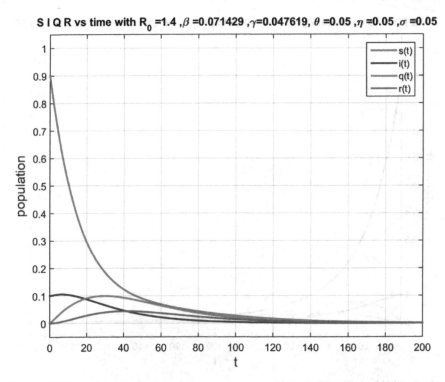

S I Q R vs time with R_0 =1.4 ,β =0.071429 ,γ=0.047619, θ =0.05 ,η =0.05 ,σ =0.05

Fig. 3 S I Q R vs time with R_0=1.4

its size after some time. After hospitalization, the number of contaminated individuals decrease and simultaneously number of individuals recovered.

Therefore from the above figurative analysis, it is observed that to minimize the spread of the disease and to prevent the total population from being infected with, effective immigration policies such as screening should be implemented. This ensures that infected individuals who might act irresponsibly may be denied entry or are exposed as to minimize their potential of infecting others. Also, it is clear that for a short term period the rate of conversion from the infective population to COVID-19 patients increase. However, in the long run, due to implementation of quarantine, there is an increasing result of reducing the COVID-19 populations which control the disease, not only decreases the endemic infective class but also lead to disease extinction forever. It means if infective becomes full-blown COVID-19 patients at a higher rate then by increasing more Quarantine and Recovery rate the infective class can be reduced. However, as more infective develop COVID-19 and pass out of the system (through COVID-19-induced death), there will be a reduction in the Recover class in the long term. The general trend of the infected population will rise first; then, it will decrease and the system becomes stable.

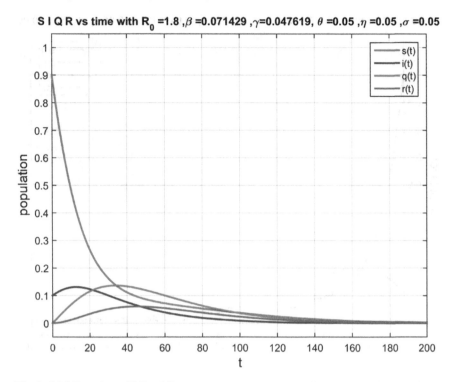

Fig. 4 S I Q R vs time with R_0=1.8

4 Conclusion

In this research paper, we have made an effort to formulate COVID-19 using a nonlinear continuous dynamic epidemic model SIQRS. For reducing the spread of disease, a technique called 'Quarantine or Isolation' is proposed and included in this study. Quarantine of infected individuals is a powerful technique and can be used to control the spreading of the epidemic. Thus, it suggests that the epidemic spreads to the whole population with the progressive time unless control measurements are taken. It is found that an endemic of infection increases in the absences of quarantine node. Also, the rate of infected immigrant enhances the spread of disease. We have discussed the local and global stabilities of the model at the disease-free equilibrium point (DFE) and an endemic equilibrium point (EE). The theory predicts that as long as $R_0 > 1$ the epidemic grows without any interruption and spreads to the whole population. Further, by using Dulac function and Poincare–Bendixson theorem it is clearly understood that for $R_0 < 1$ the nonlinear dynamic model is locally asymptomatic stable. Also, the system is globally stable when $R_0 > 1$. At last, it is observed that in 200-days, 90% individuals recovered and only a small that is 10% of the population individuals are susceptible out of the majority of the proportional population. It is interpreted that the coronavirus disease outbreak vanishes over the

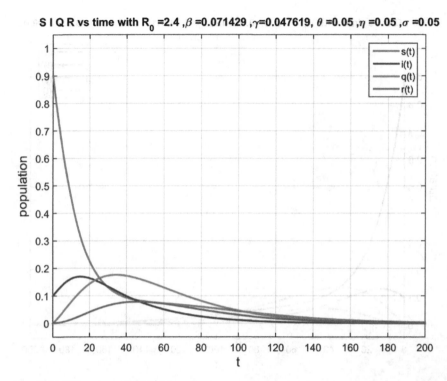

Fig. 5 S I Q R vs time with R_0=2.4

evolution of time for $R_0 < 1$ but remains alive among the population for $R_0 > 1$. After approximately in 180 days, the infected individuals decay to zero and hence from the proportional population time series, the system is stable. In the same number of days, the recovered and susceptible individuals reach their steady-state values essentially. Therefore, a complete lockdown with social distancing is needed and to be maintained to control the pandemic disease.

For the scope of future research work, this SIQRS model can be extended to different more realistic epidemic mathematical models by considering different parameters associated with the disease like infection-age group structure, incorporate age group structure and spatial structure along with the procedure of treatment, use of drugs, vaccinations and temporary immunity with vital dynamics, pre-quarantine, exposed and vertical transmission.

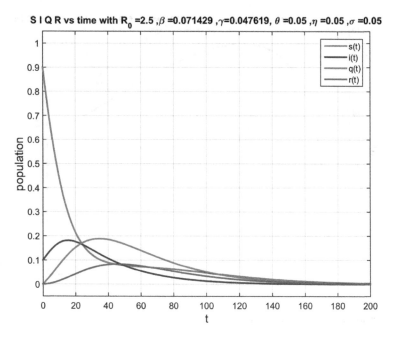

Fig. 6 S I Q R vs time with R_0=2.5

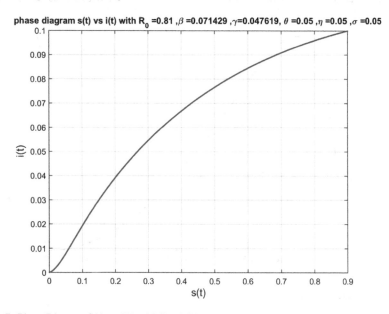

Fig. 7 Phase Diagram S(t) vs I(t) with R_0=0.81

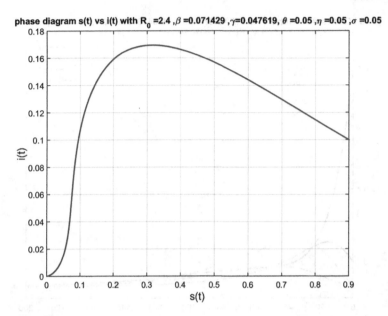

Fig. 8 Phase Diagram S(t) vs I(t) with $R_0=2.4$

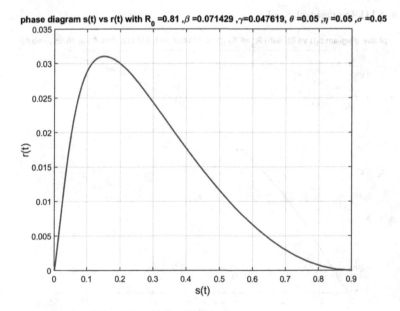

Fig. 9 Phase Diagram S(t) vs R(t) with $R_0=0.81$

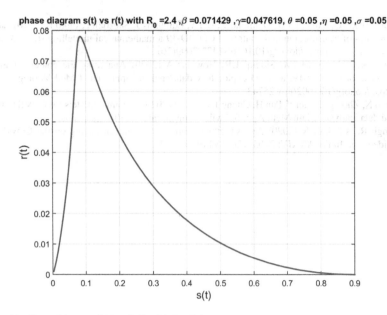

Fig. 10 Phase Diagram S(t) vs R(t) with R_0=2.4

References

1. Al-Sheikh S, Musali F, Alsolamana M (2011) Stability analysis of HIV/AIDS epidemic model with screening. Int Math. Forum 6:3251–3273
2. Horst R (2011) Thieme, global stability of the endemic equilibrium in infinite dimension, lyapunov function and positive operators. J Diff Equ 250:3772–3801
3. Ma X, Zhou Y, Cao H (2013) Global stability of the endemic equilibrium of discrete SIR epidemic model. Adv Differ Equ. Springer Open Access 42:1–19
4. Erdem M, Safan M (2017) Carlos Castillo-Chavez, mathematical analysis of an SIQR influenza model with imperfect quarantine. Bull Math Biol, Springer, pp 1–25
5. Lan G, Chen Z, Wei C, Zhang S (2018) Stationary distribution of stochastic SIQR epidemic model with saturated incidence and degenerate diffusion. Phys A 511:61–77
6. Cao Z, Zhou S (2018) Dynamical behaviours of stochastic SIQR epidemic model with quarantine adjusted incidence, discrete dynamics in nature and society, pp 1–13
7. Xia W, Kundu S, Maitra S (2018) Dynamics of delayed SEIQ epidemic model. Adv Differ. Equ. 336:1–21
8. Liu Q, Jiang D, Hayat T, Ahmed B (2018) Stationary distribution and extinction of a stochastic predator-prey model with additional food and nonlinear perturbation. Appl Math Comput 320:226–239
9. Parsamanesh M, Farnoosh R (2018) On global stability of endemic state in an epidemic model with vaccinations. Math Sci 12:313–320
10. Bin S, Sun G, Chen C-C (2019) Spread of infectious diseases modelling and analysis of different factors on spread of infectious disease based on cellular automata. Int J Env Res Publ Health 16:1–16
11. Cakir Z, Savas HB (2020) A mathematical modelling approach in the spread of the novel-2019 corona virus SARS–COV-2(COVID19) pandemic. Electron J Gen Med 17:1–3
12. Nag S (2020) A mathematical model in the time of COVID-1, March https://doi.org/10.31219/osf.io/8n22hresearchgate.net/publication/330934682

13. Kuchariski AJ, Russell TW, Diamond C, Liu Y, Edmunds J, Sabstian F, Eggo R (2020) Early dynamics of transmission and control of COVID-19 a mathematical modelling study, March 1–7, 30144–4. https://doi.org/10.1016/s1473-3099(20)

14. Dey SK, Rahman Md.M, Siddiqi UR, Howldar A (2020) Analyzing the epidemiological outbreak of COVID-19: a visual exploratory data analysis approach. J Med Virology, 1–7. https://doi.org/10.1002/jmv.25743

15. Shao N, Zhong M, Yan Y, Pan H, Cheng J, Chen W (2020) Dynamic models for COVID-2019 and data analysis. Math Meth Appl Sci wileyonlinelibrary.com/Journal/mma, 1–7

16. Singh R, Adhikari R (2020) Age structured impact of social distancing on the COVID19 epidemic in India, ARXIV: 2003. 12055VI [9-bio.PE], 1–9

Chapter 4
Mental Health Analysis of Students in Major Cities of India During COVID-19

Ashi Agarwal, Basant Agarwal, Priyanka Harjule, and Ajay Agarwal

1 Introduction

The novel coronavirus outbreak has brought the world to a standstill. The virus has clearly stopped our lives in motion. People are in high risk as this virus spreads rapidly in close proximity with other people and through community transmission [1]. The whole world is trying to contain the virus by different methods, and some of them have been unable to flatten the curve and India being one of them. The infection is spreading exponentially in India with an approximate 30,000 cases per day, and the country's overall mark has reached to 1.7 million cases [2]. Some cities of India are adversely affected by this virus such as Mumbai and Delhi. Several steps have been taken by Indian government to contain the virus such as nationwide lockdown, cancellation of flights and trains, delay in examination and many more which have caused sadness to despair among people living here. Some sections of Indian society, especially the migrant workers and students, have been affected adversely the government actions to prevent the spread of COVID-19. Millions of students were stranded in different cities and unable to reach their homes which have caused immense psychological stress to them and their parents. This outbreak

A. Agarwal
National Institute of Technology Raipur, Raipur, India

B. Agarwal (✉)
Department of Computer Science and Engineering, Indian Institute of Information Technology Kota (MNIT Campus Jaipur), Jaipur, India
e-mail: basant.cse@iiitkota.ac.in

P. Harjule
Department of Mathematics, Indian Institute of Information Technology Kota (MNIT Campus Jaipur), Jaipur, India

A. Agarwal
Department of Computer Science and Engineering, Dehradun Institute of Technology (DIT University Dehradun), Dehradun, India

© The Author(s), under exclusive license to Springer Nature Singapore Pte Ltd. 2021 51
P. K. Khosla et al. (eds.), *Predictive and Preventive Measures for Covid-19 Pandemic*,
Algorithms for Intelligent Systems, https://doi.org/10.1007/978-981-33-4236-1_4

and related events have caused immense distress among individuals and increased mental health issues like depression, stress, worry, fear, disgust, sadness, etc. [3]. The mental health issues can occur to any person affected or unaffected from coronavirus. Psychological stress can lead to depression and many other mental health issues [4]. It can lead to behavioural and psychological issues among people. A person faces several complications due to psychological stress, and increase in level of stress can lead to depression. Depression is one of the most common diseases among people worldwide. People under depression may encounter symptoms resulting to their inability to concentrate on anything, they persistently undergo the feelings of guilt, annoyance and irritation, and they suffer from less self-esteem, and experience problems in sleep. Therefore, serious consequences may result out of depression at both personal and social costs [5]. Suicidal cases were reported in India [6] and parts of world such as in Italy where two infected Italian nurses committed suicide in a period of a few days probably due to fear of spreading COVID-19 to patients.

Due to nationwide lockdown, work from home policy, shutdown of schools and colleges have created a surge on social media. People are using social media for expressing their thoughts, emotions, viewpoints to the world, and Twitter is one of the prominent used social networking sites. About 40% of consumers have spent longer than usual time on social media and messaging apps [7]. People express their views in the form of tweets. Every tweet represents a user state of mind and their viewpoint at that time. The proper analysis of these tweets may be used to find out the user's state of being, and its aggregation can lead to monitor health and provide solutions for the same [8].

It was found that there are a diverse set of quantifiable signals relevant to mental health observable in Twitter [9], due to which Twitter is widely used site for analysing depression around the world [10]. Various research works have been conducted in order to analyse depression using tweets done by users, employing machine learning algorithms [11–15]. One of the study [14] uses sentimental analysis to calculate the negativity of depressing tweets, and it was found that the negativity of sentiments has increased over period of time while the positive scores depressed.

This paper aims to examine psychological stress of the people living in major cities of India. The collected Twitter data extracted for the period of 3.5 month after the imposition of nationwide lockdown has been categorized into depressing and non-depressing tweets. This work aims at detecting psychological stress dynamics that can help government and related agencies to take appropriate steps. The primary purpose of the study is to find out the extent of the number of people that are tweeting about psychological stress and depression from major cities of India. The relationship between depressing tweets and COVID-19 cases was examined over a period of nationwide lockdown. Sentimental analysis was performed to study the negativity of tweets, and average negativity over divisions of Rajasthan, Mumbai, Bangalore and Delhi was plotted. The stress dynamics among the students stranded in Rajasthan was examined. The study gives the relation between psychological stresses of people over time period of implementation of lockdown until July 15. The paper is organized as follows: The work related to depression analysis is reviewed in Sect. 2, and the details of data are presented in Sect. 3. Sentimental analysis of depressing tweets is performed to estimate the severity range of tweets in Sect. 4. Further, the categorized data is used to examine the relationship between COVID-19 cases, depressing tweets and recovery rate for major cities of India separately in Sect. 5. In Sect. 6, dynamics between student's psychological stress and measures due to lockdown is studied along with sentimental analysis of their tweets. Finally, Sect. 7 gives conclusion.

2 Related Work

Social media is widely used as a data source for depression analysis due to the availability of data [16–19]. In Chudhury and Horvitz [16] have used Twitter as a data source for their analysis. They have used crowd sourcing methodology to build a large corpus of postings on Twitter that have been shared by individuals diagnosed with clinical depression. Their model leverages signals of social activity, emotion and language manifested on Twitter. Using the model, they introduce a social media depression index that may serve to characterize levels of depression in populations. In Rafiqul and Kabir [17] have used Facebook as a source of their data collection. They have used various machine learning algorithms for their depression analysis. They have used classification techniques such as 'decision tree', 'k-Nearest Neighbour', 'Support Vector Machine' and 'ensemble' for processing Facebook posts. They have applied these algorithms for emotion, temporal and linguistic factors independently. They have used psycholinguistic features, LIWC, a psycholinguistic vocabulary package made by psychological analysts to perceive the intellectual and etymological parts that lie on any verbal or written correspondence and convert it into numerical values. In different to these studies, special lexicology is used for depression analysis in this study. The individual tweets were processed to check if they contained lexicons [20, 21] related to depression. This was done using a string container function available in Python Pandas library. Further analysis was performed using classified tweets.

Many studies have used sentimental analysis to examine the depression level in a person. One such work of Salimath [22] uses sentimental analysis to build a metric-based depression detection model, and the sentiment was levelled up to evaluate the intensity of depression. They have used Google Cloud Natural API to process the transcripts they collected. The API inspects the transcripts and categorizes it into positive, negative and neutral sentiments along with numerical score. They developed a three-variable-based scale, i.e. X (number of negative sentences in a transcript/total number of sentences in a transcript), Y (mean of the score of all negative sentences in a transcript), Z (mean of the magnitude of all negative sentences in a transcript). The scale is the sum of three variables, i.e. X, $Y/2$ and $Z/4$. Y refers to the score of the sentiment which ranges between -1.0 and -0.25 (positive) and corresponds to the overall emotional leaning of the text. On the basis of score, they have created a range which identifies it into major depression, more severe depression for each person. In contrast to this work, we have used a text blob—simplified text processing tool of Python to perform sentimental analysis. It provides a simple API for diving into common natural language processing (NLP) tasks. Using a text blob, sentimental scores are generated for each tweet and sentiment value of each tweet, i.e. positive, negative and neutral. Apart from just examining the depression level of individual users, we have calculated depression level for major cities of India.

3 Details of Data

The source of data collection and data modification is explained in detail in this section.

3.1 Study Location

The study is conducted for the divisions of Rajasthan and three major cities of India that are Mumbai, Bengaluru and Delhi. Delhi is the capital city of India with a population of 1.9 crore. Mumbai is another densely populated city of India which has been adversely affected by COVID-19 virus. Bengaluru, the IT hub of India having population 0.8 crore is also severely affected by COVID-19. The COVID-19 dynamics for cities of Rajasthan is compared with these three major cities of India.

3.2 Data Collection

To analyse the psychological stress dynamics, we collected tweets from the different Twitter users residing in these cities. The tweets collected were from 25 March 2020 to 15 July 2020 after the announcement of nationwide lockdown. The data is collected separately for each of these cities using their geographical codes. The tweets were collected using Twitter's stream API, a verified application associated with an open stream. All the tweets were collected for a given time period. In summary, 330,841 tweets were collected with an average of 33,084 tweets from each city. Along with the tweets from Twitter datasheet having details of COVID-19 cases per day for Rajasthan, Maharashtra, Karnataka and Delhi NCT was also extracted. The data sheet so extracted had details of number of confirmed cases, dismissed cases, recovery rate per day for a period of 4 months. This data sheet was downloaded from kaggle.com.

3.3 Data Model

The data collected for a given time span was consolidated using sheet-go add inns of Google sheets. The tweets were then filtered using language classification, and all the tweets that were tweeted in English language were classified. The classified English tweets comprised about 105,750 tweets. The above counted tweets were used for further analysis. Any data obtained from any social networking contains lots of additional details which may be of little use. Therefore, data extracted from any media needs to be cleaned. For cleaning the data and to tokenize only relevant parts of the tweet natural language processing toolkit (NLTK) library was used. Natural language processing toolkit is widely used because of its high pre-processing capabilities and data normalization. It is one of the most powerful libraries available in Python for text processing and is useful for performing some of machine learning techniques like sentimental analysis.

For modelling the data, special lexicology is used. It is a branch of linguistics dealing with the vocabulary system of language. The list of lexicons relating to depression and psychological stress was created using online sources [20, 21]. The tweets were identified if it contains any of lexicons (Table 1) relating to depression. This is done using the string container function in Python Pandas library. String container function is an inbuilt function available to check the consistency of a particular word in a string. The tweets that were processed by the above function were stored in a separate data frame. The separated data frame is used for further analysis.

4 Sentimental Analysis of Tweets to Estimate the Severity of Psychological Stress

Sentimental analysis is a set of natural language processing (NLP) techniques that extract opinions in natural language text. Simply put, the objective of sentimental analysis is to categorize the sentiment of a text by sorting it into positive, neutral and negative. Sentimental analysis provides a polarity and subjectivity value to individual

Table 1 Lexical that relates to psychological stress and depression

Restless, sad, useless, crying, suffer, sleepless, afraid, unhappy, upset, unsuccessful, helpless, suffer, fail, sorrow, lonely, hate, depressed, frustrated, loser, suicidal, hurt, painful, disappoint, heartbreak, regret, dissatisfied, lost, die, sick , Anxious ,bleak, dismal, dull, fear, stress, tension, disgust, dispiriting, worried, distress

sentences after analysing it. Polarity in sentimental analysis refers to identifying sentiment orientation (positive, neutral and negative) in written or spoken language. The polarity of the sentences ranges from $[-1, 1]$, where -1 refers to most negative sentences and $+1$ refers to most positive sentences. In this study, sentimental analysis is used to find out the extent of negativity in individual tweets; the more negative the polarity of tweet, the more severe the tweet is. Sentimental analysis is performed using a text blob package available in Python. The text blob package of Python is a convenient way of doing lots of language processing tasks. The sentimental analysis for depressing tweets is plotted. The polarity range for each of the sentiments is plotted (Fig. 1). The major polarity ranges from -0.5 to 0.5. It can be observed from the Fig. 1 that polarity range for maximum number of tweet is between $[-0.3, -0.4]$

5 Analysis of Depressing Tweets

5.1 Depressing and Non-depressing Tweets

Of the processed tweets, about 3119 tweets were found out to contain keywords related to depression and psychological stress, which accounts for 2.94% of the total tweets. The pictorial representation of the same is represented using Fig. 2. Along with the words that occurred frequently in these tweets were observed. The relative use of some frequently used depression and psychological stress terms is shown using a bar graph in Fig. 3. It was observed that the word related to sadness such as sad has occurred maximum number of times followed by fear and worried with dismal being the least.

5.2 Depression Dynamics in Major Cities Along with Divisions of Rajasthan

The depression dynamics in major cities of India (Mumbai, Bengaluru and Delhi) along with cities of Rajasthan was compared with the number of confirmed cases during the study period from 1 April to 16 June. Figure 4 represents the overall depression dynamics of major cities with COVID-19 cases during study period. The number of tweets is in accordance with the lockdown timeline of India [23].

From the figure, it can be seen that number of depressing tweets was at its peak on 14 June 2020 when the numbers of COVID-19 cases were highest. It can also be seen that the depressing tweets achieved its first peak on 14 April 2020; this day marks the end of lockdown 1.0 and the announcement of 2nd lockdown [15 April to 3 May] was done by government of India on this day. The no. of depressing tweets achieve its second peak on 1 May 2020; on this day, the announcement of Lockdown 3.0[4 May to 17 April] was made. After 17 May, certain relaxations were given in

Fig. 1 Polarity value of
each depressing tweet

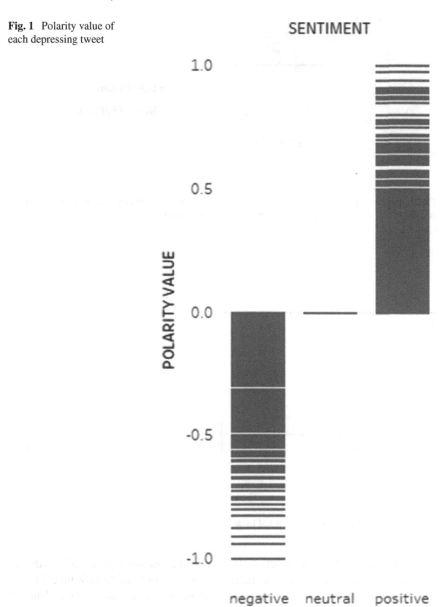

lockdown. On 30 May, the announcement of unlock 1.0 was made by Ministry of Home Affairs (MHA); on this day, the amount of depressing tweets was also less. 8 June marks the start of nationwide Unlock 1.0. Due to lockdown relaxation measures implemented by government, the cases increased rapidly and depressing tweets also increase achieving its peak on 14 June.

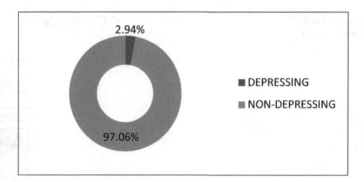

Fig. 2 Depressing tweets expressed as percentage of total tweets obtained (*2.94% of total tweets contained words related to psychological stress and depression*)

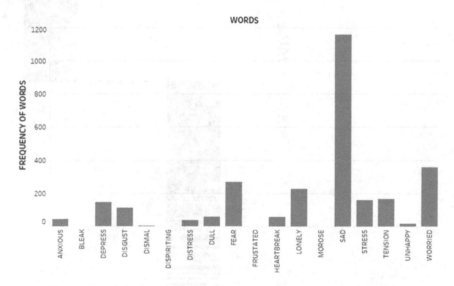

Fig. 3 Most used words in the extracted tweets

Figure 5 shows the relation between COVID-19 cases and depression level during unlock phase in India. The unlock phase [23] started in India from 7 June 2020, it was termed as unlock 1.0, after that subsequent unlock phases unlock 2.0 and unlock 3.0 for July and August were announced. During unlock phases, the COVID-19 cases began to rise exponentially in India, but various improvements in medical and healthcare facilities were done during lockdown period by MHA.

It was found that after achieving its peak on 14 June 2020 (two weeks after the relaxation in lockdown), it started to decrease even with the increase in COVID-19 cases. This may be because the people get adopted with situation and also the increase in recovery rate and improved medical facilities and health infrastructure.

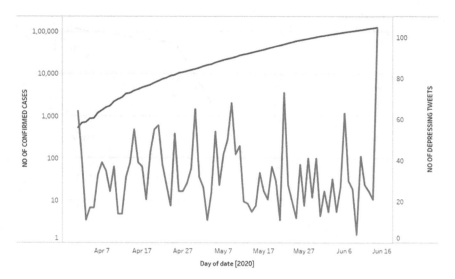

Fig. 4 Overall depression dynamics if cities of India between 1 April to 16 June (*The curved blue line represents increase in COVID-19 cases, and red line represents the number of depressing tweets. In the figure, 1 represents announcement of lockdown 2.0, 2 represents announcement of lockdown 3.0, 3 represents start of unlock 1.0*)

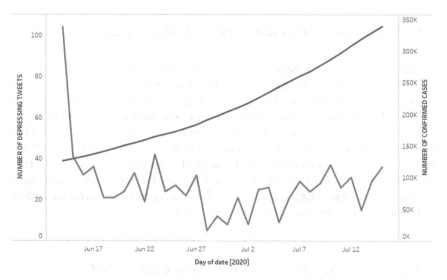

Fig. 5 Overall depression dynamics if cities of India 16 June to 15 July (*The curved blue line represents no of confirmed cases, and red line represents number of depressing tweets*)

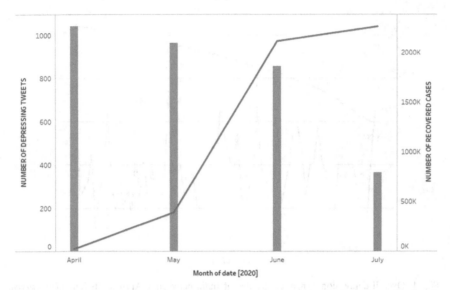

Fig. 6 Relation between number of depressing tweets and recovered cases for each month of study period (*The red line represents the no of recovered cases per month and grey bar represents number of depressing tweets.*)

5.3 Stress Level Versus Recovered COVID-19 Cases

The relationship between depressing tweets and total recovered cases was plotted for each month during our study period. The data for recovered cases per day for a period of 3.5 months was extracted from kaggle.com. It was observed that the number of depressing tweets starts to decrease with increase in recovered cases. In Fig. 6, the grey bars represent the total depressing tweets per month and black line represents increase in recovered cases. Within the start of the first lockdown, the no of recovery was very less and increased subsequently over the time, whereas the amount of depressing tweets decreased. Recovery rate increased in India due to various healthcare developments that were done during lockdown period; therefore, depression level among individuals also decreased.

5.4 Psychological Stress Level in Major Cities of India

The psychological stress level for different divisions of Rajasthan and cities like Mumbai, Delhi and Bengaluru is plotted. The average polarity is calculated for each city. The average polarity is the mean score of polarity of all tweets of each city. This average polarity is used for determining intensity of severity of psychological stress in each division. The average polarity for each division is indicated by intensity of colour. The more negative the average polarity is the more intense is

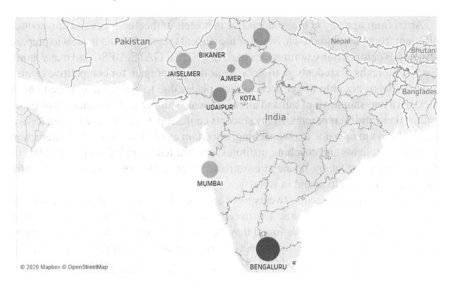

Fig. 7 Stress level in different cities of India (*The colour of the circle represents the negative average polarity of tweets, whereas the size of the circle represents the amount of depressing tweet of each city.*)

the colour of the circle. The size of the circle represents the amount of depressing tweets obtained in any division, the bigger the circle more is the volume of depressing tweets obtained from that division. The count in Fig. 7 represents scale for size of circle, and severity represents the scale for average polarity. In the interpretation (Fig. 7), the average polarity of tweets from Bengaluru find out to be most negative as compared to other divisions. Also, the amount of depressing tweets obtained is highest for Bengaluru. The number of depressing tweets is second highest for Delhi after Bengaluru, followed by Mumbai.

6   Stress Dynamics in Students Due to COVID-19 and Lockdown

For the safety of students and to prevent them from acquiring COVID-19 infection schools, colleges and universities are shut down since March. These nationwide closures are impacting over 91% of the worlds' student population. The closing of schools and universities has created an anxious situation among them. They are worried about their future and uncertainty has covered them. The lockdown obstructed the study routines, and therefore, some institutes decided to conduct online cases which had affected student's life and their thoughts towards studies [24]. Not only students, their families are also concerned about the stress level in students.

Apart from it, many of the students live in hostels of their colleges and universities different from their hometown. Many of the students stay in PG and hostels to prepare for various competition examinations like JEE, NEET, GATE, UPSC and many more. Every year lakhs of students go to Kota, Rajasthan, to prepare for competitive exams. Students were not able to get back to their places due to sudden announcement of lockdown and shutdown of rail and air movement. This created the situation of panic among them and their parents. Many students confessed that they were feeling lonely, stressed and anxious due to no coaching, uncertain exam dates, restricted interaction with other students and coaching institutes, and limited availability of food. Most of the students were facing financial constraints as they did not account for the extra time they will have to spend in Kota.

The processed depressing tweets were analysed to get the amount of depressing tweets that were from students. The tweets were categorized using lexicons such as students, exam and UGC. We found that the depressing tweets of student's account about 6.64% of total depressing tweets. It is represented from the doughnut chart below (Fig. 8). The word cloud (Fig. 9) was plotted to get the frequency of the words

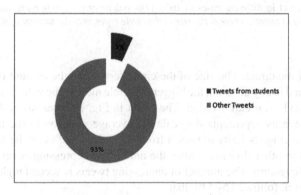

Fig. 8 Comparison of tweets by students by total depressing tweets

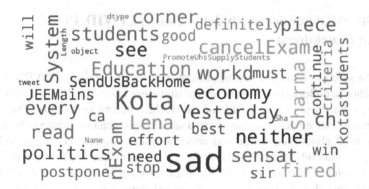

Fig. 9 Word cloud of tweets obtained by students

used by students to convey their messages to the government and institute. Around 1800 tweets were annotated manually to eliminate stress tweets other than COVID-19. The word cloud was plotted using the filtered tweets. It can be seen from the above word cloud that many of the students have appealed for cancelling exams and to promote them. Also, they have asked to send them home as they all were stranded in Kota. Sad can be seen as the most frequently used word.

6.1   Dynamics of Students Tweets

The annotated tweets of students were used to study their concern in the lockdown period. The tweets count of students that was extracted for the period of 1 April 2020 to 15 April was plotted against the lockdown timeline. The first lockdown 1.0 was announced in India from 25th March to 14th April. This is the duration when many people were away from their home, and flights and trains were cancelled and unable to reach their home. After 15 April, the lockdown was further extended in various phases. The second lockdown 2.0 was started from 14th may to 3rd May. Lockdown 3.0 extended from 4 May to 31 May. After 31 May, much relaxation was given to the people. It can be seen from the graph below (Fig. 10) that the amount of tweets was at its peak on 14 April 2020. 14/04/2020 was the last date of the first lockdown which was announced without prior information. Many students jumped to Twitter to express their problems and concerns during that time. It can also be seen that the tweets count began to decrease after that day, as the government of India took several steps to send back the stranded students to their home. It can be seen that the level of counts again started to increase a second time after June 14 2020 [25]. This is the

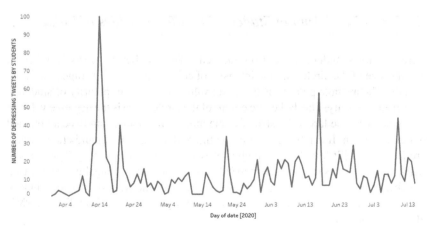

Fig. 10 Depression dynamics in students during study period (*The blue line represents amount of depressing tweets over period of time*)

Table 2 Sentiment analysis of students tweet

Tweet	Polarity	Sentiment
Stressed, depressed teens, tensions of upcoming exams, guilt of not studying, 2000 kms away from home, drastically decreased quality of food! All the other students are gone, feeling scared & alone, lonely… Not exaggerating but pls helps us	−0.21467	Negative
No one is listening to our voices. #KotaStudents #SendUsBackHome #Kota we all want to go back home	0.0	Neutral
General Promotion To MP Students Operation. No Exams In Covid successful	0.75	Positive

time when students expressed their concern regarding their exams and study issues they are facing as the uncertainty was looming due to no decision in exam date.

6.2 Sentimental Analysis of Students Tweet

Sentimental analysis was performed the annotated students tweets. The ratio of tweets of each sentiment is interpreted. Some tweets of the student are examined in Table 2. The first sentence has negative polarity as it contains words like depressed, sad, etc. The second sentence is a neutral sentence as it doesn't contain any negative or positive words. The third sentence is a positive sentence as it contains words successful. Most of the tweets from student have their average polarity range from −0.4 to 0.4. The discrete polarity range is represented in Fig. 11.

6.3 Stress Level Among Students in Different Cities of India

Figure 12 shows students tweet over each city. The number of tweets is indicated using the size of the circle, and the intensity of colour represents average polarity in each city. The average polarity is the mean value of sentiment polarity of student's tweets from each city. The darker the colour of the circle more is the negative value of average polarity, the larger the size of circle more is the depressing tweets obtained from that division. It can be seen from the figure that maximum numbers of tweets were from Kota [26], and least number of tweets was from Bikaner. The average polarity of tweets was more negative in Udaipur in contrast to Bengaluru. The reason for highest number tweets being from Kota is because the Kota is education hub of India. Every year lakhs of students go to Kota for preparation of IIT-JEE, AIPMT and other competitive exams.

Fig. 11 Polarity range of
tweets obtained from
students

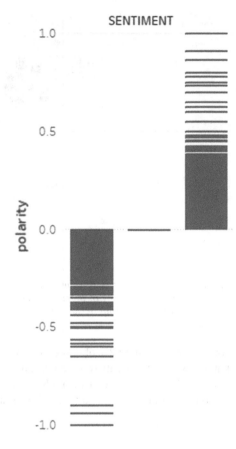

7 Conclusions

COVID-19 pandemic has affected almost all sections of society. It has caused major instability to an individual and caused psychological stress in them. Due to lockdown and other measures, people are conveying their emotions using social media. The chapter deals with the impact of COVID-19 and related events that have severely affected the mental health of people. In this study, the relation between depressing tweets and COVID-19 cases is used to estimate the level of depression among individuals and especially among students. The sentimental analysis was performed using a text blob package to get the severity of tweets, and average severity is used to define severity level in major city of India. It was observed in the analysis that the depressing tweets were at its peak as the corona cases were increasing rapidly after the relaxation of lockdown in the month of June, 2020. It was also observed that depression was decreasing with a percentage increase in recovery rate. It is evident

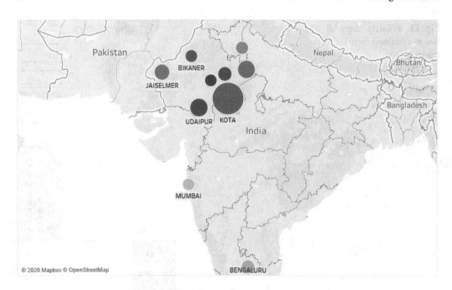

Fig. 12 Stress level among students in different cities of India (*The colour of the circle represent the negative average polarity of tweets, whereas the size of the circle represents the amount of depressing tweet from students of each cities.*)

from this study that 6.62% of depressing tweets were from students. It was also seen that the tweets of students were maximum at the end of the first lockdown. Also, the majority of tweets of students from Kota have majorly shown their concern towards uncertainty of their exam and they being stranded away from their hometown.

References

1. Surveillances V (2020) The epidemiological characteristics of an outbreak of 2019 novel corona virus diseases (Covid-19) China, 2020, China CDC Weekly 2(8):113–122
2. Mygov COVID-19 dashboard India, Available: https://www.mygov.in/covid-19/
3. Sharma A, Agarwal B (2020) A cyber-physical system approach for model based predictive control and modeling of COVID-19 in India. J Interdisc Math (Taylor Francis)
4. Bhat M, Qadri M, Beg N-U-A, Kundroo M, Ahanger N, Agarwal B (2020) Sentiment analysis of social media response on the covid19 outbreak, Brain, Behavior, and Immunity
5. Vigo D, Thorneycroft G, Atun R (2016) Estimating the true global burden of mental illness. Lancet Psychiatry 3(2):171–178
6. Goyal K, Chauhan P, Chhikara K, Gupta P, Singh MP (2020) Fear of COVID 2019: first suicidal case in India! Asian J. Psychiatry 49:101989
7. Zhou J, Zogan H, Yang S, Jameel S, Xu G, Chen F (2020) Detecting community depression dynamics due to COVID-19 Pandemic in Australia
8. Cavazos-Rehg PA, Krauss MJ, Sowles S, Connolly S, Rosas C, Bharadwaj M, Bierut LJ (2016) A content analysis of depression-related tweets. Comput Hum Behav 54:351–357
9. Coppersmith G, Dredze M, Harman C (2014) Quantifying mental health signals in twitter. In: Proceedings of the workshop on computational linguistics and clinical psychology: from linguistic signal to clinical reality, pp 51–60

10. Reece G, Reagan AJ, Lix KLM, Dodds PS, Danforth CM, Langer EJ (2017) Forecasting the onset and course of mental illness with twitter data. Scient. Rep. 7(1):13006
11. Barkur G, Vibha & Kamath GB (2020) Sentiment analysis of nationwide lockdown due to COVID 19 outbreak: Evidence from India. Asian J Psychiatry 51:102089
12. Stephen J, Prabu P (2019) Detecting the magnitude of depression in Twitter users using sentiment analysis. Int J Electr Comput Eng (IJECE) 9(7):3247–3255
13. Almouzini S, Khemakhem M, Alageel A (2019) Detecting arabic depressed users from twitter data. Procedia Comput Sci 163:257–265
14. Li S, Wang Y, Xue J, Zhao N, Zhu T (2020) The impact of COVID-19 epidemic declaration on psychological consequences: a study on active weibo users. Int J Environ Res Public Health 17:2032
15. Ramalingam D, Sharma V, Zar P (2019) Study of depression analysis using machine learning techniques. Int J Innovative Technol Exploring Eng (IJITEE) 8(7C2). ISSN: 2278-3075
16. Choudhury M, Counts S, Horvitz E (2013) Social media as a measurement tool of depression in populations. In: Proceedings of the 5th annual ACM web science conference websci'13, pp 47–56
17. Islam MR, Kabir A, Ahmed A, Kamal A, Wang, H, Ulhaq A (2018) Depression detection from social network data using machine learning techniques. Health Inf Sci Syst 6(1)
18. Chawla S, Mittal M, Chawla M, Goyal LM (2020) Corona Virus - SARS-CoV-2: an Insight to Another way of Natural Disaster. EAI Endorsed Trans Pervasive Health Technol 6(22)
19. Mittal M, Kaur I, Pandey SC, Verma A, Goyal LM (2019) Opinion mining for the tweets in healthcare sector using fuzzy association rule. EAI Endorsed Trans Pervasive Health and Technol 4(16)
20. Kumar A, Sharma A, Arora A (2019) Anxious depression prediction in real-time social data, SSRN Electron J
21. Dictionary.com, https://www.thesaurus.com/browse/depression
22. Salimath A, Thomas R, Ramalinga R, Sethuram Q, Yuhao (2019) Detecting levels of depression in text based on metrics
23. COVID-19 Pandemic Lockdown in India, https://en.wikipedia.org/wiki/COVID-19_pandemic_lockdown_in_India
24. Students stressed out due to Coronavirus, New survey founds Best Colleges.com, https://www.bestcolleges.com/blog/coronavirus-survey/
25. As uncertainty looms over examinations, The Indian Express. https://indianexpress.com/article/trending/trending-in-india/students-urge-to-cancel-exam-2020-with-memes-6458555/
26. Students stranded in Kota hoping to go back to their hometowns, duexpress.in, https://duexpress.in/students-stranded-in-kota-hoping-to-go-back-to-their-hometowns/

Chapter 5
Analyzing the Impact on Online Teaching Learning Process on Education System During New Corona Regime Using Fuzzy Logic Techniques

Neeru Mago, Jagmohan Mago, Sonia Mago, and Rajeev Kumar Dang

1 Introduction

According to World Health Organization, 2020, COVID-19 is highly infectious disease which is caused by a virus called "coronavirus." As this disease is highly infectious, it can be easily transmitted from person to another via their respiratory droplets and different contact routes like hands, nose, and mouth [1, 2]. Transmission through droplets can occur when the infected person is in close proximity with a normal individual. At such a time, the person having some respiratory symptoms like sneezing and coughing can easily pass the infection to a non-infected person with whom he is in close contact. The infection can also be transmitted through objects like utensils and clothes used by the infected person [3]. As per World Health Organization report, on June 28, 2020, the pandemic has hit around 213 countries of the world, affecting 1,61,14,449 people and 6,46,641 deaths across the world. India is not left behind. India reports 14,35,453 confirmed cases and around 32,771 deaths. The government and different communities are working worldwide to control the situation and to limit the spread of this virus. As a result of this, people are advised to stay home, and with the implementation of lockdown guidelines, people have been forced to work from home. Role of IT sector has increased manifold in ensuring the work from home culture. With non-availability of any vaccine for the coronavirus,

N. Mago
DCSA, Panjab University SSG Regional Centre, Hoshiarpur, Punjab, India

J. Mago
Department of Computer Science and Applications, Apeejay College of Fine Arts, Jalandhar, Punjab, India

S. Mago
Department of Physics, Swami Sant Dass Public School, Jalandhar, Punjab, India

R. K. Dang (✉)
UIET, Panjab University SSG Regional Centre, Hoshiarpur, Punjab, India
e-mail: dang.rajeev@pu.ac.in

© The Author(s), under exclusive license to Springer Nature Singapore Pte Ltd. 2021   69
P. K. Khosla et al. (eds.), *Predictive and Preventive Measures for Covid-19 Pandemic*,
Algorithms for Intelligent Systems, https://doi.org/10.1007/978-981-33-4236-1_5

it is anticipated that social distancing might help in limiting the spread of this virus. Different sectors, including the education sector, have seen a setback due to the COVID-19 being at a rise. The lives of every individual in the country have been largely affected due to shutting down of various organizations. As every other individual's life getting affected, the life of a student is no less affected. The schools and colleges have since a lot many years practiced classroom teaching, which includes face-to-face interaction of students and teachers. At this time of crisis, it becomes challenging to keep the education continuous and unaffected due to this disastrous pandemic.

1.1 Impact of COVID-19 in Education Sector

Distance learning is seen to have become widespread from the past 10 years [4, 5]. Various studies have been conducted where it appears that different institutions have been adopting and doing well with this new learning environment [6]. In this time of crisis, various educational organizations have come together and developed many platforms for participation in online teaching-learning projects [7]. As a result of this approach, more and more students now have the facilities to progress in their educational field while being safe in the home premises [8].

The students already working and having family responsibility can largely benefit from the online learning method as this gives them a greater flexible schedule that they can adapt and learn from [9]. Apart from the different advantages, there are certain challenges which the online mode of teaching and learning throws at faculty members as well as the students [10]. Different online courses [11] have been developed by various agencies like SWAYAM and MOOCs (Ministry of Human Resource Development, 2020). And students have been taking up different courses to gain more knowledge. But the system of taking online classes in colleges for regular course completion was never adopted by various institutions. This has led to a more digital system of teaching as well as learning.

Digitalization in the learning and teaching process has largely affected the present state of education in our country. The disruption caused by COVID-19 somehow forced the institutions to conduct classes online. As COVID-19 spread like fire in the forest, all educational institutions were shut down as the country followed quarantine policies and lockdown, which could possibly prevent the spread of COVID-19. This has led to a change of face of education from traditional classroom teaching to technology-based online teaching.

Learning has been a continuous process, and amidst the lockdown of more 100 days, the government and private institutions transformed to online teaching from classroom teaching to keep the learning process on the go. Many government and private institutions have taken a leap from conventional classroom teaching to digital teaching. They have started teaching their students through online classes so that the global COVID-19 pandemic does not affect the student's education. The campuses have been shut down, but teachers are busy working from home, preparing effective study material for their students so that there isn't any halt in the teaching-learning process. Teachers are working hard and are available for students at all times of the day in order to reduce the hardship and disruption being caused to the students across the country at this point of time due to the COVID-19 pandemic.

This shift in education from traditional classroom learning to computer-based learning might be one of the largest educational experiments. A teacher's job is not just making their students learn. Their job is to overall groom their students letting them know what is right and what is wrong. The world of education has been greatly affected by the coronavirus disease 2019 (COVID-19). Learning online through online lecture sessions has a lot of advantages over traditional classroom learning. Online learning involves the use of less paper, and it involves saving time with easy and quick access to a wide source of information. Along with this, it also saves time for traveling. Online learning gives a big advantage to the students as the student can study anywhere and at any time he wants with a few exceptions.

Digital learning has led to a reduction in cost and has taken the impact and reach of resources for students as well as teachers to another level. But there are number of challenges which learner and educator have to face during online teaching [12]. Very shortly, learning digitally will be the new face of Indian education. It will be a very useful and constructive means for both teachers and students in the coming years. The government is working with various agencies to build up new platforms where students, teachers and parents can closely connect. There has been a recent acceptance of the online teaching-learning process by the students across the country today. Teachers and students are now largely joining different platforms through which e-learning can be easily done.

As the online teaching-learning process has become more prevalent in India due to COVID-19 pandemic, it becomes particularly important to know its growth and to know whether it's actually helping the students. The present study was therefore designed to understand the student's perspective, attitudes and readiness about online classes being conducted at various educational levels.

1.2 Fuzzy Logic

The term "fuzzy logic" was coined during emergence of concept of fuzzy sets [13]. It has been explained by researchers and mathematicians in the field that fuzzy logic is a type of many-valued logic which deals with uncertainty and rationale. It is extracted from fuzzy set theory and is approximate rather than precise. It is explained [14] that fuzzy logic works on principle of artificial intelligence which combines fuzzy membership functions and set of fuzzy rules in lieu of conventional bi-valued logic. Initially, it was applied for design and development of control systems. However, with the enhancement of its capabilities and utilities, it can now be applied to varied set of applications. Steps involved in the process are as follows:

- Fuzzification is the primary stage in fuzzy inference approach. It is a process of transforming crisp values to fuzzy values equivalent to fuzzy sets expressing linguistic terms. A detailed explanation of mechanism of fuzzification and basic details of different membership functions is available in literature [15].
- Dubois et al. [16–18] explain the concept of designing and defining knowledge base and fuzzy rules using if-then format. Fuzzy sets are required for mapping each linguistic term, and it can be derived from the existing data or defined with the help of expert(s).
- The third step in fuzzy inference mechanism is applying the fuzzy rules for the evaluation. On applying fuzzy rules on the scaled input causes firing of various rules with varied strengths. Further, the conclusion is made based on the strength of the fired rules.
- The process of obtaining crisp results for the output variables is called defuzzification. The process of defuzzification is required to tell the stakeholders about the crisp output.

A FL-based expert system accepts the values of various parameters from the user as inputs which are then passed to the fuzzy inference mechanism. Depending upon the input, the multiple fuzzy rules are fired and fuzzy output is delivered. The fuzzy output is defuzzified by utilizing center of area. Various inputs may be in form of linguistic terms.

FL systems are able to deal with indefinite values or approximate concepts which permit it to emulate reasoning abilities like human beings, which may be in form of vague statements. This enables to make certain declarations such as teaching capability of a teacher is average, to be properly processed and suitable improvements suggested.

In this chapter, methodology is discussed in Sect. 2 that includes the proposed model, sample and procedure, normalized weight of skill sets and synthesis of preferences using analytic hierarchy process (AHP), fuzzy logic in inference process and its implementation in MATLAB. Section 3 describes the results and discussion on the output and its interpretation. Finally, the future scope is presented in Sect. 4, and chapter is concluded in Sect. 5.

2 Methodology

The goal of this research work is to examine the efficacy of online teaching based on different factors that affect the quality of online teaching by applying fuzzy logic. The various aspects of technical skills, professional skills, interpersonal skills and personal skills of online teaching are examined in order to provide quality education. Next, fuzzy inference mechanism as proposed by Mamdani is designed and built for assessing the probable level of execution of online teaching. The raw data is obtained through survey which is analyzed using fuzzy logic (FL), and the results are evaluated. The methodology for the proposed system is shown in Fig. 1.

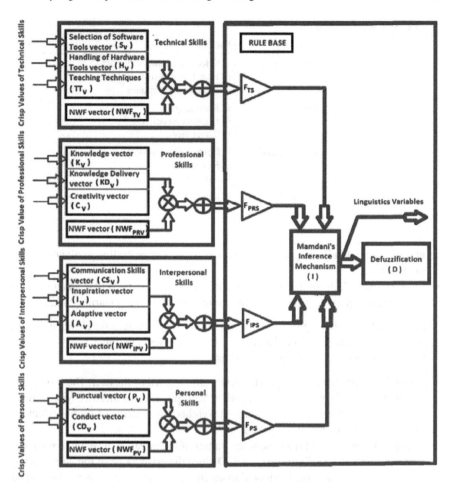

Fig. 1 Proposed model to analysis quality of online teaching

The quality of teacher is another significant factor in determining the quality of online teaching-learning process. The quality of teachers can be characterized by the **following factors/skills**:

- Technical skills of teachers comprise efficiency of selecting and handling of software and hardware tools and teaching techniques used by the teacher to impart knowledge through online mode.
- Professional skills of teachers refer to knowledge of the subject, creativity of delivering knowledge to the students and relating the subject taught to the real-world problems.
- Personal skills of teachers constitute some personal aspects of a teacher like punctuality and his/her conduct in the class. The efficacy of a teacher depends

Table 1 Skill sets and its factors

S. No.	Skill set	Factors
1	Technical	i. Selection of software tools ii. Handling of hardware tools iii. Teaching techniques
2	Professional	i. Knowledge ii. Knowledge delivery iii. Creativity
3	Interpersonal	i. Communication skills ii. Inspiration iii. Adaptive
4	Personal	i. Punctual ii. Conduct

upon the way of adjusting the classroom environment according to diverse needs of students.

- Interpersonal skills of teachers comprise communication skills, adaptation to diverse requirements of the education system and activating learning skills.

Such inputs have been given to the system in the way of values for eleven different parameters categorized in four different skill sets as shown in Table 1.

Overall system is comprised of two phases:

- **Phase 1**: Crisp values of eleven parameters are assigned by the user. These parameters are subsets of four specific categories. Multiplication of these assigned values is done with their respective normalized weights. Summation of such products is the input to fuzzy inference system.
- **Phase 2**: Using defined fuzzy sets, the values of technical, professional, interpersonal and personal skills are fuzzified. Deduce the crisp value of the output using Mamdani's inference mechanism. Further interpretation of the crisp value can be construed through linguistic terms.

2.1 Sample and Procedure

The suggested system is focused on facilitating all the stakeholders such as students, teachers and parents for determining the overall quality of online teaching mechanism. The primary step for development of fuzzy model is the collection of data for designing the fuzzy sets. For acquiring data, we require a defined team of experts. In the present work, 200 experts from different strata were made part of investigation. Set of students, teachers and parents submitted the required data for accessing the overall quality of online teaching. The teachers and students of science, commerce and arts streams were selected as each of them has its own view point about online teaching. Parent's perspective to access the quality of online teaching also plays very important role. This distribution is shown in Table 2.

Table 2 Stakeholders for data collection

Categories	No. of stakeholders
Science teachers	30
Commerce teachers	30
Arts teachers	30
Students from science	30
Students from commerce	30
Students from arts	30
Parents (at least graduate)	20
Total	200

2.2 Normalized Weight of Skill Sets (NWS) and Synthesis of Preferences Using Analytic Hierarchy Process (AHP)

Analytic hierarchy process (AHP) is a systematic methodology for analysis and organization of intricate decisions on the basis of psychology and mathematics [19]. The group decision making is the core area of application of AHP and thus can be applied to variety of decision-making situations in the areas of business, health care and education. The methodology of utilizing the AHP may be outlined as:

- Problem must be modeled as a hierarchy that contains decision objective, alternatives to achieve the goal and the criteria to evaluate the alternatives.
- Pair-wise comparison matrix of parameters must be defined to make the decision about the priorities of the parameters.
- In order to produce the overall priorities for the hierarchy of parameters, synthesis of judgments is being done.
- Consistency of the judgments is evaluated.

In this research, AHP is used to verify the consistency of input received from stakeholders.

- **Collection of data reference to ranking of skill sets from experts**: List of 200 experts from different streams including parents (who are at least graduate) has been given in Table 2. This has been done for finding weights and arranging the skill sets as per priority of skill set. Maximum priority is to be assigned as "1", and least priority is to be represented by "4". The cumulative representation of records has been expressed in Table 3. Technical skills were kept on rank 1 by 56 experts, while 31, 67 and 46 experts kept it at second, third and fourth ranks, respectively.
- **Computation of the weighted mean of all the frequencies**: Weighted mean (WM) of the skill set (WSK) affecting the characteristic of online teaching can be calculated by Eqs. (1) and (2).

Table 3 Priority of factors

Skill set	Rank			
	1	2	3	4
Technical	56	31	67	46
Professional	79	52	38	31
Interpersonal	64	53	37	46
Personal	67	56	41	36

Table 4 Skill sets and their weights

Skill set	Technical skills	Professional skills	Interpersonal skills	Personal skills	Total
Weighted mean (WM)	49.7	57.9	53.5	55.4	216.5
Weight (WSK)	2.30	2.67	2.47	2.56	10

$$\text{WM}[i] = \sum_{wt=4, j=1}^{wt=1, j=4} (\text{Fq}[i][j] \times wt) / \sum_{wt=1}^{4} wt \tag{1}$$

where WM[i] is the weighted mean and Fq[i][j] is the frequency of the preference of skill set i. Here, i and j vary from 1 to 4 and wt varies from 4 to 1. A "1" is kept as minimum weight, while "4" is assigned as maximum weight.

$$\text{WSK}[i] = \frac{\text{WM}[i] \times 10}{\sum_{j=1}^{4} \text{WM}[j]} \tag{2}$$

where WSK[i] is the weight of the skill set i. It is calculated out of 10. WSK of the skills which influences the online teaching quality has been given in Table 4.

In this sample, AHP has been used for analyzing the consistency of measure. As per AHP, eigenvector and maximum eigenvalue ($\lambda_{\max}$) have been computed by using pair-wise comparison matrix. Relative importance among different factors is represented by eigenvector, while $\lambda_{\max}$ has been used for measurement of consistency ratio. Step-by-step details have been given as below:

- Step 1: Defining pair-wise comparison matrix (CM)

    WSK(Professional Skills)-WSK(Personal Skills) = 0.11
    WSK(Professional Skills)-WSK(Technical Skills) = 0.37
    WSK(Interpersonal Skills)-WSK(Technical Skills) = 0.17
    WSK(Personal Skills)-WSK(Technical Skills) = 0.26
    WSK(Professional Skills)-WSK(Interpersonal Skills) = 0.20
    WSK(Personal Skills)-WSK(Interpersonal Skills) = 0.90

Matrix R depicts the difference matrix of the weights of the skill and $R^T = 1 - R$.

Table 5 Skill sets and their priority weights vector

Skill set	Technical	Professional	Interpersonal	Personal
Priority weight vector (PWV)	0.1235	0.3906	0.2121	0.2738

$$R = \begin{pmatrix} 0 & 0.11 & 0.20 & 0.37 \\ & 0 & 0.90 & 0.26 \\ & & 0 & 0.17 \\ & & & 0 \end{pmatrix} \quad R^T = \begin{pmatrix} 1 & 0.89 & 0.80 & 0.63 \\ & 1 & 0.10 & 0.74 \\ & & 1 & 0.83 \\ & & & 1 \end{pmatrix}$$

$$R - R^T = \begin{pmatrix} -1 & -0.78 & -0.60 & -0.26 \\ & -1 & -0.80 & -0.48 \\ & & -1 & -0.66 \\ & & & -1 \end{pmatrix} = \begin{pmatrix} 1 & 0.78 & 0.60 & 0.26 \\ & 1 & 0.80 & 0.48 \\ & & 1 & 0.66 \\ & & & 1 \end{pmatrix}$$

$$\text{Pairwise Comparison Matrix (CM)} = \begin{pmatrix} 1 & 0.78 & 0.60 & 0.26 \\ 1.28 & 1 & 0.80 & 0.48 \\ 1.67 & 1.25 & 1 & 0.66 \\ 3.85 & 2.08 & 1.52 & 1 \end{pmatrix}$$

- Step 2: Computation of priority weights or eigenvector.

Let $\text{Wt} = (\text{wt}_1, \text{wt}_2, \text{wt}_3, \ldots \text{wt}_n)^T$ be the priority weights of comparison matrix and can be calculated by Eq. (3). The priority weights of various skill sets are shown in Table 5.

$$\text{wt}_i = SS_i \Big/ \sum_{i=1}^{n} SS_i \tag{3}$$

where $SS_i = \sqrt[n]{\prod_{j=1}^{n} a_{ij}}$, $i = 1, 2, 3, \ldots, n$ and a_{ij} is the values in CM.

- Step 3: Calculation of maximum eigenvalue ($\lambda_{\max}$). It can be calculated by Eq. (4)

$$\lambda_{\max} = \frac{1}{n} \sum_{i=1}^{n} \frac{(\text{AW})_i}{W_i} \tag{4}$$

The value of $\lambda_{\max}$ computed to be 4.0201.

- Step 4: Consistency Index (CIn) for the comparison matrix can be calculated by Eq. (5)

$$\text{CIn} = (\lambda_{\max} - n)/(n - 1) \tag{5}$$

- Step 5: Compute consistency ratio (CRo) using Eq. (6)

$$CRo = CIn/RI \qquad (6)$$

From Eqs. 5 and 6, we can compute Consistency Index CIn= 0.0067 and Consistency Ratio CRo = 0.0074, respectively. Normally, the comparison matrix can be considered consistent if CRo < 0.1 which is acceptable in this example, and it shows fine degree of the consistency.

2.3 Fuzzy Logic in Evaluation Process

In the proposed model, fuzzy logic has been used for the evaluation of the performance of online teaching based upon their technical, professional, interpersonal and personal skills. The stakeholders provide the vague values of various parameters between 0 and 10. These values are fuzzified, and fuzzy if-then rules are applied from the knowledge base. The multiple rules are fired, and then, defuzzification is applied to compute the crisp value depicting the quality of online teaching.

Suppose we have to evaluate n teachers on the basis of Selection of Software Tools (S), Handling of Hardware Tools (H) and Teaching Techniques (TT). Domain experts assign the scores of Selection of Software Tools (S), Handling of Hardware Tools (H) and Teaching Techniques (TT) in the range 0 to 10. Combining Selection of Software Tools Vector (S_v), Handling of Hardware Tools Vector (H_v) and Teaching Techniques Vector (TT_v), we get the Technical Skills Matrix (TSM) of the order 3 × n,

$$TSM_{3 \times n} = \left[TS_{ij} \right]_{3 \times n}$$

where $i = 1$ represents S_v, $i = 2$ represents H_v, $i = 3$ represents TT_v and $j = 1$ to n represents teachers' number, $[TS_{ij}] \in [0,10]$ represents the Technical Skills of teacher j.

Priority weight (PW) of technical skills is 0.1235 as shown in Table 5 and is used for computing weighted mean of various factors influencing technical skills such that the maximum sum of factor of online teaching i satisfies

$$\sum_{i=1}^{3} F_{TS}(i) = 10$$

Similarly, we can compute Professional Skills Matrix (PRM), Interpersonal Skills Matrix (IPSM) and Personal Skills Matrix (PSM). Based on these matrices and their respective PWV as shown in Table 5, crisp values of overall performance levels of teacher j are computed and are denoted by F_{TS}, F_{PRS}, F_{IPS} and F_{PS} respectively.

- Step 1. Fuzzification

- $\mu F_{TS}(j)$ represents the fuzzy input membership value of overall performance level based upon technical skills of teacher j such that $\mu F_{TS}(j) \in [0,10]$.
- $\mu F_{CS}(j)$ represents the fuzzy input membership value of overall performance level based upon conceptual skills of teacher j such that $\mu F_{CS}(j) \in [0,10]$.
- $\mu F_{PRS}(j)$ represents the fuzzy input membership value of overall performance level based upon professional skills of teacher j such that $\mu F_{IPS}(j) \in [0,10]$.
- $\mu F_{PS}(j)$ represents the fuzzy input membership value of overall performance level based upon personal skills of teacher j such that $\mu F_{PS}(j) \in [0,10]$.

Here, fuzzy membership functions having five levels related to technical skills have been used, where level = 1 represents the linguistic term "Poor", level = 2 represents "Fair", level = 3 represents "Good", level = 4 represents "Very Good" and level = 5 represents "Excellent". Their membership functions have been described in Fig. 2. Similarly, these identical five fuzzy membership functions have been incorporated for professional, interpersonal, personal skills and for the output variable that is quality of online teaching (QS).

- **Step 2. Inference Mechanism**

In second step, overall quality of online teaching is evaluated on the basis of fuzzy input values of technical $\mu F_{TS}(i)$, professional $\mu F_{PRS}(i)$, interpersonal $\mu F_{IPS}(i)$ and personal skills $\mu F_{PS}(i)$ of teacher i and the fuzzy rules (FR). We can obtain the fuzzy sets for defuzzification by max–min inference mechanism, which can be expressed in Eq. (7)

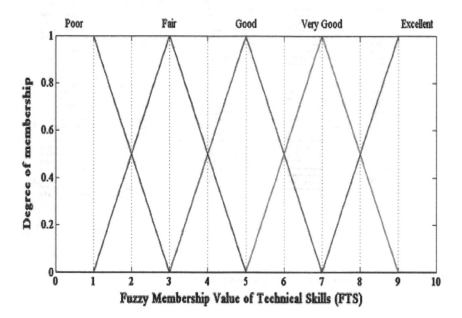

Fig. 2 Fuzzy functions having five levels

$$y_{ij} = \max\{\min(\mu_{F_{\text{TS}}}(i)m_1, \mu_{F_{\text{IPS}}}(i)m_2, \mu_{F_{\text{CS}}}(i)m_3, \mu_{F_{\text{PS}}}(i)m_4)\} \qquad (7)$$

where γ_{ij} is the output of inference of quality of online teaching i in the fuzzy set j.

- **Step 3. Defuzzification**

This step quantifies the output on the basis of the given fuzzy sets and the membership values. In this chapter, quantification of quality of online teaching i has been done by applying the Center of Area—CoA(QS) method and is written in Eq. (8).

$$\text{CoA}_i = \frac{\int (x \times \mu(x)\mathrm{d}x}{\int \mu(x)\mathrm{d}x} \qquad (8)$$

CoA refers to a reasonably acceptable crisp value of quality of online teaching i. Quality of online teaching is decided by checking:

if CoA(QS) $\in$ [0, 2] then Quality of Online Teaching is *Poor*.
if CoA(QS) $\in$ (2, 4] then Quality of Online Teaching is *Fair*.
if CoA(QS) $\in$ (4, 6] then Quality of Online Teaching is *Good*.
if CoA(QS) $\in$ (6, 8] then Quality of Online Teaching is *Very Good* and
if CoA(QS) $\in$ (8, 10] then Quality of Online Teaching is *Excellent* (Fig. 3).

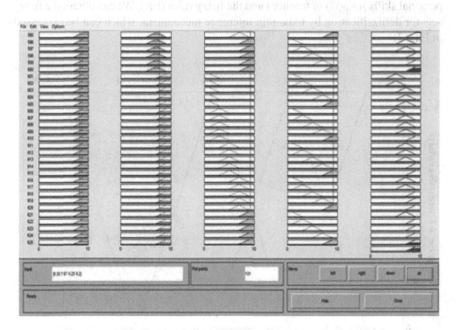

Fig. 3 Rule base view of online teaching-learning quality

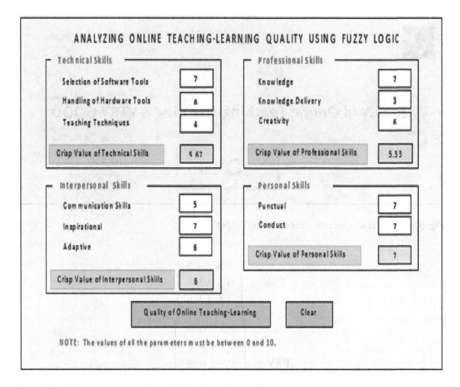

Fig. 4 Rule base view of online teaching-learning quality

2.4 Implementation Process

MATLAB has been used for designing and developing the graphical user interface (GUI), which is used for receiving the input parameters from the stakeholders and for displaying the overall probable quality of online teaching as shown in Figs. 4 and 5. All the values for these parameters vary from 0 to 10 and are sent to the fuzzy inference system (FIS) for processing inputs and delivering outputs. Lowest value is represented by '0' and highest value by '1'.

3 Results and Discussion

The use of fuzzy logic is significant due to the intrinsic inaccuracy ambiguity in the evaluation of the quality of online teaching. However, such inaccurate information is represented by the fuzzy logic with the mathematical model. Proposed system has been illustrated with the following example.

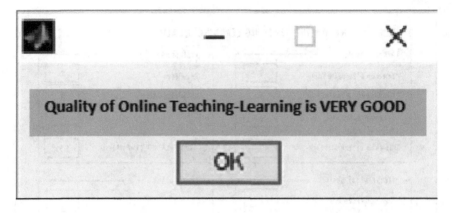

Fig. 5 Graphical user interface for receiving output

$$TSV = \begin{bmatrix} 7\ 8\ 2\ 4\ 8 \\ 6\ 5\ 3\ 5\ 8 \\ 4\ 6\ 1\ 5\ 9 \end{bmatrix}$$

$$PSV = \begin{bmatrix} 7\ 9\ 3\ 6\ 9 \\ 8\ 8\ 4\ 5\ 8 \\ 6\ 8\ 5\ 6\ 8 \\ 7\ 9\ 2\ 6\ 9 \\ 7\ 9\ 3\ 7\ 10 \end{bmatrix}$$

$$IPSV = \begin{bmatrix} 5\ 7\ 3\ 6\ 9 \\ 6\ 8\ 4\ 7\ 10 \\ 6\ 7\ 4\ 6\ 9 \\ 7\ 9\ 2\ 7\ 9 \end{bmatrix}$$

$$PRSV = \begin{bmatrix} 7\ 8\ 3\ 6\ 8 \\ 3\ 6\ 2\ 5\ 7 \\ 6\ 6\ 2\ 5\ 8 \end{bmatrix}$$

Their respective normalized weight factor vector is

- PWV = [0.1235 0.2121 0.3906 0.2738]
- $F_{TS} = \mu F_{TS}(i) = [5.67\ 6.33\ 2\ 4.67\ 8.33]$
- $F_{PRS} = \mu F_{CS}(i) = [5.33\ 6.67\ 2.33\ 5.33\ 7.67]$
- $F_{IPS} = \mu F_{IPS}(i) = [6\ 7.75\ 3.25\ 6.5\ 9.25]$
- $F_{PS} = \mu F_{PS}(i) = [7\ 8.8\ 3.4\ 6\ 9.2]$.

Scores of five teachers have been shown in Table 6.

These inputs were used as measure for evaluating the quality of five teachers and inference mechanism concluded that the overall quality of online teaching of

Table 6 Scores of five teachers

Skill set	Teachers				
	Teacher 1	Teacher 2	Teacher 3	Teacher 4	Teacher 5
Technical	5.67	6.33	2	4.67	8.33
Professional	5.33	6.67	2.33	5.33	7.67
Interpersonal	6	7.75	3.25	6.5	9.25
Personal	7	8.8	3.4	6	9.2

five teachers, are "Very Good", "Excellent", "Fair", "Very Good", and "Excellent" respectively. As the input values are to be from 0 to 10, instead of 0 to 1, stakeholders can easily assume the value as per their experience.

Illustration: The first teacher scores are 5.67, 5.33, 6 and 7 in technical, professional, interpersonal and personal skills, respectively. Figure 3 represents the rule base view of online teaching-learning quality based on the rules fired from the knowledge base. The defuzzified value (CoA) of the *Online Teaching-Learning Quality* inferred lies between (6, 8). Thus, the quality of student comes out to be "VERY GOOD".

R_{75}: If (FTS is VGood) and (FIPS is VGood) and (FPRS is VGood) and FPS is Good) then (QS is VGood).

R_{86}: If (FTS is VGood) and (FIPS is Good) and (FPRS is VGood) and (FPS is VGood) then (QS is VGood).

R_{95}: If (FTS is Good) and (FIPS is VGood) and (FPRS is VGood) and (FPS is VGood) then (QS is VGood).

4 Future Scope

The proposed fuzzy logic-based system provides acceptable and accurate results for analyzing the quality of online teaching. Therefore, the aim of developing a system to analyze the online teaching-learning process is achieved. There are still many issues that need to be addressed. These issues are discussed as below.

Firstly, the system that is proposed in this chapter is a prototype. One can implement this system as a database solution to keep track of online teaching-learning process. Further mobile application can be developed so that stakeholders in education actually participate in the evaluation of the performance of online teaching. The mobile devices use wireless communication technology, and its reach covers almost every nook and corner of India; therefore, the access to the system will be cost-effective and instant. We used MATLAB to implement the proposed system. The proposed system can be developed using agent and multiagent system. Java Agent Development Environment (JADE) can be used as an agent framework, and Java Expert System Shell (JESS) can be used to incorporate reasoning capabilities in agents.

The efficacy of other soft computing techniques like Bayesian networks, neuro-fuzzy logic, genetic algorithms, multiagent system, etc., can also be verified in this problem domain. In future, we would also like to have fusion of database and soft computing techniques so that the results produced can be saved for guiding the students and teachers in the right direction. This will help in maintaining high standards in teaching-learning process and producing directly employable youth.

5 Conclusion

The chapter describes the state of education system in this time of COVID-19 pandemic where online or virtual classes are the only medium to provide quality education to students. This research was conducted to analyze the quality of online teaching-learning process using artificial intelligence technique, i.e., fuzzy logic (FL). The proposed system utilizes the power of fuzzy logic and is producing desired results. The quality of education system can be improved by integrating it with the innovations of information technology for the evaluation of online teaching. For that we need a system that exhibits features such as knowledge-sharing, self-sufficiency and human reasoning. It is not worthwhile to apply Boolean logic in such type of applications because of its inability to emulate human reasoning. However, fuzzy logic is a mathematical technique for developing a decision support system and for interpreting such vague information.

The objective of the chapter is to demonstrate the strength of fuzzy logic in dealing with the problems of analyzing and evaluating teachers and students in higher education system. The system is to provide assistance to various stakeholders in analyzing the performance of online teaching-learning process and taking timely measures so as to improve the quality of education.

One aspect of this chapter deals with the selection, categorization and analysis of various factors for the evaluation of the quality of online teaching-learning process. Literature in the field suggested eleven such parameters for the evaluation of online teaching. Opinions gathered from the stakeholders and literature further suggested four broader categories for classifying the selected parameters for the evaluation of online teaching. We have designed a framework for receiving the data from the stakeholders, examining its consistency and analyzing it.

Further, we have also designed and developed individual decision support systems based on Mamdani's fuzzy inference system. The stakeholders use the graphical user interface designed in MATLAB to enter the values of various factors. The fuzzy inference system thus produces the required defuzzified output about the quality of online teaching-learning process.

The conclusion derived from the results of the proposed model suggests that the performance of the proposed systems is consistent to stakeholders' intelligent predictions. It can be further concluded that the developed models are capable enough to support various stakeholders in evaluating the performance of online teaching-learning process.

The system proposed in this research system offers alternative opinion to the stakeholders to check the online teaching-learning environment in the education system, and thus, right and timely steps in the right direction can be taken to provide quality education to the students. The soft computing techniques especially fuzzy logic have immense potential to solve such imprecision in the problems of analyzing, interpreting and evaluating the online teaching-learning process.

References

1. Lall S, Singh N (2020) CoVid-19: unmasking the new face of education. Int J Res Pharm Sci 11(SPL1):48–53
2. Lin et al (2020) A conceptual model for the coronavirus disease 2019 (COVID-19) outbreak in Wuhan, China with individual reaction and governmental action. Int J Infect Dis 93:211–216
3. Ong et al (2020) Air, surface environmental, and personal protective equipment contamination by severe acute respiratory syndrome coronavirus 2 (SARS-CoV-2) from a symptomatic patient. JAMA J Am Med Assoc 323(16)
4. Cheney R, Muralidharan (2005) India education profile, National center on education and the economy new commission on the skills of the american workforce November 2005
5. Harper C, Yen DC (2004) Distance learning, virtual classrooms, and teaching pedagogy in the Internet environment. Technol Soc 26(4):585–598
6. Oblinger D, Kidwell J (2000) Distance learning: are we being realistic? Educause Rev 35(3):30–34
7. Dutton D, Perry J (2002) How do online students differ from lecture students. J Asynchronous Learn Network 6(1)
8. Wojciechowski A, Palmer L (2005) Individual student characteristics: can any be predictors of success in online classes? Online J Distance Learn Adm
9. Mansour B, Mupinga DM (2007) Students' positive and negative experiences in hybrid and online classes. Hybrid and Online Courses
10. Palloff RM, Pratt K (2003) The virtual student. A profile and guide to working with online learners. Jossey-Bass Higher Adult Edu Ser
11. Ataizi M (2005) Online Communication courses: new trend for communication education
12. Howell W, Lindsay NK (2003) Thirty-two trends affecting distance education: an informed foundation for strategic planning. Online J Distance Learn Adm
13. Bellman RE, Zadeh LA (1977) Local and fuzzy logics. In: Dunn JM, Epstein G (eds) Modern uses of multiple-valued logic. Episteme (A Series in the Foundational, Methodological, Philosophical, Psychological, Sociological, and Political Aspects of the Sciences, Pure and Applied), Volume 2. Springer, Dordrecht
14. Ross TJ, Sellers KF, Booker JM (2002) Considerations for using fuzzy set theory and probability theory. In Fuzzy logic and probability applications, Society for Industrial and Applied Mathematics, pp 87–104
15. Siler W, Buckley JJ (2005) Fuzzy expert systems and fuzzy reasoning. Wiley
16. Dubois D, Lang J, Prade H (1991) Fuzzy sets in approximate reasoning, part 2: logical approaches. Fuzzy Sets Syst 40(1):203–244
17. Dubois D, Prade H, Testemale C (1988) Weighted fuzzy pattern matching. Fuzzy Sets Syst 28(3):313–331
18. Devi BB, Sarma VVS (1985) Estimation of fuzzy memberships from histograms. Inf Sci 35(1):43–59
19. Safian M, Ezwan E, Nawawi A (2011) The evolution of analytical hierarchy process (AHP) as a decision making tool in property sectors

Chapter 6
Healthcare 4.0 in Future Capacity Building for Pandemic Control

Jagjot Singh Wadali and Praveen Kumar Khosla

1 Introduction

COVID-19 has been declared by World Health Organization as a global pandemic with affecting almost every human on this planet. It is the outbreak of third coronavirus after Severe Acute Respiratory Syndrome (SARS) and Middle East Respiratory Syndrome (MERS) that the world has seen in the past two decades. The latter two types of coronavirus (SARS and MERS) were confined to small regions, whereas the outbreak of novel coronavirus from Wuhan, China has created havoc in almost every country in the world [1]. The world has witnessed several calamities like earthquakes, tsunami but never experienced this type of disaster which has reached almost every country whether it is developed or developing. It is going to push millions below the poverty line and ruin major economies. The viral transmission of this virus from person-to-person has suddenly brought several challenges not only for health care but for almost all the sectors. The technology world is accepting those challenges and applying problem-solving and critical thinking in designing new technological innovative applications to take a stab at this pandemic [2].

The evolution of pandemic has proved that technology is vital for human lives. The outbreak of COVID-19 has disconnected people from all over the world due to several restrictions imposed. But still, technology has enabled people to connect with each other. Normal life came to a halt due to several issues caused due to this pathogen. Technology advancements in various sectors have acted as a backbone of the economy and played a crucial role during this era of pandemic. It has enabled work for home culture, as well as money-making business for the worldwide populace. Moreover, the technologies are also being used to deal with the challenges caused

J. S. Wadali (✉) · P. K. Khosla
Centre for Development of Advanced Computing (C-DAC), Ministry of Electronics & IT, Mohali, Punjab, India
e-mail: jagjotwadali@gmail.com

© The Author(s), under exclusive license to Springer Nature Singapore Pte Ltd. 2021
P. K. Khosla et al. (eds.), *Predictive and Preventive Measures for Covid-19 Pandemic*,
Algorithms for Intelligent Systems, https://doi.org/10.1007/978-981-33-4236-1_6

due to this pathogen. The rapid spread of the pandemic has forced each country to use every technological possibility to deal with this deadly virus [3].

However, there are some drawbacks to technological advancements also. Despite various breakthrough technological systems in various sectors still humans suffer from natural calamities like earthquakes, pandemic, or tsunami. With the support of technological advancements like airports and railways, this pathogen finds its presence across the globe in 213 countries affecting 80 million humans [4]. The humans are fighting the battle with the invisible enemy. The rapid evolution, emergence, and spread of this deadly pathogen proved that technological advancements act as a shelter or a savior of human lives from the natural calamities; however, it does not have the capability to stop or halt the calamities. Moreover, the technology does not reach the masses due to cost and several other factors. Furthermore, people do not invest much in technologies dealing with natural calamities as the probability of occurrence is quite low. The world populace has never witnessed this sudden outbreak which had brought forward enormous challenges not only in the health sector but in every sector. The biggest challenge is to protect the non-effected and cure the affected.

The healthcare sector has witnessed this pandemic on a large scale that it has exposed its strengths as well as weaknesses [5]. Healthcare service providers are overburdened with the responsibility as they have to provide the services and also safeguard themselves from this viral transmission. There is a tremendous change in healthcare services since the spread of the pandemic. With the support of technology, the healthcare industry has moved from a conventional system to a modern technology-driven system [6]. That is one of the five pillars of Atmanirbhar Bharat announced by the Prime Minister of India. The epidemic brought forward several challenges and issues for health care; however, technology-driven health care had enabled healthcare providers to address these challenges. Since the outbreak of this disease, various technological solutions have been developed which have slowed down the spread of disease to some extent as well as safeguarded the providers. Moreover, the solutions also enabled non-COVID patients to get treatment without being infected. In addition, various existing technologies and new avatars of technologies had strengthened the healthcare system and prepared the world for future calamities.

Each country has used its strengths in tackling these difficult times. Various technological solutions are designed to address the specific challenges depending upon the use-case and problem statement. Out of various technological systems, telemedicine has emerged as one of the essential technologies in enabling healthcare care services post-emergence of COVID-19. Patients and doctors are using it to connect with each other [7]. From tertiary care hospitals to primary care centers, most of the health facilities had turned to an Internet-based telemedicine system. It is quite effective in dealing with COVID as well as non-COVID patients. Digital health technologies and various telemedicine-based systems are developed or designed accordingly to address the specific requirements of the patients. The usage of telemedicine system has rapidly increased across nations since the spread of the pathogen. Various countries had implemented this technology as it has the following benefits:-

1. Providing medicine at a distance,
2. Reducing point of contact,
3. Avoiding visits to the hospital and reducing the load.

There are various barriers in adoption of telemedicine and still if adopted widely has the vast potential in creating a digital future for faster diagnosis and treatment.

2   Evolution of Healthcare

The sole purpose of the healthcare sector is to improve the health of humans. It is the aggregation of different organizations that provides services to the patients with curative, preventive, rehabilitative, and palliative care [8]. The United Nations International Standard Industrial Classification (ISIC) categorizes the healthcare industry as generally consisting of

1. Hospital activities,
2. Medical and dental practice activities,
3. Other human health activities.

The healthcare sector is evolving with a span of time too. Healthcare 1.0 was formed during the industrial revolution and focused on public health. Later on, the emergence of technology brought forward the concept of Healthcare 2.0 with bigger hospitals and better medical education. The introduction of computer-based devices for the health care led to Healthcare 3.0. With the advent of new technologies and new avatars of previous technologies led to the emergence of Healthcare 4.0, which had further strengthened the healthcare system [9].

As technology had connected the world, people are migrating and traveling to different places. Nowadays, patients are consulting doctors from different places for better healthcare services. Keeping in view, the primary focus of Healthcare 4.0 is on wider aspects which include interoperability, virtualization, decentralization, real-time capability, service orientation, and modularity [10].

Healthcare 4.0 is focusing on the 360° view of the consumers benefitting stakeholders. The healthcare service providers are enabling technology-driven solutions including early and faster diagnosis, remote patient monitoring, self-assessment tools, and virtual care [11].

2.1   Digital Healthcare

World Health Organization (WHO) published a framework known as the Tanahashi framework in 1978, which demonstrates the performance gaps in the healthcare system and the ways they prevented quality and mass coverage. Digital health interventions can possibly fill those gap areas in providing better health care [12].

Digital health care refers to the use of information and communication technologies to aid healthcare professional and their clients manage illnesses and health risks. Since the last decade, there is enormous development of healthcare technologies, which are benefitting healthcare providers as well as patients. These includes

1. Electronic health record (EHR),
2. Mobile health (mHealth),
3. Telemedicine/telehealth,
4. Portal technology,
5. Self-service kiosk,
6. Remote monitoring tools,
7. Sensors and wearable technology,
8. Wireless communication,
9. Real-time locating services,
10. Pharmacogenomics/genome sequencing [13].

Moreover, to further improve the digital healthcare system as well as to maintain interoperability, accessibility and keeping in view several other factors, various standards and protocols were defined in digital health care for viewing, sharing, transferring, and storing of digital health data of patients. There are several standards and protocols which were defined including DICOM, HL7, SNOMED, etc. [14].

2.2   Transition from Digital to Advanced Healthcare Systems

The new avatars and new versions of technologies are not only strengthening the healthcare system but also making it efficient and affordable. Previously, digital technologies replaced the analog machine, whereas, nowadays, advanced digital technologies are replacing modern digital technologies. New avatars of technologies including AI, Big Data, and IoT are transforming digital health care to advance digital health care which will be the future of health care. This will enable faster diagnosis, rapid testing, quick self-assessment and self-diagnosis, and a lot more [15]. Moreover, it will enable healthcare services in rural areas as well as make it affordable and accessible for under-privileged.

There are mainly two types of healthcare services including preventive and corrective measures for a particular disease. Further, each type of healthcare service has multiple options as shown in Table 1. The technologists, researchers, and healthcare workers are trying every technological possibility to develop solutions for each of the healthcare services. The advanced technologies are strengthening every healthcare services in a unique way as listed in Table 1:

The use of technology has provided several benefits to the stakeholder which includes sharing of digital records at different locations, consulting doctor without visiting hospital, early disease detection, etc. [16].

Table 1 Types of healthcare services and technology-driven solutions

S. No.	Healthcare service/methods	Types	Technology-driven healthcare
1	Preventive (The steps or initiatives or processes taken to prevent the disease from spread or occurrence) Hospital visit is not necessary	Physical examination/diagnosis/testing	1. To diagnose the patients remotely or at same location with no contact using digital and sensor technology and wearable devices 2. Rapid and faster diagnosis using AI and Big data
		Awareness and education	1. To spread awareness using Web sites, mobile application, and social media 2. To provide education using chatbots
		Self-assessment and self-diagnosis	1. To identify the symptoms without intervention of doctor using mobile apps 2. Patients can do self-diagnosis through mobile apps
		Tracing of infected patients	1. Tracing the infected patients using location-based tracking technologies, AI, and big data
2	Corrective measures (The steps or initiative or processes taken to cure the patient from the disease) Hospital visit depends upon the type of illness	Physical examination/diagnosis/testing	1. To identify the symptoms faster and quicker using image scanning technologies, AI, and Big Data
		Treatment	1. Using robotics for delivery of medical equipments to patients 2. Using telemedicine for remotely monitoring the patients through no contact 3. Using robotics, IoT for remotely monitoring the patients

(continued)

Table 1 (continued)

S. No.	Healthcare service/methods	Types	Technology-driven healthcare
		Follow-up	1. Using teleconferencing or virtual care to monitor the health status of the patients
3	Other	Analysis	1. Using AI, Big Data for statistics and analysis of infected patients

3 Healthcare in the Era of Pandemic

The healthcare system was designed to deal with different types of diseases but not for the purpose to deal with sudden abrupt of the global crises in the form of a pandemic. The world has witnessed how easily obscure animal virus has turned into a human threat and had exposed the weaknesses of the healthcare system [5]. This pandemic had affected the healthcare system of every country including the world's largest spending healthcare system in the USA and advanced healthcare system in European countries [17]. The deadly pathogen did not come alone but brought several challenges for the healthcare providers along with it. Three of the major challenges for the healthcare providers include (1) treatment of COVID patients, (2) treatment of non-COVID patients and safeguarding from viral transmission of coronavirus, and (3) safeguarding their own health workers.

Every country's healthcare system is designed to cater to the needs of its citizens. The emergence of COVID-19 has realized the strengths as well as weaknesses of the healthcare system of each country [18]. The eruption of this pathogen not only affected the existing healthcare system but also came as a new disease to deal with [19]. It has brought forward several issues. Firstly, due to its faster spreading rate, several countries imposed restrictions on movement based on their own laws and regulations [20]. Many countries including India imposed a complete lockdown for 49 days making healthcare services less accessible to its citizens. Secondly, tracing, tracking, and testing of the COVID infected patient is another set of challenge for healthcare providers. As the virus spread at faster rate, healthcare providers are focusing on mass testing, rapid diagnosis, and isolating the infected. Thirdly, every human has suffered badly due to coronavirus. With the economic slowdown and limited access, many of the humans suffered diseases like depressions and anxiety which added fuel to the existing problems. Especially it was difficult for migrants and travelers to get access to health care. In this scenario, health services were required at home. Fourthly, based on demographics and population, the healthcare system has to deal with crisis depending upon the country. Challenges in one country can be different from challenges in other countries [21]. For India, the second-largest populated country in the world has different challenges with respect to European countries. With 65% of the populace living in rural areas and around 25% living below poverty live, the challenges to deal with coronavirus in India are quite different and there was a requirement to develop low-cost technological solutions to tackle the pandemic.

3.1 Challenges with Respect to COVID Patients

There are various challenges faced by healthcare providers to deal with the pandemic. Firstly, the pathogen spread at a faster rate and transmits from person-to-person. Secondly, it is difficult to trace or test based on symptoms as it takes around 14 days for the symptoms to appear. Thirdly, symptoms do not appear in most of the patients. Fourthly, there is no vaccination for this disease. Mostly, healthcare providers are doing first-level diagnosis or screening based on body temperature. Fever is one of the symptoms for this disease, however, for the second level diagnosis, separate testing is required that is time-consuming. The prime objective of the healthcare providers is to trace, track, and treat the infected patients as well as isolate them to stop its spread. Various challenges faced by healthcare workers while providing the services to deal with COVID patients are explained in Table 2.

3.2 Challenges with Respect to Non-COVID Patients

There is another set of challenges for non-COVID patients. Firstly, there are patients who are suffering from various non-communicable diseases other than COVID-19. They are not getting treatment due to restrictions imposed due to pandemic. Secondly, there are new patients who suffered from various other diseases including depression, and others after emergence of coronavirus. The healthcare providers are looking for the ways to deal with these challenges as shown in Table 3. They are looking for ways to provide the healthcare services in the midst of the pandemic.

4 Technology-Driven Health Care—Preparing for the Next-Generation Health Care

Technologies had played a vital role in strengthening the healthcare system. Various technological developments in healthcare took pressure off over the overworked health workers. Now, these technologies are opening new doors for healthcare workers to deal with the pandemic. Based on the capabilities and strengths, each country is trying every possible way to use technology against dealing with pandemic including treating COVID as well as non-COVID patients [2].

Table 2 Challenges for COVID patients

S. No.	Healthcare services/methods	Types	Challenges
1	Preventive measures	Testing the COVID patient	1. Chances of healthcare workers getting infected 2. Requirement of personal protective equipments while testing 3. Large scale testing required
		Awareness	1. Mostly, people do not have knowledge about the disease and there are more rumors. It is challenging for providers to spread right information to the public
		Self-diagnosis and self-assessment	1. It is the responsibility of healthcare providers to provide the information regarding self-diagnosis and self-assessment to raise awareness among public
		Tracing the contacts of COVID patients	1. Difficulty in tracing the close contact of COVID patients as it takes minimum 1–14 days for the symptoms to appear 2. Difficult to diagnose asymptomatic patients
		Isolating close contacts of COVID patients	1. Previously, there were no separate wards in the hospital. However, since the outbreak of pandemic, it was mandatory for the hospitals to have quarantine centers and isolation wards to keep the close contacts of infected patients as well as infected patients, respectively
2	Corrective measures	Testing the COVID patient with symptoms	1. Chances of healthcare workers getting infected 2. Issues in rapid as well as mass testing 3. Wearing of protective kits while physical examination of infected patients

(continued)

Table 2 (continued)

S. No.	Healthcare services/methods	Types	Challenges
		Treatment of COVID patient	1. Requirement of separate wards 2. Difficulty in delivering medical care like medicine
		Follow-up	1. Difficult to follow-up with COVID cured patients

Before the outbreak of coronavirus, technology was playing a crucial role in strengthening the health care, but post-coronavirus, it became an integral part of the healthcare services. Now, the technology is driving health care and transforming into the future generation health care. Various technologists along with healthcare providers are developing and designing new solutions/applications to use technology in its full potential to design modern, advanced, and robust healthcare systems. Their prime focus is on contact-less examination or diagnosis, remote patient monitoring, and protecting their own health workers. Although, this coronavirus, may fade away due to effective vaccination in the future, but it will certainly prepare the health care to deal with future calamities [4].

Various researchers and technologists are focusing on designing technology-driven healthcare systems for tracking, tracing, and treating COVID patients. Their main purpose is to develop smart devices for faster diagnosis, contact-less monitoring, rapid testing, and remote patient monitoring to prevent the disease from spreading. Incorporating several advanced technologies like machine learning, AI, and Big Data algorithms, technologists are focusing on affordable and efficient healthcare services [22].

Various studies are published to discuss various technologies, innovative technological solutions, and applications developed to address the challenges brought forward by a coronavirus. The author identified and categorized technologies into two types. The first type of technologies supports diagnostic processes and case-findings including non-contact thermometers, AI, drones, self-assessment applications, and virus genome sequencing. The second type of technologies supports therapeutic and logistic applications that include pharmaceutical tech, robots, telemedicine, GIS, IoT, Big Data, and blockchain [23].

The various technologies are strengthening the healthcare services as shown in Table 4. These technologies are preparing the healthcare system to next-generation healthcare system driven by technology [22]. In addition, this technology-driven healthcare system will be able to fill the existing gap area in health sector.

Table 3 Challenges for non-COVID patients

S. No.	Healthcare services/methods	Types	Challenges
1	Preventive measures	Testing the non-COVID patient	1. Requirement of personal protective equipments while physical examination of patients 2. Sanitizing medical equipment's and hands frequently
		Awareness	1. It is challenging for the healthcare workers to provide health-related information to the patients during lockdown 2. It is essential for the healthcare providers to raise awareness about all the necessary precautions while getting treatment
		Self-diagnosis	1. Non-COVID patients were unable to visit hospitals during lockdown 2. Patients were in dilemma as they were not able to differentiate between common flu and coronavirus
		Tracing the contacts of COVID patients	1. Difficult to find close contacts of COVID infected patients 2. Dealing with patients suffering from other disease as well as COVID also 3. Requirement of separate wards to isolate the close contacts of COVID infected patients
		Isolating close contacts of COVID patients	1. Requirement of separate quarantine centers 2. Requirements of healthcare workers to monitor the patients in quarantine centers
2	Corrective measures	Testing the non-COVID patient with symptoms	1. People not getting treatment due to lockdown 2. Limited healthcare facilities 3. Chances of getting infected

(continued)

Table 3 (continued)

S. No.	Healthcare services/methods	Types	Challenges
		Treatment of non-COVID patient	1. To treat the patients without getting infected 2. Treating patients in lockdown 3. Providing care to the non-COVID patients with or without hospital visit
		Follow-up	1. Challenging to monitor the patients remotely

4.1 Technological Solutions to Deal with COVID Patients

For treating COVID patients, the healthcare provider is turning their faces toward technology to find suitable innovative technological systems which should provide various solutions including contact-less physical examination/diagnosis, remote patient monitoring, teleconferencing, robotics for contact-less delivery of medical services, chatbots for awareness among people, wearable devices for remote patient monitoring [24], etc. Various solutions have been developed in a short span of time to trace, test, and treat COVID patients [25, 26] as shown in Table 5.

4.2 Technological Solutions to Deal with Non-COVID Patients

COVID-19 has significantly disrupted the healthcare services for the non-communicable disease. It has become difficult for healthcare service providers to treat the non-COVID patients in the midst of this pandemic [32]. Various solutions have been developed by the technologists to deliver healthcare services for the diseases other than COVID as shown in Table 6.

5 Telemedicine—A Priceless Boon for Healthcare System

Telemedicine refers to providing medicine at a distance. It is quite efficient in dealing with almost all types of diseases, especially communicable diseases that are transmitted from person-to-person [46]. The final solution to the COVID-19 disease will be a multifaceted system with each face of the system representing a specific technology-driven solution. This multifaceted system will not only tackle the pandemic but will

Table 4 Technologies for dealing with pandemic

S. No.	Technologies	Advantages
1	Artificial intelligence	1. For self-assessment and self-diagnosis of the various diseases 2. For tracing and tracking COVID patients
2	Big Data	1. For tracking and tracing COVID patients
3	Drones	1. For disinfecting various places 2. For street patrols and monitoring 3. For medicine delivery
4	Robotics	1. To provide medical services to people in quarantine and isolation 2. For providing medicines to the COVID affected patients
5	IoT	1. For patrolling and surveillance of isolation wards 2. Remote patient monitoring
6	Blockchain	1. Useful in various ways including tracking the spread of the disease, managing insurance payments, maintaining sustainability of medical supply chain, and tracking pathways
7	Open-source technologies	1. As the coronavirus spread in almost every country, it is essential for healthcare providers to share information between each other in a rapid way 2. In this scenario, open-source projects are developed facilitating access to research data and scientific publication which help in developing customized solution according to own needs
8	Imaging techniques	1. For detection of coronavirus through X-ray
9	Sensors and wearable devices	1. No contact physical examination of COVID patients
10	Telemedicine and telehealth	1. For teleconsultations 2. For remote monitoring 3. For virtual care, etc
11	3D printing	1. With the high risk of healthcare workers getting infected, there is huge shortage of ventilators, face masks, and other medical equipment's. Three-dimensional (3D) printing can play an important role as a disruptive digital manufacturing technology

(continued)

Table 4 (continued)

S. No.	Technologies	Advantages
12	Gene-editing technologies	1. At the moment, there are no approved medicines to protect people from or treat them for COVID-19, although some antiviral therapies are being tested. Researchers are working to use this technology in the diagnosis and treatment of coronavirus
13	Nanotechnology	1. Nano-based products are currently being developed and deployed for the containment, diagnosis, and treatment of COVID-19. An experimental nano-vaccine has become the first vaccine to be tested in a human trial
14	Synthetic biology	1. In response to the current pandemic, synthetic biologists are applying cutting-edge tools to speed up the development of a successful vaccine. Their efforts illustrate synthetic biology's potential to design, build, and test solutions for an unanticipated challenge such as COVID-19
15	Positioning or GIS	1. For tracing and locating and monitoring infected patients on real-time basis
16	Augmented reality/virtual reality	1. For remotely monitoring patient 2. Virtual home care

also save the life of common people and healthcare workers. The telemedicine will be the major component in this multifaceted system.

Telemedicine has emerged as a boon for health care in several ways [7, 47]. Firstly, it enabled healthcare services for dealing with COVID patients as well as patients who were suffering from other diseases. Secondly, it also enabled the reach of health care in the time of the spread of pandemic when the moment was restricted or limited due to the spread of the pandemic. Thirdly, it enabled healthcare workers to provide services in the low-resource areas or the areas having less accessibility. Fourthly, it enabled common people to seek consultation at the comfort of their houses during a pandemic.

There are a plethora of advantages offered by telemedicine, especially for general-purpose diseases which can be cured without testing/physical diagnosis as well as for situation where the patient presence is not necessary [48]. Some of the modalities do not require visiting hospitals and can be cured from the distance. This enables reducing overload on the healthcare system as well as saving additional costs for personal protective equipment.

There is tremendous growth in telemedicine since the outbreak of coronavirus [49]. Governments of various countries had taken initiatives to deploy telemedicine solutions to deal with pandemic [50, 51]. There are several barriers to the adoption of telemedicine [49], but still, it has grown exponentially since the outbreak of the pandemic.

Table 5 Technological solution for COVID patient

S. No.	Healthcare services/methods	Types	Technological solution/applications
1	Preventive measures	Testing the COVID patient	1. Sensor-based digital thermometer to detect diseases without physical contact
		Awareness	1. WHO started with WhatsApp-based chatbot to provide information regarding epidemic [27]
		Self-diagnosis and self-assessment	1. Self-diagnosis mobile app launched by various healthcare providers [28]
		Tracing the contacts of COVID patients	1. Various countries had developed mobile apps to trace COVID patients [29]
		Isolating close contacts of COVID patients	1. For monitoring the patients in quarantine centers [29]
2	Corrective measures	Testing the COVID patient with symptoms	1. Technological applications and solution for rapid testing [30]
		Treatment of COVID patient and follow-up	1. Non-contact treatment of COVID patients [31] 2. Monitoring the patients remotely and virtual care

5.1 Telemedicine for Tacking Pandemic

Various authors published articles about the effect of telemedicine in dealing with pandemic and found that it was quite efficient in dealing with healthcare crisis during a pandemic [52]. Telemedicine not only reduced the point of contact between patient and doctor but also provided continuous care to a community which helped reducing mortality and morbidity in the outbreak of COVID-19.

Telemedicine offers various solutions depending upon the use-case scenario. There are several aspects of telemedicine as shown in Fig. 1 [53]. Firstly, there are various modes of telemedicine including real-time, store and forward, remote patient monitoring, and mobile health. Secondly, there are several streams in telemedicine like telediagnosis, teleconsultations, telesurgery, telerehabilitation, etc. Thirdly, myriad streams are there in telemedicine to address different modalities including teleradiology, telepathology, telephysciatry, etc. Fourthly, there are different telemedicine models and solutions addressing specific need of the patients.

Moreover, telemedicine is quite effective in reducing the workload from the healthcare workers as well as reducing the patients visiting hospitals by providing them service at their home. Generally, for hospitals, they serve two divisions which include

Table 6 Technological solution for non-COVID patients

S. No.	Healthcare services/methods	Types	Technological solution/applications
1	Preventive measures	Testing the non-COVID patient	1. Using technology-driven solutions for diagnosis of various diseases without physical contact [33, 34]
		Self-awareness and self-diagnosis	1. Mobile applications like Ada for self-assessment and self-diagnosis for various diseases [35] 2. Various applications including chatbots and social media for raising awareness for various diseases among citizens
2	Corrective measures	Testing the non-COVID patient with symptoms	1. Using technology-driven solutions for physical examination of various diseases without no contact [33, 34]
		Treatment of COVID patient and follow-up	1. Use of various technologies to remotely monitor and treat the patients 2. Use of telemedicine for treating non-communicable diseases [36, 37]. Solution for various modalities includes chronic disease [38], celebral palsy [39], neurology [40], spine surgery [41], pysicatry [42], alzehimer disease [43], eye diseases [44], dental disease [45], etc

(a) outpatient division (OPD) and (b) inpatient division (IPD) for various diseases. Telemedicine has enabled healthcare services for both the divisions as shown in Table 7.

5.2   Telemedicine Initiative in Various Countries

The use of telemedicine systems has grown exponentially since the outbreak of coronavirus. Various countries including developed and developing countries are using telemedicine solution to deal with COVID patients as well as non-COVID

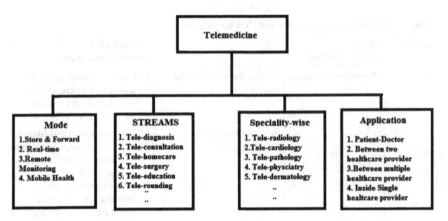

Fig. 1 Different aspects of telemedicine

patients. Various telemedicine initiatives by various countries are [54–61] shown in Table 8.

5.3 Future of Telemedicine

The world has witnessed that the telemedicine has emerged as one of the essential technology which has a capability to bring medical care to the patient. There are several opportunities in the field of telemedicine and if scaled up it can act as a boon for mankind. Telemedicine solution if adopted widely can not only have the capability to deal with pandemic but will create several opportunities and jobs for technologists, researchers, and healthcare practitioners.

According to the report by Verified Market Research, telemedicine market will grow exponentially and expected to reach USD 75 billion by 2025 [62]. Various companies started investing in telemedicine companies for future generation [63]. The paradigm shift from "hospitals" to "virtual hospital" using telemedicine will change the future of health care [64]. Healthcare services will be provided to the patients without least intervention of doctors and from distance.

Moreover, according to WHO, there are around 1.5 million medical devices till now ranging from low-cost devices like thermometers to expensive device like chemotherapy machines [65]. To operate these complex devices, there is a huge demand for medical device softwares to operate these devices. These hardware devices as well as software's are strengthening the telemedicine system in a better and efficient manner.

Various technologies are also strengthening telemedicine systems [66]. Technologists are using various technologies like robotics in telerehabilitation, Artificial intelligence in telediagnosis, IoT in remote patient monitoring, drones and robots

Table 7 Telemedicine for various divisions in hospitals

S. No.	Type of division in hospitals	Definition	Telemedicine solutions
1	OPD	1. The department provides diagnosis, treatment, and follow-up for patients who does not want to stay overnight. The department provides facilities for several different diseases 2. Patients looking for OPD's generally visits hospitals for minimum three times for (a) diagnosis/physical examination, (b) treatment, (c) follow-up	1. Telemedicine offers several solutions for dealing with OPD patients to minimize transmission 2. Telemedicine supports multiple modalities including teleradiology, teledermatology, teleophthalmology, etc., for dealing with patients suffering from various diseases 3. Telemedicine-enables telediagnosis, teleconsultation, etc., for treatment of disease 4. Telemedicine enables tele-education for sharing information between doctors 5. Telemedicine enable teleconsultation and reducing patient in the hospitals
2	IPD	1. The department provides diagnosis, treatment, and follow-up for patients who wants to stay overnight 2. The patient needs a bed and should be kept under medical observation for minimum 12 h 3. The department provides facilities for several different diseases	1. Telemedicine offers various solutions to deal with IPD patients including tele-robotics, telerounding, and telerehabilitation 2. Telemedicine enables virtual care and remote patient monitoring and reduces point of contact 3. Telemedicine enables remote monitoring through wearable devices

for telerounding. These technologies are making telemedicine system reliable and efficient for patients as well as user-friendly for doctors.

Table 8 Telemedicine solutions in various countries

S. No.	Country	Telemedicine solution
1	India	1. eSanjeevaniOPD for Indian citizens to consult doctor at home without traveling to hospitals
2	China	1. Chunyu doctor 2. Ping an good doctor
3	USA	1. Doctor on demand and HeyDoctor offer free coronavirus risk assessments
4	Canada	1. CloudMD app 2. Ontario Telemedicine network
5	Russia	1. Moscow telemedicine center
6	France	1. Covidam app to monitor COVID infected patients
7	Italy	1. Virtual hospital in Italy for providing healthcare to citizens
8	Brazil	1. AI-powered detection of COVID using chest scanning 2. AI-enabled chatbots for educating people about COVID
9	UK	1. Doctorinthehouse.net telemedicine service started for the people
11	Australia	1. HotDoc 2. Australian healthcare providers took initiatives to start telemedicine services at various centers

6 Discussion

Technology had strengthened the healthcare system in various ways. It has not only provided better healthcare but also provided services to the areas where there are limited access and fewer resources [67]. Especially during the time of crisis, it has played a vital role in fighting against coronavirus [68]. It has not only fought against the pandemic but also acted as the backbone of the economy. If coronavirus had brought several challenges for mankind, then technologies had offered several innovative technology-driven solutions to deal with these challenges. Technology-driven solutions enabled faster diagnosis, rapid testing, and tracing of COVID patients and also offered various solutions for other non-communicable diseases.

Furthermore, technology had also restored the healthcare services which was badly affected due to coronavirus. Most of the populace took advantage of technology-driven solutions to get care at home without visiting hospitals. Coronavirus had left several challenges for mankind and the innovative solutions developed out of these challenges will prepare the world for the next natural calamities.

7 Conclusion

It is concluded that technology-driven innovative solutions helped fighting coronavirus. Telemedicine emerged as the critical technology of utmost importance in the time of the pandemic. Still, it is underutilized due to several issues related to adoption. If escalated properly, it has the potential to provide healthcare service in an innovative way that the future generation healthcare services will be totally based on self-diagnosis, self-assessment, and technology-driven operated by health-care providers. The existing telemedicine solutions have to move beyond mere audio video chat and provide vitals of the patient to the consultant. There is a need to automate the acquisition of these vitals.

References

1. The New England Journal Of Medicine. https://doi.org/10.1056/NEJMp2003762
2. The economic times. https://economictimes.indiatimes.com/tech/software/how-countries-are-using-technology-to-fight-coronavirus/articleshow/74867177.cms
3. Healthcare IT news. https://www.healthcareitnews.com/news/europe/covid-19-has-accelerated-adoption-non-contact-patient-monitoring-technology-says-frost
4. Worldometers. https://www.worldometers.info/coronavirus/
5. Stat news. https://www.statnews.com/2020/03/02/the-coronavirus-exposes-our-health-care-systems-weaknesses-we-can-be-stronger/
6. Geospatial world. https://www.geospatialworld.net/blogs/how-technology-innovation-is-boosting-healthcare-systems/
7. World economic forum. https://www.weforum.org/agenda/2020/05/telemedicine-covid-19-game-changer/
8. Wikipedia. https://en.wikipedia.org/wiki/Healthcare_industry
9. Chen C, Loh E, Kuo KN et al (2020) The times they are a-Changin'—Healthcare 4.0 is Coming! J Med Syst 44:40
10. Estrela VV, Monteiro AC, França RP, Iano Y, Khelassi A, Razmjooy N (2018) Health 4.0 as an application of industry 4.0 in healthcare services and management. Med J Technol 2:1
11. Deloitte. https://www2.deloitte.com/global/en/pages/life-sciences-and-healthcare/articles/global-health-care-sector-outlook.html
12. WHO guideline recommendations on digital interventions for health system strengthening. https://apps.who.int/iris/bitstream/handle/10665/311941/9789241550505-eng.pdf?ua=1
13. Beckers Health IT. https://www.beckershospitalreview.com/healthcare-information-technology/10-biggest-technological-advancements-for-healthcare-in-the-last-decade.html
14. ISO. https://www.iso.org/ics/35.240.80/x/
15. The Medical Futurist. https://medicalfuturist.com/ten-ways-technology-changing-healthcare/
16. AIMS education. https://aimseducation.edu/blog/the-impact-of-technology-on-healthcare/
17. The economic times. https://health.economictimes.indiatimes.com/news/industry/coronavirus-is-a-global-crisis-and-the-biggest-challenge-we-have-faced-in-our-life-time/74962917
18. Stat news. https://www.statnews.com/2020/03/02/the-coronavirus-exposes-our-health-care-systems-weaknesses-we-can-be-.stronger/
19. HealthManagement.Org. https://healthmanagement.org/c/healthmanagement/issuearticle/towards-post-covid-19-lessons-and-challenges-for-hospitals-and-healthcare-infrastructures
20. BBC News. https://www.bbc.com/news/world-51737226
21. Innohealth magazine. https://innohealthmagazine.com/2020/trends/analysis-of-challenges-covSid-19-on-indian-healthcare-industry/
22. Ten technologies to fight coronavirus. https://www.europarl.europa.eu/RegData/etudes/IDAN/2020/641543/EPRS_IDA(2020)641543_EN.pdf
23. Mastaneh Z, Mouseli A (2020) Technology and its solutions in the Era of COVID-19 crisis: a review of literature. Evidence Based Health Policy, Manage Econom 4(2):138–149

24. HealthTech. https://healthtechmagazine.net/article/2020/02/5-ways-healthcare-tech-helping-tackle-coronavirus
25. Mobihealthnews. https://www.mobihealthnews.com/news/roundup-techs-role-tracking-testing-treating-covid-19
26. ICTworks. https://www.ictworks.org/digital-health-solutions-covid-response/#.XyJXIZ4zaUk
27. Socialmediatoday. https://www.socialmediatoday.com/news/whatsapp-launches-world-health-organization-chatbot-to-answer-covid-19-quer/574617/
28. Geospatialworld. https://www.geospatialworld.net/blogs/popular-apps-covid-19/
29. DW. https://www.dw.com/en/coronavirus-tracking-apps-how-are-countries-monitoring-infections/a-53254234
30. Kgpchronicle. https://kgpchronicle.iitkgp.ac.in/iit-kharagpur-researchers-develop-novel-technology-for-covid-19-rapid-test/
31. Premier Inc. https://www.premierinc.com/newsroom/press-releases/premier-inc-real-time-technology-solution-tracks-manages-and-supports-treatment-of-covid-19-patients-across-the-country
32. World Health Organization. https://www.who.int/news-room/detail/01-06-2020-covid-19-significantly-impacts-health-services-for-noncommunicable-diseases
33. TytoCare Introduces New Portable Telemedicine Device. https://www.tytocare.com/news-and-events/tytocare-introduces-new-portable-telemedicine-device/
34. GOMD. https://gomd.care/field-kits/
35. https://play.google.com/store/apps/details?id=com.ada.app&hl=en_IN
36. Azarpazhooh MR, Morovatdar N, Avan A, Phan TG, Divani AA, Yassi N, Stranges S, Silver B, Biller J, Belasi MT, Neya, SK (2020) COVID-19 pandemic and burden of non-communicable diseases: an ecological study on data of 185 countries: COVID-19 and non-communicable diseases. J Stroke Cerebrovasc Dis 105089 (2020)
37. Da Silva Rodrigues RJ, Mendes IP, de Souza WL (2020) MyHealth: a system for monitoring non-communicable diseases. In: 17th international conference on information technology–new generations (ITNG 2020). Springer, Cham, pp 439–444
38. Nouri S, Khoong EC, Lyles CR, Karliner L (2020) Addressing equity in telemedicine for chronic disease management during the Covid-19 pandemic. NEJM Catal Innovations Care Del 1(3)
39. Ben-Pazi H, Beni-Adani L, Lamdan R (2020) Accelerating telemedicine for cerebral palsy during the COVID-19 pandemic and beyond. Front Neurol 11:746
40. Ganapathy K (2020) Telemedicine and neurological practice in the COVID-19 Era. Neurol India 68(3):555
41. Tan KA, Thadani VN, Chan D, Oh JYL, Liu GKP (2020) Addressing coronavirus disease 2019 in spine surgery: a rapid national consensus using the Delphi method via teleconference. Asian Spine J 14(3):373–381
42. Torous J, Wykes T (2020) Opportunities from the coronavirus disease 2019 pandemic for transforming psychiatric care with telehealth. JAMA Psychiatry
43. Takeda C, Guyonnet S, Ousset PJ, Soto M, Vellas B (2020) Toulouse Alzheimer's clinical research center recovery after the COVID-19 crisis: telemedicine an innovative solution for clinical research during the coronavirus pandemic. J Prev Alzheimer's Dis 1
44. Saleem SM, Pasquale LR, Sidoti PA, Tsai JC (2020) Virtual ophthalmology: telemedicine in a Covid-19 era. Am J Ophthalmol
45. Giudice A, Bennardo F, Antonelli A, Barone S, Fortunato L (2020) COVID-19 is a new challenge for dental practitioners: advice on patients' management from prevention of cross infections to telemedicine. Open Dentistry J 14(1)
46. Smith AC, Thomas E, Snoswell CL, Haydon H, Mehrotra A, Clemensen J, Caffery LJ (2020) Telehealth for global emergencies: Implications for coronavirus disease 2019 (COVID-19). J Telemed Telecare, 1357633X20916567
47. Chauhan V, Galwankar S, Arquilla B, Garg M, Di Somma S, El-Menyar A, Krishnan V, Gerber J, Holland R, Stawicki SP (2020) Novel coronavirus (COVID-19): leveraging telemedicine

to optimize care while minimizing exposures and viral transmission. J Emergencies, Trauma Shock 13(1):20

48. Bokolo AJ (2020) Exploring the adoption of telemedicine and virtual software for care of outpatients during and after COVID-19 pandemic. Irish J Med Sc (1971):1–10

49. The medical futurist. https://medicalfuturist.com/covid-19-was-needed-for-telemedicine-to-finally-go-mainstream/

50. Bain & company https://www.bain.com/insights/covid-19-accelerates-the-adoption-of-telemedicine-in-asia-pacific-countries/

51. The economic times. https://health.economictimes.indiatimes.com/news/health-it/covid-19-lockdown-2-0-telemedicine-in-india-to-see-continued-growth/75172147

52. Monaghesh E, Hajizadeh A (2020) The role of telehealth during COVID-19 outbreak: a systematic review based on current evidence

53. Evisit. https://evisit.com/resources/what-is-telemedicine/

54. Esanjeevaniopd. esanjeevaniopd.in

55. Fisk M, Livingstone A, Pit SW (2020) Telehealth in the context of COVID-19: changing perspectives in Australia, the United Kingdom, and the United States. J Med Internet Res 22(6):e19264

56. Pharmaphorum. https://pharmaphorum.com/news/free-telemedicine-service-in-uk-will-connect-patients-to-at-home-doctors/

57. NPR. https://www.npr.org/2020/04/29/847171229/in-paris-a-new-app-is-helping-doctors-monitor-covid-19-patients-remotely

58. Center for disease control and prevention. https://www.cdc.gov/coronavirus/2019-ncov/global-covid-19/telehealth-covid19-nonUS.html

59. Ultraspecialisti. https://www.ultraspecialisti.com/

60. Hospital and healthcare management. https://www.hhmglobal.com/industry-updates/press-releases/radlogics-expands-deployment-of-its-ai-powered-solution-to-support-chest-imaging-for-covid-19-patients

61. World bank blogs. https://blogs.worldbank.org/digital-development/after-coronavirus-telemedicine-here-stay

62. Scientect. https://scientect.com/uncategorized/690618/telemedicine-market-to-witness-huge-growth-by-2027-top-manufacturers-aerotel-medical-systems-intouch-technologies-amd-global-telemedicine-obs-medical-cisco-systems-cerner-corporation-allscripts/

63. CNBC. https://www.cnbc.com/2020/08/24/google-to-invest-100-million-in-amwell-at-ipo-in-cloud-deal.html

64. Electronichealthreporter. https://electronichealthreporter.com/how-are-virtual-hospitals-changing-the-future-of-healthcare/

65. Orthogonal. https://orthogonal.io/insights/the-increasing-importance-of-software-in-medical-devices-html/

66. Ting DSW, Carin L, Dzau V, Wong TY (2020) Digital technology and COVID-19. Nat Med 26(4):459–461

67. Wadali JS, Sood SP, Kaushish R, Syed-Abdul S, Khosla PK, Bhatia M (2020) Evaluation of free, open-source, Web-based DICOM viewers for the Indian national telemedicine service (eSanjeevani). J Dig Imag 1–15

68. https://www.mygov.in/aarogya-setu-app/

Chapter 7
Preventive Behavior Against COVID 19: Role of Psychological Factors

Richa Singh and Anurag Upadhyay

1 Introduction

The COVID 19 pandemic is being caused by a new strain of corona virus, which can cause fever, dry cough, etc., and in serious cases, it can cause difficulty in breathing. Some people infected with the novel corona virus remain asymptomatic and do not show any symptoms, but they can transmit the disease. This novel corona virus is highly contagious and can be transmitted directly from one person to another through the droplets emitted by coughing and sneezing or indirectly through touching the contaminated surfaces and then touching eye, nose, or mouth with the contaminated hands. Millions of people are affected across the globe since its outbreak in December 2019 in Wuhan, China [1]. Thereafter, the cases of COVID 19 have increased at an unprecedented magnitude and led to the public health crisis globally. World Health Organization [2] declared COVID 19 a pandemic on 11 March, 2020, as it has affected millions of people throughout the globe.

Scientists and health professionals across the world are under their way to develop vaccine and pharmaceutical treatment for COVID 19. Due to lack of vaccine and pharmaceutical treatment along with high rate of transmission, the novel coronal virus has created a serious challenge to control the spread of the disease [3]. However, the spread of COVID 19 can be mitigated by following the preventive measures being suggested by health officials and professionals. To overcome this disease, adoption of preventive behavior and the compliance with the guidelines issued by health officials by the general public is necessary to slow the spread of the virus [4].

R. Singh
Department of Psychology, Vasanta College for Women, Rajghat Fort, Varanasi, India
e-mail: richasingh.bhu@gmail.com

A. Upadhyay (✉)
Department of Psychology, Udai Pratap Autonomus College, Varanasi, India
e-mail: dr.anuragwits@gmail.com

The preventive public health measures suggested by health officials and professionals include personal protection practices such as frequently washing the hands or using sanitizers, reducing face touching, using face masks, disinfecting frequently touched surfaces, staying at home when feeling sick, social distancing, etc.

Despite emphasis on preventive behavior against COVID 19 by governments and health officials across the world, people are ignoring these recommendations and fail to engage in preventive behaviors. Since adoption of preventive behavior requires behavioral change, psychological factors need to be considered in context to the preventive behavior against COVID 19.

1.1   Preventive Health Behavior and COVID 19 Pandemic

Preventive health behavior is defined as adoption of behavior or activities for preventing disease by those who consider themselves to be healthy in an asymptomatic stage [5]. For a longer and healthier life, preventive health behavior must be followed, for example, taking a balanced diet, exercise regularly, avoid smoking, alcohol, etc. Pandemics are public health crisis, in which adoption of preventive health behavior suggested by health authorities becomes even more important for both, those who are well and those who are ill. Preventive health measures taken by those who are well to prevent infection and those who are infected to prevent the spread of the virus to others are very crucial in any public health emergency [6].

Preventive health behavior during COVID 19 is inexpensive and readily available and acts as effective primary prevention till the vaccine or pharmacological treatment comes. During the present COVID 19, pandemic health authorities have recommended preventive health behavior for COVID 19. It includes the practice of hand hygiene, respiratory hygiene (e.g., using face mask), social distancing, and disinfections for preventing the spread of the novel corona virus. Despite the fact that at present in the absence of vaccine and pharmacological treatment, preventive behavior is the only way to slow down the spread of virus, and most people fail to adhere to the recommended guidelines.

World Health Organization [7] has suggested four main methods to manage the spread of infection during any pandemic. These methods include risk communication or public education, vaccine and antiviral therapies, hygiene practices, and social distancing. For the current COVID 19 pandemic, since vaccines and antiviral therapies are not available till date, the focus is on the rest three measures in which psychological factors play a crucial role.

1.2   Risk Communication

Giving information to the public to make a well-informed decision about how to protect their health during a pandemic is referred to as risk communication [8].

Effective risk communication plays a crucial role in controlling the outbreak of any pandemic. World Health Organization [9] has discussed the important elements of risk communication. Careful consideration of the psychological issues involved in risk communication will make it more effective. During this present COVID 19 pandemic, importance of effective risk communication has become more important due to the unavailability of vaccine and pharmacological treatment. This will help the people in adoption health and safety guidelines to protect themselves from corona virus and will also help the authorities in the management of COVID 19.

1.3 Hygiene Practices

Hygiene practices play a very important role in protecting against infection. During any pandemic, it becomes even more important. Hygiene practices recommended during the present pandemic includes washing hands with soap and water frequently for 20 s especially when coming from outside or using alcohol-based sanitizers, using face masks, covering mouth, and nose while sneezing or sneezing into the crook of one's arm, reducing face touching, and disinfecting frequently touched surfaces. During this current COVID 19 pandemic, many governments are making it mandatory to wear the masks and are imposing fines if they do not wear it. The effectiveness of facemasks was known previously and was widely used during Spanish flu pandemic [10]. Hand washing is generally acceptable among general public to reduce the spread of infection, but it does not mean that it is actually translated into washing behavior [8]. People's perception of risk is likely to affect their engagement in hygiene practices. Individuals who perceive themselves at low risk of infection from corona virus are less likely to adopt hygiene practices as compared to those who perceive themselves more susceptible to infection. Therefore, the psychological factors involved in hygiene practices need to be explored.

1.4 Social Distancing

During the early phase of COVID 19, many countries imposed lockdown to ensure social distancing to reduce the spread of disease. Social distancing includes isolating or quarantine of infected person, school, and workplace closure, closing recreational facilities, cancelling mass gathering, imposing travel restrictions, self-imposed isolation of uninfected persons, etc. It also includes keeping an interpersonal space of 1–2 m from the people who shows sign of infections. During any pandemic outbreak, social distancing measures must be applied immediately, rigorously, and consistently for it to be effective [11]. Although social distancing measures helps in decreasing the spread of infection, it also leads to economic hardships and adverse effect on the mental health of people which creates hindrance in adherence to it. Non-adherence to the recommendations by the health authorities is a major problem, and we will discuss this later in the chapter.

2   Psychological Factors and Preventive Health Behavior

Preventive health behaviors are beneficial for health, and in the current pandemic situation, it is believed to reduce the transmission of infection. A number of factors determine preventive health behavior. It includes individual's cognition (believes, attitude, decision making, etc.), socio-cultural, environmental, and economic factors. We will be focusing on the psychological factors because that can be intervened through health-related education and persuasive communication. Psychologists have tried to explain whether an individual will adopt preventive behavior based on cognitive and social factors. These cognitive and social factors have been used to build models, which suggest that evaluation of perceived risk of a disease, consequences of adopting preventive behavior and assessing one's self-efficacy will determine the engagement in preventive health behavior. Therefore, it is important to look into the psychological factors that contribute to behavior change during pandemic.

Various theoretical models have been used to explain preventive health behavior. In context to COVID 19, in the present chapter, we will discuss the applicability of Rosenstock's health belief model [12], Roger's protection motivation theory [13], and Azen's theory of planned behavior [14] to explain the adoption and engagement of preventive health behavior by people. In all these model, it is assumed that while making a decision related to preventive health behavior, people analyzes the consequences rationally. Now, we will discuss each of these theories in context to adoption of preventive behavior during COVID 19.

2.1   Health Belief Model

One of the most influential models used to explain preventive health behavior is Rosenstock's health belief model [12]. The model focuses on how the attitudes and beliefs individual holds for a particular disease influence their engagement in preventive behavior. The model specifies how health behaviors is cognitively represented and what are the components of self-protective health behavior [15]. The model focuses on the psychological factors involved in the beliefs individual hold regarding a disease that influence their decision regarding preventive behavior. The model assumes that people will adopt preventive health behavior if they perceives the risk of disease and believes that the recommended preventive behavior will help to reduce the risk of contracting the disease.

According to this model, two factors determine whether an individual will adopt preventive health behavior. These factors include *risk perception* or *threat perception*, i.e., whether a personal health threat from a disease is being perceived, and *health-related behavioral evaluation*, i.e., whether the perceived threat will be reduced after engagement in preventive health behavior. The model suggests that whether a person will adopt the preventive behavior for COVID 19 can be predicted on the basis of person's belief in personal threat from corona virus along with the person's belief that using mask, hand washing, staying at home, etc. will be effective in reducing the threat of getting infected. Perceived susceptibility and perceived severity of a disease indicates threat perception and health-related behavioral evaluation is being indicated by the evaluation of perceived benefits associated with adoption of preventive and perceived barriers or obstacles in performing a preventive behavior.

2.1.1 Components of Health Belief Model

The original health belief model proposed that individual's willingness to engage in health behavior is being determined by four main factors. These factors are perceived susceptibility of a disease, perceived severity of a disease; perceived benefits associated with health behavior and perceived barriers in performing the health behavior [16]. The model predicts that an individual will adopt a preventive behavior if they consider themselves to be vulnerable to a disease, perceive that the disease is severe and can cause disability or death or can have severe social consequences, believes that adopting preventive behavior will be beneficial in reducing the threat of the disease and can overcome the barriers. These four components of the model significantly contribute to the prediction of preventive health behavior.

Perceived Susceptibility

Perceived susceptibility is the belief about being infected or getting a disease. It is the subjective perception by the individual that he or she is at the risk of acquiring a disease, for example, my chance of getting infected with corona virus is high or low. There are variations in the feeling of vulnerability or susceptibility toward a disease. During the current pandemic young children, older adults, persons with preexisting medical conditions, and healthcare professionals are more at risk of getting infected in comparison with the young healthy adults. So, the perceived susceptibility of both groups will be different.

Perceived Severity

It refers to the feeling of seriousness of contracting a disease. It basically reflects the cognition about the consequences of disease. Both medical (e.g., disease or disability) and the possible social consequences (how the disease will affect the work or family life, social relationships) are being considered. Perceived susceptibility combined with perceived severity is termed as perceived risk.

Perceived Benefits

Individual's perception or the beliefs about the benefits or effectiveness of preventive measures available to reduce the risk of a disease is referred as perceived benefits. An individual's belief regarding the beneficial effect recommended preventive behavior in reducing the perceived risk of a particular disease influences the decision involving the implementation of preventive behavior.

Perceived Barriers

Perceived barriers refer to the perceived obstacles in the adoption of recommended preventive health behavior. Individuals compare the effectiveness of a recommended action with how expensive or painful it will be to adopt and the time involved in it. Thus, people make a cost–benefit analysis and if the perceived benefits are more than the perceived barriers, then there is greater chance of adoption of preventive behavior.

Cues to Action

Later on another component was added to the model which was called *cues to action,* i.e., when certain belief sets are held; these are the strategies to activate readiness for preventive behavior or reminders about potential health problem. It can be both external (e.g., media advertisement or social influences) or internal (e.g., symptom perception). External cues to action are relevant for preventive health behavior as there are no symptoms.

Apart from the above mentioned components, General Health Motivation was added to the model to indicate the person's readiness for the health related matter for themselves [17]. Later on, the theory developers also added age, gender, ethnicity, personality, and socioeconomic status as the modifying factor to the model to predict health behavior.

2.1.2   Health Belief Model and COVID 19

The health belief model is important in context to COVID 19 as it identifies a number of key and modifying factors which will help in the prediction of an individual's engagement to recommended preventive health behavior. Also the components in the model and specially the beliefs can be intervened or changed which can lead to change in behavior. So, in the present COVID 19 situation, this model can used to identify the factors which are creating hindrance in the adoption of recommended preventive behavior. If the people perceive that they are not susceptible and consequences of corona virus infection are not severe, there are fewer chances that they will engage in preventive behavior. In such cases, beliefs of the people need to be changed or intervened. If the risk perception is high but people believe that there are barriers in adoption of preventive behavior, then the authorities should make arrangement to eliminate those barriers.

Thus, in the present COVID 19 health crisis, health belief model can provide useful insight in understanding the decision-making process related to adoption of preventive health behavior. It identifies that in forming a decision related to health behavior, an individual simultaneously compares a number of cognitive factors which includes a cost–benefit analysis of threat perception of disease and what are the advantages and disadvantages of a particular preventive behavior for the individual [15].

2.2 Protection Motivation Theory

Individual's attitude and subsequent behavior toward preventive behavior can be influenced by the fear appeals. In any pandemic like COVID 19, the aim is to make general public aware about the risk of experiencing a negative health outcome if they do not adopt the recommended preventive behavior. To identify the role of fear and threat experiences in attitude change and subsequent behavior modification through persuasive communication, Rogers [13] developed a model, and it was named as protection motivation theory. The theory focuses on how the fear appeals can influence the modification of health behavior. The significant cognitive factors which mediate arousal in fear experience and ultimately influence behavior are being identified by the model. According to protection motivation theory, the information related to a disease received from various sources activates two appraisal processes, i.e., threat appraisal and coping appraisal. Both the appraisal processes involves cognitive factors that mediate the relationship between experience of threat and subsequent behavior change and operates in parallel to each other [15].

2.2.1 Components of Protection Motivation Theory

There are three key components of protection motivation theory, i.e., threat appraisal, coping appraisal, and protection motivation. Threat and coping appraisal determines protection motivation which in turn arouses the person to engage in preventive behavior.

Threat Appraisal

Threat appraisal is concerned with the factors which are important to understand the basis of threat. It involves two components (i) *perceived severity* of a threat or seriousness of a disease and (ii) *perceives vulnerability* of a threat or chance of getting a disease. Individuals will perceive severe health threat when they will perceive that they are vulnerable to a severe disease and this perception will help the individuals to take preventive health behavior. For example, during the current COVID 19 pandemic, those people are more likely to adopt the recommended preventive health behavior who perceives that it is a serious disease which will affect the health adversely, and they are vulnerable to get infected due to corona virus.

Coping Appraisal

An individual's assessment of their capacity to face the threat or risk of a disease is referred as coping appraisal [18]. It also involves two components: (i) *Response efficacy,* i.e., belief that one can face the threat through a recommended preventive behavior. (ii) *Self-efficacy,* i.e., the ability of an individual to face the threat or the confidence in their skill that they can engage in the preventive health behaviors. The theory predicts that likelihood of preventive behavior to be undertaken increases with high level of response efficacy and self-efficacy.

Protection Motivation

Protection motivation is the central factor in this theory. It can be defined as an individual's intent to engage in preventive behavior to lessen the threat associated with a disease. It is a mediating variable which emerges when individuals engage in the thinking of threat appraisal and coping appraisal. Protection motivation emerge as a consequences of the comparisons when the perceived severity and vulnerability of a disease is more and when the response efficacy and self-efficacy is greater than the costs linked with engaging in preventive behavior. Meta-analysis [19] of different studies on protection motivation theory has shown that perceived severity and vulnerability of a disease, response efficacy, and self-efficacy were positively related with protection motivation; therefore, protection motivation can be predicted based on these components.

2.2.2 Protection Motivation Theory and COVID 19

Protection motivation theory can be useful in predicting whether people will adopt the preventive measures or not during COVID 19. As the theory states, high level of perceived risk influences the adoption of preventive behaviors by the public. So during this ongoing pandemic, focus should be on increasing the awareness about corona virus risk based on the information received from public health professionals and health authorities. Different media platforms can be utilized to increase the awareness about the actual risk involved if a person gets infected. At the same time, individuals should also be made aware that they are capable of protecting themselves from corona virus if they adopt hand hygiene, use mask, and maintain social distancing, and other recommended preventive measures.

In a recent study [20] conducted on the healthcare workers of Iran to predict the preventive behavior during COVID 19, the result revealed that threat and coping appraisal were significant predictors of protection motivation to adopt COVID 19 preventive behavior. The protection motivation significantly predicted the COVID 19 preventive behavior.

2.3   Theory of Planned Behavior

Another popular explanatory model of preventive health behavior is the theory of planned behavior. Theory of planned behavior was developed by Ajzen [14] to understand how the health attitude held by an individual affects their subsequent behavior. The model states that people holds expectations regarding the consequences of their specific health-related behavior and the value of each consequences for themselves. This theory has been developed from their previous theory of reasoned action. Theory of reasoned action suggested that intention to engage in a preventive behavior predicts the actual behavior. This intention to engage in preventive or health behavior can be predicted from (i) *attitude* toward such behavior, i.e., belief about perceived consequences of engaging in preventive behavior and the evaluation of the consequences, and (ii) *perceived or subjective norms*, i.e., perceived expectations to engage in preventive behavior and the motivation to comply with those norms. But this initial model does not included any important aspect, i.e., the control people have on their own behavior. So, the model was revised, and a new component, i.e., perceived behavioral control, was added to the model, and it was called as theory of planned behavior.

2.3.1   Components of Theory of Planned Behavior

Theory of planned behavior assumes that health behavior is the result of behavioral intentions, or in other words behavioral intention is the antecedent condition, and health behavior is the consequence. Behavioral intention can be anticipated on the basis three psychological elements. These elements represent the components of this theory, which include attitude toward specific health action, subjective norms, and perceived behavioral control.

Attitude Toward Specific Action

It is the belief about the outcome of behavior and the evaluation of those outcomes. For example, during this corona virus pandemic, if individuals believe that using masks, hand washing, and social distancing will protect them against the infection (outcome expectancy), this will help them to remain healthy. Being in good health is a good thing (value association). Then, people will have positive attitude toward recommend preventive behaviors, and it may result in engagement in preventive behaviors.

Subjective Norms

It is the belief about what other people (those who are important to us) thinks how we should behave (normative belief) and the motivation to comply (i.e., doing what significant others wants us to do) with those normative beliefs. For example, if wearing mask in public places becomes a subjective norm, then most of the people will comply with this norm and will be motivated to wear masks if they go out in public places.

Perceived Behavioral Control

It is the belief regarding a person's control on his or her behavior, i.e., the feeling that one is able to perform recommended health behavior and that behavior will have the intended effect. This concept is very similar to the concept of self-efficacy. For example, if a person believes that wearing mask or frequent hand washing is under their own control, then they are more likely to form an intention to wear mask and do frequent hand washing.

The attitude, normative beliefs, and perceived control along with the expectancy value evaluation predicts a person's intention and subsequently predicts the actual behavior [15]. According to this theory, preventive behavior can be predicted on the basis of intention moderated by perceived behavioral control. The intention is influenced by attitude toward preventive behavior and subjective norms.

2.3.2   Theory of Planned Behavior and COVID 19

Theory of planned behavior suggests that individual's decision regarding the acceptance of the recommended preventive health measure for COVID 19 will depend upon three things. At first, they analyze their beliefs regarding the potential consequences of preventive behavior (social distancing, face masks, or hand washing, etc.) which is reflected in their attitude toward preventive behavior against COVID 19. Simultaneously, the person also analyzes what the significant others think about their engagement in preventive behavior (subjective norm) and their willingness to comply with those norms. Finally, the person will look for any difficulty to perform preventive behaviors, for example unavailability of sanitizer or soap and water at workplace, etc. These three components will decide the intention to comply with recommended preventive behavior against COVID 19 and finally influence the behavior.

3 Risk Perception and COVID 19

Since psychological and behavioral factors play an important role in managing pandemic, determining how perceived risk is linked to engagement in preventive behavior is very important. The psychological evaluation of the probability and consequences of an adverse outcome is referred as risk perception [21]. Risk perception is a complex phenomenon which is affected by various factors such as probability, severity, controllability, dread, catastrophic potential, and unfamiliarity with a hazard [22]. Due to the importance of risk perception in any epidemic or pandemic, it is a major component of many health behavior theories. In health belief model and protection motivation theory, risk perception primarily involves two types of beliefs, i.e., perceived susceptibility or vulnerability and perceived severity.

Besides susceptibility and severity, there are other factors which can influence the perception of risk for disease. Worry is an important factor associated with risk perception. Pandemics are associated with fear and worry among people. Public worry over getting infected with the disease affects their risk perception. When facing a risk of being infected with a disease during a pandemic, individual's emotional response to it is referred as worry and can also predict the adoption of preventive behavior [23]. Worry about a pandemic is affected by an individual's values, social context, and socio-demographic characteristics like age, sex, education, income, etc. [24].

3.1 Risk Perception and COVID 19

Due to COVID 19, lockdown has been imposed, and people are advised to remain in quarantine or in isolation if get infected with corona virus. This has led to worry, anxiety, and perception of risk among people. Risk perception among people is an important factor that determines engagement in preventive behavior. Authentic and clear information related to any pandemic (e.g., COVID 19) must be communicated to the general public which in turn will facilitate engagement in preventive behavior. During the COVID 19 pandemic, perception of risk will trigger the engagement in social and physical distancing, personal, hand hygiene, use of mask, and other recommended preventive behaviors [25].

Higher level of perceived risk and susceptibility is associated with compliance to preventive health recommendations [26]. Role of psychological factors in predicting preventive behavior against COVID 19 has been studied recently by Yildrim, Gecer, and Akgul [25]. They reported that preventive behavior related to COVID 19 can be predicted on the basis of individual's perceived vulnerability, perceived risk, and fear of disease. In their study, they also reported that in comparison with male participants, females were more susceptible and reported higher level of risk and fear. Therefore, there are more chances of females to adopt preventive behavior in comparison with males.

Another study [27] conducted during the initial stage of COVID 19, United States examined the influence of risk perception on engagement in preventive behavior. They reported that perceived likelihood of becoming infected significantly predicted hand washing and social distancing measures while perceived severity of illness does not significantly predicted preventive behavior. The study concluded that higher level of perceived risk can predict engagement in preventive behavior.

Risk perception of a pandemic is a significant factor that can affect the number of new positive cases [28]. Relatively higher level of risk perception of COVID 19 among people [27] is indicative of the fact that people are well informed and aware of the risk of COVID 19. Awareness of risk associated with corona virus infection is very important as this will help people to understand seriousness of the infection and to adopt and engage in preventive behavior.

4   Adherence to Preventive Behavior

Adherence is a complex phenomenon related to health behavior. During a pandemic, adherence to preventive measures recommended by the health officials and the government is very crucial in mitigating the spread of the disease. In the present, public health crisis due to COVID 19 requires people to make behavioral changes and comply with the recommended preventive behavior and reporting voluntary if there is any symptom and go for testing.

Adherence refers to a situation when individual's behavior confirms with the recommended behavior and advice proposed by health practitioner [15]. Adherence in health care takes two forms, i.e., behavioral and medical. Medical adherence concerned specially with medication like taking the prescribed correct dosage, at correct time, etc. Behavioral adherence refers to the health behaviors like adoption of exercise, hand hygiene, wearing masks, etc. Earlier the term compliance was used to indicate the confirmation of patient's behavior toward physician's advice. Because compliance implied a passive role of the patient and an authoritarian role of physician, the term compliance was replaced with adherence as it reflects active management or self-regulation of treatment advice.

Haynes [29] defined adherence as the degree to which an individual's behavior matches with medical or health advice. Adherence is a complex concept, and it varies across different forms of recommended behaviors. Majority of people does not comply with health advice, and there are varieties of factors responsible for non-adherence. Non-adherence to health advice is a significant problem in the management of chronic or infectious diseases. Non-adherence can be of two types (i) *passive*, i.e., that results from the miscomprehension of treatment advice, and (ii) *active*, i.e., when patients deliberately and intentionally makes a decision not to follow the treatment regime [30].

Positive health outcome is associated with adherence with recommended health advice, while non-adherence is related to negative health outcomes [31]. Non-adherence has negative effect on the health of both the individual and the society.

In a pandemic situation like COVID 19, non-adherence to recommended preventive behaviors will lead to spread of infection at a higher rate, thus creating hindrance in its management. Non-adherence with health advice is associated with large number of factors ranging from economic, social, interpersonal, and personal factors like age, gender, education, etc. Individual's decision to adhere to the treatment or recommended preventive is also influenced by cognitive and affective factors. Therefore, these factors need to be explored in order to understand non-adherence.

4.1 Factors Associated with Non-adherence

Various reasons for non-adherence to recommended health behavior have been identified. Previous studies have suggested that social and economic factors (e.g., social support, socioeconomic status), therapy-related factors (e.g., presence of adverse effects, duration of treatment, and drug effectiveness), presence of symptoms, and disease severity, and patient-related factors (e.g., age, gender, and education) affects non-adherence to recommend health behavior [32].

4.1.1 Patient Characteristics

Studies have shown that patients with less social support and more socially isolated are less compliant. Meichenbaun and Turk [33] divided the patient's characteristics on three dimensions which are associated with compliance or adherence. These are (i) *Social characteristics*: which includes characteristics of individual's social situation, lack of social support, family instability, competing or conflicting demands, residential instability, and lack of resources, (ii) *Personal characteristics*: it includes demographics (age, sex, education, etc.), sensory disabilities, forgetfulness, and lack of understanding, and (iii) *Health beliefs*: it includes inappropriate or conflicting beliefs, competing sociocultural and ethnic folk concept of disease and treatment and inherent models of illness.

4.1.2 Disease Characteristics

Certain characteristics of the disease like severity of disease and the visibility of symptoms have been found to be associated with adherence. Studies have reported that asymptomatic chronic disease patients do not comply with treatments frequently [34]. Patients may comply with the treatment, when the symptoms are apparent and unwanted.

4.1.3   Treatment Characteristics

Various treatment factors have been identified which are associated with compliance or adherence. Meichenbaun and Turk [33] categorized the treatment factors into four categories. These are: (i) *Preparation for treatment*: Before starting actual treatment, the patient has to take appointment with doctor, and this may involve long waiting time, lack of individual appointments, etc., which may lead to frustration and non-adherence. (ii) *Immediate characteristics of the treatment*: It involves complexity and duration of treatment regimen, and more complicated and lengthier treatment regimen are associated with less adherence. More is the degree of behavior change, inconvenience and expenses involved less adherence is being observed. (iii) *Administration of treatment*: Inadequate supervision by the professional, absence of continuity of care, and failure to supervise drug administration is associated with non-adherence, and (iv) *Consequences of treatment*: It involves physical and social side (e.g., stigma) effects of treatment. Lower levels of physical side effects are associated with higher level of adherence. Decreased adherence was observed in.

4.1.4   Interpersonal Factors

The nature of doctor–patient relationships affects the adherence to treatment regimen. Patient-centered or affiliative style which promotes positive friendly and caring relationship leads to better adherence [35] as compared to authoritarian or control-oriented relationship.

4.1.5   Social and Organizational Setting

The social and organizational setting where the consultation of patient with doctor takes place also affects adherence. Various setting characteristics have been identified by the researchers [33] which potentially affects adherence. Adherence is more when waiting times are reduced, and appointment is individualized, when care involves follow up and is personalized, when treatment is supervised through home visits, etc. Apart from immediate medical setting, the social setting in terms of friends and family also play important role in adherence.

Different theoretical health models have been used to explain adherence and non-adherence. Based on the models of health belief and planned behavior, relationship between adherence rate and the perceived susceptibility has been reported. According to these models, adherence behavior can be predicted on the basis of beliefs held by the individuals. Studies have reported that higher level of perceived susceptibility, perceived severity is associated with greater level of compliance with hygiene practices [36].

4.1.6 Preventive Behavior Adherence and COVID 19

During COVID 19 pandemic, health officials across the globe are recommending people to adopt and engage in social distancing, hand hygiene, using masks, restrict mass gathering, travel restrictions, etc. To maintain social distancing, lockdown has been imposed, and people have been advised to remain in quarantine or in isolation if get infected with corona virus. If people infected with corona virus follow the instruction for quarantine, then only it will help in preventing the spread of virus to other people. Awareness about the disease and the isolation procedures is significant predictors of adherence to quarantine.

In a recent review [37], researches reported that there a number of factors during a pandemic outbreak that determine adherence to quarantine. Based on the studies being reviewed, they suggested that to improve adherence to quarantine health official should provide timely and strong reasoning for quarantine along with the code of behavior that should be followed during isolation. Emphasis should also be given to the social and cultural norms to improve adherence. Perceived benefits of quarantine, i.e., engagement in quarantine if got infected will reduce the spread of infection to others, should be highlighted. They further reported that sufficient supply of food, medicines, and other essentials will lead to better adherence to quarantine.

Thus, to improve adherence with preventive behavior during the present COVID 19 situation, various factors must be considered. These include identifying the predictors for adherence, knowledge about preventive behaviors for COVID 19, and perception of severity and vulnerability of public toward corona virus. All these factors must be considered when communicating and persuading with the general public and designing intervention programs to improve adherence with the preventive behavior for COVID 19.

5 Conclusion

At present, the world is facing the biggest health crisis in terms of COVID 19. Management of COVID 19 largely depends on preventive behavior till the vaccine or pharmacological treatment comes. Preventive behaviors recommended by health officials to combat with corona virus are very crucial as it will reduce the rate of transmission of highly contagious disease. For the management of any pandemic, World Health organization has recommended four things, i.e., risk communication, vaccine and antiviral treatment, hygiene practices, and social distancing. Since vaccine and antiviral treatments are not available right now, the focus is on rest three factors in which psychological factors play a very crucial role.

Psychological factors play a very important role risk communication. Clear and accurate risk perception facilitates engagement in preventive behavior. Besides this, there are large numbers of psychological factors that mediate the decision regarding the engagement in preventive behavior. Factors like attitude, beliefs, decision making, and other socioeconomic factors determine the engagement to preventive behaviors regarding COVID 19.

Various theories and models in health psychology have tied to explain the factors that determine the indulgence in preventive health behavior. Health belief model states that perceived risk and health-related behavioral evaluation, i.e., if individual perceive that corona virus is severe and he or she is susceptible to it, and more benefits are associated with social distancing, hand hygiene, and wearing masks as compared to barriers in adoption to it. So, the strategy to enhance preventive behavior in public should consider both, i.e., demographical variables and the individual's psychological characteristics to increase the perceived risk and stimulate the behavioral evaluation. Identification of barriers in adopting the preventive behavior needs to be resolved by the authorities and will help in engagement and adherence with preventive behavior recommended for COVID 19. Protection motivation theory emphasizes that protection motivation is a function of threat appraisal and coping appraisal and helps in the prediction of engagement to preventive behavior. According to the theory of planned behavior attitude, normative beliefs and perceived behavioral control determines the engagement to preventive behaviors. Therefore, all these variables identified by different models need to be considered while designing the intervention programs for adoption of preventive measures for general public.

Another very important psychological aspect with COVID 19 is non-adherence or non-compliance with the recommended preventive behavior like quarantine, hand hygiene, etc. Identifying the predictors of adherence, perceived susceptibility, and severity of COVID 19 and the knowledge about preventive behavior must be considered in designing the intervention programs and persuading general public to engage in preventive behaviors recommended for COVID 19.

Since, psychological factors play a very important role in the adoption of preventive behavior against COVID 19, these factors must be considered while designing the intervention programs to improve the adherence and engagement of people with preventive behaviors recommended for COVID 19.

References

1. Huang C, Wang Y, Li X, Ren L, Zhao J, Hu Y et al (2020) Clinical features of patients infected with 2019 Novel Corona Virus in Wuhan, China. The Lancet 395(10233):497–506
2. World Health Organization: Corona virus disease (COVID 19) technical guidance: Infection prevention and control. https://www.who.int/emergencies/diseases/novel-coronavirus-019/technicalguidance/
3. Lai CC, Shih TP, Ko WC, Tang HJ, Hsueh PR (2020) Severe acute respiratory syndrome Corona Virus 2 (SARA-CoV-2) and corona virus disease 2019 (COVID-19): the epidemic and the challenges. Int J Antimicrob Agents 55(3):105924
4. Anderson RM, Heesterbeek H, Klinkenberg D, Hollingsworth T (2020) How will country based mitigation measures influence the course of COVID 19 epidemic? the Lancet. 395(10228):931–934
5. Cobb K (1966) Health behavior, illness behavior and sick role behavior. Arch Environ Health 12:246–266

6. Katz R, May L, Sanza M, Johnston L, Petinauk B (2012) H1N1Preventive health behavior in a university setting. J. Am College Health 6(1):46–56
7. World Health Organization (2008) WHO outbreak communication planning guide. Author, Geneva
8. Taylor S (2019) The psychology of pandemics: preparing for the next global outbreak of infectious diseases. Cambridge Scholars Publishing, U.K.
9. World Health Organization (2005) WHO checklist for influenza pandemic preparedness planning. Author, Geneva
10. Arnold C (2018) Pandemic 1918: eyewitness account from the greatest medical holocaust in modern history. St. Martin's Press, New York
11. Maharaj S, Kleczkowski A (2012) Controlling epidemic spread by social distancing: do it well or not at all. BMC Public Health 12:679
12. Rosenstock IM (1974) The health belief model and preventive health behavior. Health Educ Monograph 2:354–368
13. Rogers RW (1975) A protection motivation theory of fear appeals and attitude change. J Psychol 91:93–114
14. Aizen I (1985) From intentions to actions: a theory of planned behavior. In: Khul J, Beckman (eds) Action control: from cognition to behavior. Springer, Heidlberg, pp 11–39
15. Albery IP, Munafo M (2008) Key concepts in health psychology. Sage, New Delhi, pp 50–51
16. Norman P, Corner M (1993) The role of social cognition model in predicting attendance at health checks. Psychol Health 8:447–462
17. Strecher VJ, Rosenstock LM (1997) Health Belief Model. In: Baum A, Newman S, Weinman J, West R, McManus C (eds) Cambridge handbook of psychology, health and medicines. Cambridge University Press, Cambridge, pp 113–117
18. Carolina W (2011) The Determinants of preventive health behavior: literature review and research perspective. HAL-00638266 (2011)
19. Floyd DL, Prentice-Dunn S, Rogers RW (2000) A meta-analysis of protection motivation theory. J Appl Soc Psychol 30:407–429
20. Bashirian S, Jenabi E, Khazaei S, Barati M, Karimi-Shahanjarini A, Zareian S, Rezapur-Shahkolai F, Moeini B (2020) Factors associated with preventive behaviorof COVID19 among hospital staff in Iranin 2020: an application of the Protection Motivation Theory. J Hosp Infect 105:430–433
21. Sjoberg L (2000) Factors in risk perception. Risk Anal 20(1):1–11
22. Slovic P (1987) Perception of risk. Science 236:280–285
23. Khosravi M (2020) Perceived risk of COVID-19 pandemic: the role of public worry and trust. Electron J Gen Med 17(4):em203
24. Vaughan E, Tinker T (2009) Effective health risk communication about pandemic influenza for vulnerable population. Am J Public Health 99(S2:S3):24–32
25. Yildirim M, Gecer E, Akgul O (2020) The impact of perceived vulnerability and fear on preventive behavioragainst COVID 19. Psychol Health Med 10:1–9
26. Brug J, Aro AR, Richardus JH (2009) Risk perception and behaviortowards pandemic control of emerging infectious diseases. Int J Behav Med 16:3–6
27. Wise T, Zbozinek TD, Michelini G, Hagan CC (2020) Changes in risk perception and protective behaviorduring the first week of the COVID 19 pandemic in the United States. Psy Ar Xiv Preprints. /https://doi.org/10.31234/osf.io/dz428
28. Cori L, Bianchi F, Cadum E, Anthonj C (2020) Risk perception and COVID 19. Int J Environ Res Public Health 17(9):3114. https://doi.org/10.3390/ijerph17093114
29. Haynes RB (1979) Introduction. In: Haynes RB, Sackett DL, Taylor (eds) Compliance in health care. John Hopkins University Press, Baltimore, MD, pp 1–10
30. Marteau TM, Weinman J (2004) Communicating about health threats and treatments. In: Sutton S, Baum A, Johnston (eds) The Sage handbook of health psychology. Sage, London, pp 270–298
31. DiMatteo MR, Giordani PJ, Lepper HS, Croghan TW (2002) Patient adherence and medical treatment outcome: a metaanalysis. Med Care 40(9):794–811

32. Kardas P, Lewek P, Matyjaszczyk M (2013) Determinants of patient adherence: a review of systematic reviews. Front Pharmcol. 4:91
33. Meichenbaum DC, Turk D (1987) Facilitating treatment adherence: a practioner's guidebook. Plenum Press, New York
34. Miller NH (1997) Compliance with treatment regimens in chronic asymptomatic diseases. Am J Med 102(2):43–49
35. DiMatteo MR, DiNicola DD (1982) Achieving patient compliance. Pergamon Press, Elmsford, New York
36. Kwok KO, Li KK, Chan HH, Yi YY, Tang A, Wei WI, Wong YS (2020) Community response during the early phase of COVID 19 epidemic in Hong Kong: risk perception, information exposure and preventive measures. Med Rxiv
37. Webster RK, Brooks SK, Smith LE, Woodland L, Wessely S, Rubin GJ (2020) How to improve adherence to quarantine: Rapid review of the evidence. Public Health 182:163–169

Chapter 8
Impact of the COVID-19 on Consumer Behavior Towards Organic Food in India

Anamika Chaturvedi, Md Rashid Chand, and Mujibur Rahman

1 Introduction

India is a developing country, the economy is growing fast thus people of India is also changing their life style. They are ready to eat anything to save time like readymade food, frozen food, fast food that is not good for health. There fast & unbalanced life style giving them various deceases like obesity, sugar, cholesterol problem, blood pressure etc. Lack of time & increased income is a catalyst in causing health problem. Gradually the consumer of Indian market especially affluent class and upper-middle class is moving towards healthy life style, which starts with healthy food means organic food. People want a trusted healthy food, which is free from chemical, fertilizer & certified by govt. Organic food is a new food section for Indian consumer. They are showing a positive attitude towards organic food buying. Organic food is produce without any artificial fertilizer and chemical. The food industry in India is on boom due to several facilities provided by government in recent year. The organic food market is also gating boon in this year due to health education awareness and increasing disposable income of middle class because the middle class is the biggest part of the consumer market. There is a big opportunity to sell the organic product in domestic market as well as well international market because there is huge gap between demand and supply in organic food market. The GDP of our country in 2019 was 7.3, and it is assumed that in 2020 it will be 7.5 after a storm of GIST. The global organic food market in year 2017 was about 210.25 $ billion and it is assumed that it will grow by 262.85 $ till 2022. In India the growth of organic food market in the year 2018–19 370 $ million to 515 $ million is proposed which is good sign for Indian organic food market as well as for economy of the

A. Chaturvedi (✉)
UP Institute of Design, Noida, India
e-mail: c.anamika@upidnoida.ac.in

M. Rashid Chand · M. Rahman
Galgotias University, Greater Noida, India

country. Knowing the consumers attitude towards organic food is key to success in the market. Some demographic factors, which can affect the buying attitude of consumers like age, gender, income, education, marital status etc. In India the big part of consumers are changing their eating behavior completely as organic. Organic beverages like herbal and organic tea sharing the highest value, which is followed by bread, bakery items, pulse and dairy products. Delhi-NCR is the most prominent region for consumption of organic food because affluent and educated class belongs to this region. Here the customers are health conscious and they are ready to pay a big amount for their good health because the organic food is the healthiest and safe food product as we compare it with normal food available in market. Objective of the study is to examine & identify the factors that influence the consumer's attitude towards organic food in India especially in NCR during COVID-19 time slot. How people are thinking over healthy eating and pure eating at this Corona time.

Purpose of the Study

To identify the factor which influence the behavior & attitude of consumers at this COVID-19 rough time.
To analyze the impact of demographic characteristics on consumer's attitude towards organic food in the COVID-19 era.

2 Literature Review

Ashraf et al. [1] explore about the non-consumption behavior of consumer towards organic food It includes several factors like individual beliefs, trust toward organic food quality and utility. They link between the actual purchase behavior and social pressure, which make them purchase the organic food products. To find out the answer there is theoretical framework was established (TBP), which includes the measurement scales for different factors like attitude, perceived behavioral control (PBC) and subjective norms. The result that all the factors make an impact on purchasing behavior like attitude and perceived behavior only subjective norm doesn't play a role in purchasing behavior. They also find that income is the important factor for less consumption of organic food in by consumers [22]. In his, paper "Awareness Attitude And Perception Analysis As Strategies Of Consumer Buying Behaviour towards Organic Food Products Among The College Students In Coimbatore District" found that in south India people are more aware about organic food like 96% people were aware about the organic food while 51.6% public buy food from organic product store. Rather, Anitha [15] in her paper "Marketing strategy and consumer buying behavior of organic food in Rajasthan" explore that in Rajasthan consumer behavior towards organic food is directly linked with education and income. In Rajasthan, most of the females are between the age of 25–35 shop for their home and the workers preferred the organic food, which is followed by the post graduate and graduate women who are aware about the advantages of using organic food. The income group of 15–20 lacks people is buying the organic good frequently and the category is 10–5 lacks income group who buy the organic food less frequently [17]. In her research, "A study on consumer awareness and buying the green products in Chennai city" Explored that 80 percent people were aware about the green products and their benefit. She found with help of The Duncan Multiple Range test (DMRT) that age group of below 25 and above 55 are out of the line and the age group 26–35, 36–45, and 45–55 are the considerable for the green products buying. She also explore that there is big impact of education and income group on buying behaviour of customer 36.5% of people were post graduate and the income group of 29.2% op consumer were more than 75,000, 27.1% of consumer were between 25,000–50,000. Patel [13] have explore about, the analysis of consumers' awareness and preferences for green building practices which were carried out by cross-tabulations between six demographic characteristics, viz. city, gender, age, qualification, occupation, and income of consumers versus twelve green buildings practices. The research says that there is relationship with age and education regarding the green learning practices according to researcher 40% of consumer between the age of 31–45 were accepted that they have learn about green practices during their schooling and college education. "A Study on Consumer Behavior towards Organic Food Products in Pondicherry" by [18] found that in Pondicherry Indian and foreigners both were aware about the organic products and 60 percent of consumers were buying the organic food item. There finding says that only 10–20% shops are available to sell the organic food at the premium prices. Their willingness to buy the organic food was motivated by their occupation and knowledge most of the consumers were graduate. The researcher Maheswari had explored about awareness of green marketing and its influence on buying behavior of consumers: special reference to Madhya Pradesh, India. They found that consumers behavior about organic products are based on awareness and good marketing strategy because by using a questionnaire based on HEP-NEP questions [23], they found that 60% of consumer were aware about the eco friendly products and other hardly recognize the organic products. They also explored that 80% of consumers were strongly agree that they should buy the organic products [14]. In their paper titled, "Consumer awareness of green products and its Impact on Green Buying Behavior." The number of respondents was 533. They found the result that there is significance relationship between consumer behavior and green product awareness. There is huge lack of awareness of green products the level of knowledge about the green products in J&K is average. In the paper, it is suggested that there is a urgent need of consumer awareness in Jammu and Kashmir about the advantages of green products and their availability because it is observed that higher the awareness level higher the buying behavior of green products and low level of knowledge about the green products little spend on green products buying [11]. The researcher has explore the consumer awareness and preferences towards organic vegetables in Belgavi District of Karnataka which was surprisingly very positive 90% of customer were told that they were aware about the organic vegetables are good for health and they use organic vegetables. The researcher collected the data from 60 consumers through structured questionnaire. There was 81.67% consumer agreed that organic vegetables were very testy in comparison with normal vegetables grown with the help of fertilizer. It was also found that 86.67% of consumer were gave their opinion that organic vegetables have long shell life and it be long time fresh, where all the consumer were agreed on that statement that organic veggies are healthier than normal vegetables. In his research for university, student's awareness perception and green purchase intention towards eco-friendly products in Delhi-NCR explored that now students are becoming aware about the green products,they are sincerely thinking about the environmental issues also search regarding eco-friendly products,they are moving towards buying of green products like organic foods, eco-friendly products. The students of GGSIP University in Delhi-NCR participated in survey. It was explored that 40% of students were learning from social media and 29% from print media. The researcher also found that male students are more concern in compression to female while doing shopping. Karpagavalli and Nathiya [6] explore about the consumer awareness and attitude towards purchasing organic products. Researcher mainly considers the consumer behavior factors like education, income, and gender. The researcher has taken the sample size of 500 in the sample area Tripur Districts in Karnataka. He found that there is a lack of awareness in consumer regarding organic products also explores that there is a relation between education and buying behavior of organic products the consumers more educated they are having more tendency to buy organic food, there is also a gender relation and female were more aware about organic products in comparison with male [2].

Chiciudean [2] at has been explored that organic food is following a positive trend in market but growth is steady and slow in comparison to europian countries and the reason is mistrust, high price etc. Dhanalakshmi [3] found that students or young age children are very much aware about the organic food and they want to purchase it but due to high price and unavailability in market they have to shift for some other option. Gumber [4] explore that male and female has no difference regarding awareness of organic food also there is no impact of age difference in buying behaviour this modern age everybody is aware about the organic food. Guzy [5] found that 94% of public is aware about the organic food but lack of interest is developed due to non lebling and high price. Melovic et al. [10] analyse that price, food quality, distribution system and modern media as a promotional tool is the best factor to impact on consumer buying behaviour, Muttalageri and Mokshapathy [11] explored that in the Balgavi district that there is lack of govt. support for farmer consumers are not getting enough organic food in market, another factor is premium price of the product is also a factory for low market growth and less active behaviour of consumers. Nguyen et al. [12] has explored that there is significant impact of awareness, price and safety and health consciousness on consumer attitude towards organic food. Sri Rithi et al. [21] in her paper explored that most of the working female with income group 600000 income group prefer organic food mostly other also accepted that high price is the most difficult barrier in buying organic food. Sundaresh [22] explore that most of the young age from the 19–22 age group graduate are interested in buying of organic food, which shows that young generation is showing a positive attitude towards organic food.

3 Research Methodology

Research methodology is a way to systematically solve the research problem. Here to solve the research problem, we design a questionnaire and the validity and reliability were tested by Cronbach's Alpha and KMO and Bartlett's test. Statistical method includes frequencies, cross-tabulation from descriptive statistics and factor analysis. Nonparametric test used for the statistical analysis to find the significant relation between demographic variables for attitude towards organic food of consumers. The demographic variables were statistically analyzed by Kruskal Wallis like age, income, education and profession to find out the significant impact on consumer attitude towards organic food. For all the variables, level of significance was $\alpha = 0.05$ for all test.

3.1 Survey Method and Research Design

There was a questionnaire having 50 questions for collection of data. Questionnaire was pretested on 20 individuals with demographic characteristics. Due to the COVID-19 and lockdown condition, the data were collected by online data collection method. Data were mostly collected from tier 1 city of Delhi-NCR, India during the period of March to July 2020. Only above 18 years of people were selected for online survey. There were 300 mails sent to collect the data but only 250 have returned and only 180 were completed. The sample sizes of current study were 180 respondents.

3.2 Questionnaire Development

The study on organic food can be influenced by several factors like knowledge, awareness, culture, habit, and motivation. The questionnaire is constructed to measure the above variable by the questions from 1 to 10 questions are framed for the demographic characteristics of respondents like age, income, education, gender, marital status, children, family members, and profession. Questions from 11 to 20-measure variable such as awareness and knowledge, questions from 21 to 51 measure the measure the attitude and behavior of consumers. There was a five-point Likert scale was used measure the attitude, behavior, awareness and knowledge of consumers. Response options were ranged from most disagree (1) to most agreed (5).

132

Table 1 Reliability statistics

Cronbach's Alpha	No. of items
0.916	40

Table 2 KMO and Bartlett's test

Kaiser–Meyer–Olkin measure of sampling adequacy		0.807
Bartlett's Test of Sphericity	Approx. Chi-Square	4677.115
	Df	465
	Sig	0.000

3.3 Reliability and Validity of Questionnaire

The questionnaire was tested SPSS 24.0 version for reliability and validity testing. For each questionnaire, there was Cronbach's alpha coefficient estimated, and its values were (Cronbach's α) 0.916, which is indicating the validity and reliability of the questions (Table 1).

The principal component analysis with varimax applied to measure the reliability of questionnaire. The (MSA) measuring of sampling adequacy for the questionnaire was 0.807 which above than the accepted value of 0.45. Due to exceed, the MSA level most of the variables are collectively meeting the threshold of sampling adequacy with an MSA value of 0.807 and statistically significant. There are some variables tested but they were not up to the mark so reduce the number of variables based on communality and anti-image correlation (Table 2).

3.4 Respondents Profile

There were 180 questionnaire were filled correctly online by the respondents out of 250 submitted questionnaire. The age group of 26–35 is showing more awareness in buying organic food with great percentage. As we can see in table, three our respondents are quite young (51%) and postgraduate (54%), young generation can give present and future both picture very clear. Most of the respondents are male (75.6%) and service class (57%) which says that grocery for the home mostly purchased by male when they retune from the office. Our respondents are belongs to middle class based on their income group Rs. 50,000–1, 50,000 (51%). There are 56% married respondents, and 44% unmarried has been participating in filling of online questionnaire. The details are given in Table 3.

Table 3 Respondent's profile

Profile		Frequency (N)	Percent (%)
Age	18–25	44	24
	26–35	91	51
	36–45	31	17
	46–55 & Greater than 55	14	8
Gender	Female	44	24.4
	Male	136	75.6
Profession	Unemployed	8	4
	Business	22	12
	Service	102	57
	Student	39	22
Education	Professional	8	4
	Graduate	38	21
	Post-graduate	97	54
	Professional	16	9
	Undergraduate	21	12
Income	Less than Rs. 50,000	17	9
	Rs. 50,000–1, 50,000	92	51
	More than 1, 50,000	71	39
Marital status	Married	101	56
	Unmarried	79	44

4 Analysis and Result

The analysis of data based on the information collected through questionnaire. The questions were calculated on Varimax rotation for the construction of component. There were seven principal components constructed by the technique varimax rotation, and it is explained 74.7 of the total variance (Table 4). There was principal component analysis and exploratory factor analysis utilized to identify the dimensions for attitude towards organic food. The factor loading threshold was 0.55 [16], and all the variables below 0.55 were eliminated from the analysis. The scree plot suggested seven factors. 31 factors were selected. KMO–MSA for these variables was 0.807, which was more than 0.45 MSA level. Thus, all the selected variables are statistically significant. As we can see Table 4.

Principal component analysis extracted seven factors where all seven factors segregated based on good factor loading and communalities (Table 5). The first component is perception towards organic food accounted for 19.006 of the variance. Some other statements, like organic meat buying, future buying due to income increase, were having the factor loading was less like 0.45 or 0.50, thus, they eliminated from further analysis. Cronbach's alphas of all the factors are mention below

Table 4 Total variance explained

Component	Initial eigenvalues			Extraction sums of squared loadings			Rotation sums of squared loadings		
	Total	% of variance	Cumulative %	Total	% of Variance	Cumulative %	Total	% of variance	Cumulative %
1	10.711	34.55	34.55	10.71	34.55	34.55	5.892	19.006	19.006
2	4.677	15.087	49.637	4.677	15.087	49.637	5.28	17.031	36.037
3	2.359	7.61	57.247	2.359	7.61	57.247	3.68	11.871	47.908
4	1.651	5.326	62.573	1.651	5.326	62.573	3.124	10.077	57.985
5	1.434	4.626	67.199	1.434	4.626	67.199	2.493	8.042	66.028
6	1.21	3.904	71.103	1.21	3.904	71.103	1.351	4.357	70.385
7	1.116	3.598	74.702	1.116	3.598	74.702	1.338	4.317	74.702
8	0.829	2.675	77.376						
9	0.768	2.478	79.854						
10	0.733	2.364	82.218						
11	–	–	–						
31	0.055	0.178	100						

Extraction Method: Principal Component Analysis

Table 5 Varimax rotated component analysis factor matrix

Factors	Factor loading	Communalities
Factor 1—Consumer's perception towards organic food (Cronbach's α = 0 0.893)		
It is free from chemical fertilizer and pesticides	0.835	0.834
This is good for me and my family health	0.809	0.810
It increase immune system at this scenario	0.772	0.805
It save environment from pollution	0.715	0.722
It is nutritive and testy	0.703	0.730
It is a new trend in modern food style	0.702	0.695
It is fresher than conventional food	0.695	0.762
Factor 2—Consumer's health Consciousness (Cronbach's α = 0.756)		
I choose food item carefully to ensure health safety	0.734	0.627
I think that I am a health conscious consumer	0.667	0.687
I often read about health update in newspaper and magazines	0.655	0.845
Human beings are upsetting the balance of nature	0.649	0.815
Factor 3—Consumer's knowledge about organic food (Cronbach's α = 0.826)		
I know that organic foods are natural way to protect the environment	0.693	0.651
I know how environmental and health benefit of organic food	0.661	0.748
I know that organic foods are nutritive and tasty	0.650	0.638
I know that organic foods are free from chemical fertilizers and sprays	0.640	0.670
Factor 4—Consumer's future buying behavior (Cronbach's α = 0.793)		
If appearance and test will be better	0.714	0.734
if variety and assortment will be increased	0.681	0.680
if I have more time to look for organic food	0.676	0.730
if It becomes cheaper	0.641	0.573
It will be available in local store and market	0.613	0.699
Factor 5—Consumer's preferred Brand for organic food (Cronbach's α = 0.893)		
24 Mantra	0.816	0.631
Farm2Kitchen	0.790	0.800
Organic Garden	0.733	0.822
Organic Tattva	0.707	0.793
Just Organics	0.706	0.851
Factor 6—Consumer's buying habits of organic foods (Cronbach's α = 0.860)		
Pulses & cereals	0.687	0.727
Spices & herbs	0.685	0.818

(continued)

Table 5 (continued)

Factors	Factor loading	Communalities
Bread & bakery products	0.632	0.817
Milk & milk products	0.645	0.830
Factor 7—Consumer's trust regarding organic food (Cronbach's α = 0.785)		
I trust on organic food and production	0.759	0.822
The quality of organic foods is best	0.756	0.792

all are having the value more than (70%). The selected components are based on their relation with factors. All components under seven factors discussed below.

4.1 Factors Discussion

Factor 1—Consumer's perception towards organic food determines the association importance attitude towards organic food. As the value of the factor is highest then person come in these criteria will be definitely positive attitude towards organic food. Higher the association leads higher consumption. With help of this factor, we can get the real picture of consumer attitude towards organic food. *Factor 2—Consumer's health Consciousness* is the eating habit of consumers. It shows the readiness of consumer to adopt organic food. If the consumer is health, conscious then organic food will be his or her first choice. This factor will give an overview of health conscious consumer and their relation with organic food. Health conscious consumer is a prime consumer of organic food, and it is most important factor that increases the positive attitude towards organic food. *Factor three—Consumer's knowledge about organic food* towards organic food make new customer and retain old customer of organic food. The aware customer can make a beneficial decision towards organic food because he knows the benefits of organic food, which can influence positive approach towards organic food. For the information and knowledge about label of the product, certifications of the product, etc., are important. A knowledgeable customer can convert into a loyal customer of organic food. *Factor 4—Consumer's future buying behavior identifies* the future aspects of consumers. Consumers are the future of the market so it is important to understand the consumers thinking for future buying. There are several reasons that are play as barriers for consumer buying. The consumers are not buying the organic food in current situation, and there are certain variable like availability, variety, premium price, income (during COVID-19) can show us the reason behind why people are not buying organic food. *Factors 5—Consumer's preferred Brand for organic food identify* the most liked brand by the consumers in market. There are some brands famous in India especially in Delhi-NCR who is providing organic food. These variables can lead us the most preferred brand by the consumers and why. This factor can help marketer to understand the buying pattern of consumers, the preferences chosen by consumers can give a base to other marketer. *Factor 6—Consumer's buying habits of organic foods* includes all the type of organic food but due to less value of KMO (less than 0.45) two variables (meat and meat product) and (baby product) were removing from the analysis. It can lead us the opportunity that what the customer want and what are their choice in organic food category. With the help of this, marketer can segregate the most demanded organic food product by the consumers. *Factor 7—Consumer's trust regarding organic food* is also an important factor because many people think that there is no possibility that people are not using pesticides in organic food so they cannot trust on organic food that why they don't buy organic food. The variables lead us towards trust factor of organic food.

4.2 Demographic Impact on Consumer Behavior Towards Organic Food

The demographic characteristics like age, income, education, marital status showed significant relationship with consumer attitude towards organic food. There were nonparametric test (Kruskal–Wallis Test) applied to analyze the relation with consumer attitude and demographic characteristics. Gender did not shown a significant impact on consumer attitude towards organic food. The Mann–Whitney test applied but the p value was greater than the significant value ($p > 0.05$). That is why we can conclude that there is no impact of gender on consumer attitude towards organic food male and female both equally purchase organic food. In NCR, both male and female do shopping and both are conscious about their health that is the reason gender does not affect the buying attitude of consumers during COVID-19. Factors like marital status positively affect the buying attitude of consumers, some component like health consciousness, increase immune system, best quality free from fertilizer. All component showed $p < 0.05$. The other analysis shown that most of the married consumer were interested in buying the organic food rather than unmarried consumers. Thus, we can conclude that married consumers can be the prospects for the organic food products. Other factors are analyzed, and the results are shown in table below with their explanation income (Table 6), education (Table 7), age (Table 8), and profession (Table 9.)

4.3 Income (Refer Table 6)

Kruskal–Wallis test used to analyze the impact of income on factor identified. Only those variable which were significant at $p < 0.5$ were taken in Table 6. Factor one (perception towards organic food) and factor four (future buying behavior) shown significant impact of income. Consumers are willing to pay for healthy food which is free from fertilizer with $p < 0.05$ which is 0.005 and chi square value 10.622 with

Table 6 Income

Income		N	Mean rank	Chi-Square	df	Asymp. Sig
Factor 1						
It is free from chemical fertilizer and pesticides	Less than Rs. 50,000	17	54.74	10.622	2	0.005
	Rs. 50,000–1, 50,000	92	92.39			
	More than 1, 50,000	71	96.62			
It increase immune system at this scenario	Less than Rs. 50,000	17	62.47	6.131	2	0.047
	Rs. 50,000–1, 50,000	92	93.41			
	More than 1, 50,000	71	93.44			
It is fresher than conventional food	Less than Rs. 50,000	17	48.65	14.034	2	0.001
	Rs. 50,000–1, 50,000	92	96.82			
	More than 1, 50,000	71	92.33			
This is good for me and my family health	Less than Rs. 50,000	17	55.32	10.377	2	0.006
	Rs. 50,000–1, 50,000	92	95.73			
	More than 1, 50,000	71	92.15			
Factor 4—Consumer's future buying behavior						
It becomes cheaper	Less than Rs. 50,000	17	58.32	8.912	2	0.012
	Rs. 50,000–1, 50,000	92	97.35			
	More than 1, 50,000	71	89.33			
Buying in future if variety & assortment will be increased	Less than Rs. 50,000	17	53.56	11.404	2	0.003
	Rs. 50,000–1, 50,000	92	92.43			
	More than 1, 50,000	71	96.84			
Appearance & test will be better	Less than Rs. 50,000	17	53.74	10.117	2	0.006
	Rs. 50,000–1, 50,000	92	94.02			
	More than 1, 50,000	71	94.74			

Table 7 Education

Education		N	Mean rank	Chi-Square	Df	Asymp. Sig
Factor 1						
I like to buy It increases immune system at this scenario	Under Graduate	8	4.50	29.5	3	0.000
	Graduate	38	96.00			
	Post Graduate	97	79.75			
	Professional	16	81.25			
This is good for me and my family health	Under Graduate	8	4.50	31.809		
	Graduate	38	95.20			
	Post Graduate	97	82.40		3	0.000
	Professional	16	67.13			
Factor 2—Consumer's health Consciousness						
I think that I am a health conscious consumer	Under Graduate	8	4.50	31.457	3	0.000
	Graduate	38	90.41			
	Post Graduate	8	4.50			
	Professional	38	90.41			
Factor 5—Consumer's preferred Brand for organic food						
Preferred brand Organic Garden	Under Graduate	8	98.75	10.174	3	0.017
	Graduate	38	66.86			
	Post Graduate	97	79.31			
	Professional	16	106.00			

2 degree of freedom. The other factors of consumer perception towards organic food also were shown significant impact of income, and we can say that consumer are willing to pay for the food which is fresh, healthy and can increase the immune system. In factor 4, we can see consumer prefer to pay for variety of organic food from future buying with the chi square value 11.404, p value 0.003 that is less than, 05 p values. The consumers are willing tom buy in future if the product becomes cheaper (chi square value 8.912 and p value 0.012), consumer will buy more in future. There are another significant influence of income with consumers test and appetence towards organic food in future want to spend on test and packaging which can be fruitful information for the companies. We can see from the chi-square value all the consumers having income from above 500,000 showing good significance. There is no significance difference between consumer from 50,000–100,000 and more than 1, 50,000. Both are cause equal significance on consumer buying behavior.

Table 8 Age

Age		N	Mean rank	Chi-Square	df	Asymp. Sig
Factor 1—Consumer's perception towards organic food						
It is free from chemical fertilizer and pesticides	26–35	8	5.00	8.8	2	0.012
	36–45	38	95.32			
	46–55 or Greater than 55	97	80.95			
It is a new trend in modern food style	26–35	8	4.50	8.5	2	0.015
	36–45	38	85.80			
	46–55 or Greater than 55	97	83.21			
It is fresher than conventional food	26–35	8	4.50	7.4	2	0.025
	36–45	38	96.00			
	46–55 or Greater than 55	97	79.75			
Factor 4—Consumer's future buying behavior						
It will be available in local store and market	26–35	38	90.41			
	36–45	8	4.50	7.3	2	0.025
	46–55 or Greater than 55	8	4.50			
I have more time to look for organic food	26–35	8	4.50	8.7		
	36–45	38	97.28			
	46–55 or Greater than 55	97	82.55		2	0.013

4.4 Education (Refer Table 7)

As we can see in the table education significantly, influence the perception of consumer towards organic food. From factor one, the consumer who is graduate shown higher value towards increasing immune system for chi- square test 29.5 with degree of freedom 3 and significant p value < 0.05. Family health is almost equally important for the graduate and post-graduate consumers with the chi-square value 31.80. Graduates and professionals shown a great response to health consciousness (factor 2) with the chi-square value 31.45 and p value is less than 0.05 with 3 degree of freedom. The consumers especially graduates and professional shown a great association with "Organic India" brand preference (factor 5) with the chi-square vale 10.17, p value 0.017 which is less than 0.05. Therefore, we can conclude that graduate and postgraduate consumers are having a perception of health consciousness and family health is important and want to buy a food product that can increase their immune system at this crucial corona time that is a very good combination for marketer to market their organic food. On the other side, brands like Organic Tattva, 24 Mantra, form to kitchen can study the product profile of organic garden why it is most preferred brand by consumers.

Table 9 Profession

Profession		N	Mean rank	Chi-Square	df	Asymp. Sig
Factor 1—Consumer's perception towards organic food						
It increase immune system at this scenario	Unemployed	8	4.50	27.53	4	0.001
	Business	22	84.23			
	Home Maker	7	106.86			
	Service	102	95.70			
	Student	39	90.58			
Factor 2—Consumer's health consciousness						
I choose food item carefully to ensure health safety	Unemployed	8	4.50	26.323		
	Business	22	90.64			
	Home Maker	7	101.50		4	0.001
	Service	102	93.94			
	Student	39	92.53			
Factor 3—Consumer's knowledge about organic food						
I know that organic foods are nutritive and tasty	Unemployed	8	4.50			
	Business	22	83.75	26.011	4	0.000
	Home Maker	7	103.43			
	Service	102	94.51			
	Student	39	94.58			
Factor 5—Consumer's preferred Brand for organic food						
Preferred brand Organic Tattva	Unemployed	8	89.63	12.331	4	0.015
	Business	22	81.50			
	Home Maker	7	88.79			
	Service	102	99.64			
	Student	39	67.60			

4.5 Age (Refer Table 8)

There is only two factors (1 and 4) showed the significant relation with age group. As we can see in table, age group 36–45 showed great response ((95.32%) to chemical and fertilizers free food product perception towards organic food with mean of 2.92 and std. deviation 1.096 (it is free from chemical fertilizer and pesticides). The p value is $p < 0.05$ that is 0.012, chi-square value 8.8 with the degree of freedom 2. We can conclude that middle age group people are more interested in buying organic food, and in future, they can be prospect for companies. Another statements (it is new trend in modern food style) and (it is fresher than conventional food) are also having the mean of, respectively, 3.3 and 3.7 with the Std. Deviation 1.5 and 1.5. The p value is less than 0.05 which is 0.015 and 0.025, respectively, and the chi-square value is 8.5, 7.4. Based on all the values, we can say age group 36–45 is the best target group for the companies to market their organic products because this group prefer fresh, fertilizers free and trendy food products that is specialty of organic food. There is no significant relationship with age group 18–25 with other age group. Another factor 4 future buying has two components showed positive relation with age group. The availability of local store showed a significant relation with the age group 18– 26 (90.41%) with mean and std. deviation is, respectively, 3.4, 1. 6. The chi-square value is 7 and $p < 0.5$ concluded that youngsters are ready to buy in future if it is easily available in market. The future buying has another component affected by age group is availability of time (I have more time to look for organic food) showing the significant relationship with age group 36–45 (97%). The variable having p value at $p < 0.05$ (0.013) and Chi-square value is (8.7) which means. Marketer has to found a new way to make organic food available smoothly and quickly because people want to buy but they do not have time for it.

4.6 Profession (Refer Table 9)

As we can see in the table, there are four factors that show the influence on profession and buying behavior of consumers. Factor 1 (increasing immune system) is having significant relation with all the profession except unemployed. The variable having p value is $p > 0.05$ 0.001 with mean 3.71 and Std. Deviation of 1.47. The chi-square value 27.53 with 4 degree of freedom gives a food item that can increase their immune system at the time of COVID-19 because this is only internal medicine can prevent from corona virus. This is the excellent opportunity for the organic product seller to offer organic food. The other variable health consciousness (from Factor 2) also having significant relationship with the statement (I think that I am a health conscious consumer) and (I choose food item carefully to ensure health safety) shows a positive influence on profession business and service class other do not' have any significant relation. The mean is 3.05 and 3.80 with the Std. Deviation 1.08, 1.52, respectively. All the above factors are showing significant relationship with the Chi-square value of 21.10 and 26. 32. The above values explained that consumers are more conscious about their health, and they choose carefully food item so there is a chance to buy organic food by customers, which means future is bright for organic food. At factor, 3 consumers are aware about the nutrition and test of organic food the p value of this statement is $p < 0.05$, which is 0.000 accepted ranges, and chi-square 26.011 explained a significant relation with profession. The service, professional, homemaker, and students are more aware about organic food than businesspersons are. There is a scope to make businessperson aware about benefits of organic food. In factor 5, consumers (service, professionals & homemakers) preferred brand is organic Tattva with the mean of 2.64 and Std. Deviation of 1.46. The chi-square value 12.33 with p value 0.015 establishes a significant relation with the consumer profession and preferred brand. Thus, marketer can explore that why they prefer the Organic Tattva, what is its USP and how they can attract consumer for their own organic brands.

4.7 Overall Frequencies and Agreement & Non-agreement Percentage

See Table 10.

4.8 Discussion

There were seven components that were selected to led the information as consumer's perception towards organic food, buying habits of consumers, health consciousness, consumer knowledge about organic food, preferred brand of organic food, future buying reason of organic food and trust. Thirty-one variables were selected for the analysis. The analysis says that male and female both ware aware about the organic food, and they want to buy the organic food; there are two most important perception factors free from chemical and increase immune system. Perception was the basic criteria to select the respondent for organic food' 87% of consumers are agreed that organic foods are free from chemical fertilizers, 89% of them agreed on the good quality of the organic food. Sixty percent consumers want to buy organic food increasing immune system at the time of COVID-19. All the other variables chosen by the consumers above 70% but being organic food trendy is only liked by 49% of consumers so if marketer want to focus, they should positioned the organic food like good eating habit food. Consumer's frequency table showed us that consumers of India are health conscious because more than 70% of consumers agreed that they choose item carefully which good for health and self for that they also keep them update. The awareness level of consumers are good in India about organic food because frequency table showed that more than 75% of consumers know about all the characteristics of organic food(free from fertilizer 76%, natural products 80%, good for health 76%). In the frequency table, consumers showed an interesting behavior towards future buying 80% of consumers need time to buy organic food, and availability in local store in future (73.3%) will bring the consumer in buying basket. There is no preferred brand by consumers all are having more than 60% agreed consumers. Therefore, there is an opportunity for new marketer to explore the market. The frequency table explains itself that most of the consumers buy organic bread and bakery products (60%).

4.9 Managerial Implication

The frequency table can help the marketer to understand the important aspects of research. The marketer can make marketing, promotional, and positioning strategy based on result. The research outcomes can help the companies to understand the

Table 10 Frequency

		Agree		Disagree or neutral	
		N	%	N	%
Factor 1—Consumer's perception towards organic food					
1	It is free from chemical fertilizer and pesticides	157	87.2	23	12.7
2	This is good for me and my family health	161	89.4	19	10.6
3	It increase immune system at this scenario	107	60.0	38	21.1
4	It save environment from pollution	128	71.1	52	28.9
5	It is nutritive and testy	125	69.4	55	30.5
6	It is a new trend in modern food style	89	49.4	91	50.5
7	It is Fresher than conventional food	134	74.4	46	25.5
Factor 2—Consumer's health consciousness					
8	I choose food item carefully to ensure health safety	144	79.9	36	20
9	I think that I am a health conscious consumer	143	79.4	37	20.5
10	I often read about health update in newspaper & Magazines	109	60.5	71	39.5
11	Human beings are upsetting the balance of Nature	136	75.6	44	24.4
Factor 3—Consumer's knowledge about organic food					
12	I know that organic foods are natural way to protect the environment	147	81.6	33	18.3
13	I know how environmental & health benefit of organic food	138	76.7	42	23.4
14	I know that Organic Foods are Nutritive and tasty	117	65	63	35

(continued)

Table 10 (continued)

		Agree		Disagree or neutral	
		N	%	N	%
15	I know that organic foods are free from chemical fertilizers and sprays	146	81	34	18.9
Factor 4—Consumer's future buying behavior					
16	If Appearance & test will be better	124	68.8	56	31.1
17	If Variety & assortment will be increased	149	82.8	31	17.1
18	If I have more time to look for organic food	107	59.4	73	40.5
19	If It becomes cheaper	132	73.3	48	26.6
20	It will be available in local store and market	154	85.5	26	14.4
Factor 5—Consumer's preferred Brand for organic food					
21	24 Mantra	128	71.1	52	28.9
22	Farm2Kitchen	120	66.7	60	33.3
23	Organic Garden	138	76.7	42	23.4
24	Organic Tattva	120	66.7	60	33.3
25	Just Organics	133	73.9	47	26.1
Factor 6—Consumer's buying habits of organic foods(Cronbach's $\alpha = 0.860$)					
26	Pulses & cereals	128	71.1	52	28.9
27	Spices & Herbs	109	60.6	71	39.5
28	Bread &bakery products	112	62.2	68	37.8
29	Milk & Milk products	105	58.4	55	30.6
Factor 7—Consumer's trust regarding organic food (Cronbach's $\alpha = 0.785$)					
30	I trust on organic food and production	121	67.2	59	32.7
31	The quality of organic foods are best	146	81.1	34	18.8

perception and future buying behavior of consumers; these two can lead the companies to know about the thinking and choice of consumers. It also helps in finding the problems of consumer facing towards organic food like unavailability of organic food in convenience store, premium price. It can also give an overview about the customer's preference towards organic food item through buying habits like which products customers liked more to buy. For the managerial implications, outcomes of health consciousness and knowledge level of consumers can also help organic food companies to plan their advertising strategy.

4.10 Limitation and Further Scope of Study

Due to COVID-19, the size of the data is low and it can mostly target north India especially in Delhi-NCR and only online survey; after the situation being normalize, there can be research based on big size and big population area.

5 Conclusion

The above analysis clearly stated that service class male with age group of 36–45 years with the annual income of 50,000–1,50,000 are the buyer of organic products. However, marketer fails to make organic product available for consumers easily. The consumers are lacking due to unavailability of organic food because in future buying most of the respondent selects the availability on local store and in variety. Premium price is another important factor that people are ready to buy if food products will be cheaper. This is current study in Delhi-NCR during COVID-19. As per various literature review, there are very few work done in Delhi-NCR over organic food especially at this COVID-19 times. The conclusion is that COVID-19 a golden era for the marketer to increase the sale of organic food by smooth delivery facility, and in future, the demand will increase. The demographic characteristics have significant relation with consumer's attitude towards organic food. Overall conclusion is this due to COVID-19 people are attracted towards a healthy life style and healthy food if we talk about the positive aspect of COVID-19, we can say there is a positive impact on consumer attitude towards organic food due to COVID-19 in India.

References

1. Ashraf MA, Joarder MH, Ratan SR (2018) Consumers' anti-consumption behavior toward organic food purchase: an analysis using SEM. Br Food J, 19–20
2. Chiciudean GO, Harun R, Ilea M, Chiciudean DI, Arion FH, Ilies G et al (2019) Organic food consumers and purchase intention: a case study in Romania. Agronomy 9(145):1–13

3. Dhanalakshmi A (2018) A study of consciousness and perception towards organic food products among college studdents in Salem District. Ph.D. Thesis, Periyar Institute of Management Studies (PRIMS) Periyar University, Management, Tamil Nadu
4. Gumber G (2018) Consumer buying behaviour towards organic food a study in Delhi NCR National Capital Region, pp 204–205
5. Guzy MJ (2018) Obstacles to the development of the organic food market in Poland and the possible directions of growth. Wiley Food Sci Nutrition, 1–11
6. Karpagavalli DR, Nathiya MS (2016) A study on consumer awareness, attitudes and motivational factors towards purchasing organic products in Tirupur District. Peer Rev J 1(18):141–146
7. Kumar P (2107) Consumer's perception and purchase intention towards organic products. Ph.D. Thesis, Guru Jambheshwar University of Science & Technology, Business Management, Hisar
8. Mahmood SM (2018) Religiosity among Muslim Consumers and its impact on consumer buying behaviour towards food products in Delhi and NCR. Aligarh Muslim University, Commerce. Aligarh Muslim University, Aligarh, UP, India
9. Mehra S, Ratna P (2014) Attitude and behaviour of consumer towards organic food: an exploratory study in India. Int J Bus Excellence 7(6):677–700
10. Melovic B, Cirovic D, Dudi B, Vulic TB, Gregus M (2020) The analysis of marketing factors influencing consumers' preferences and acceptance of organic food products—recommendations for the optimization of the O. Foods 9(259):1–25
11. Muttalageri M, Mokshapathy S (2015) Constraints in production and marketing of organic vegetable growers in Balagavi District in Karnatka. Asian J Manag Res 5(4):558–564
12. Nguyen HV, Nguyen N, Nguyen BK, Lobo A, Vu PA (2019) Organic food purchases in an emerging market: the influence of consumers' personal factors and green marketing practices of food stores. Int J Environ Res Public Health 16(1037):1–17
13. Patel CP (2016) The impact of green marketing: an upcoming power with special reference to consumer preferences and green marketers opportunities. Shodhganga, 327
14. Rather RA, Rajendran D (2014) A study on Consumer awareness of green products and its impact on green buying behaviour. Int J Res (IJR) 1(8):1483–1493
15. Rathore A (2017) Marketing strategy and consumer buying behaviour of organic food in Rajasthan. IIS University, Jaipur, Department of Management, Shodhganga, Jaipur
16. Ratna P, Mehra S (2014) Attitude and behaviour of consumers towards organic food: an exploratory study in India. Int. J. Bus. Excellence 7(6):677–700
17. Aruna S (2018) A study on consumer awareness and buying behaviour towards the green products in Chennai City. University of Madras, Madras
18. Sarumathi S (2015) A study on consumer behaviour towards organic food in Pondicherry City. Ph.D. Thesis, Pondicherry University, Department of International Business, Pondicherry
19. Soni MP (2017) Organic food industry: problems & prospect. Ph.D. Thesis, Mohanlal Sukhadia University, Department of Banking & Business Economics Faculty of Commerce, Udaypur
20. Soni P (2015) Indian consumer's adoption of a 'green' innovation & social identity—the case of organic food. J Comm Econ Comput Sci 01(4):1–23
21. Sri Rithi K, Subarna N, Latha P, Balaji DM (2018) Challenges and Issues faced in buying and selling organic products: perspectives of Consumers and entrepreneurs. Int J Pure Appl Math 119(17):2519–2526
22. Sundaresh K (2018) A study on awareness attitude and perception analysis as strategies of consumer buying behaviour towards organic food products among the college students in Coimbatore District. Department of BSMED, Bharathiar University, Coimbatore
23. Van Liere KD, Dunlap RE (1981) Environmental Concern. Environ Behav 13(6):651–676

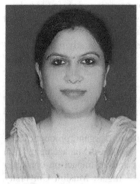

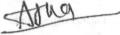

Anamika Chaturvedi is currently working as an Assistant Professor with the department of Business Administration UP Institute of Design Noida. She is M.Sc, PGDCA, & MBA from AKTU Lucknow & pursuing PHD from Galgotias University. She is having more than 12 years experience of teaching.

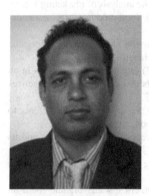

Dr. Md Rashid Chand is currently Associate Professor in Galgotias University Greater Noida. He is Ph.D. from Banasthali University, MBA (Jamia Millia Islamia, Delhi), UGC-NET (Management), PGD IRPM, BVB Delhi, Advance Diploma in Mass Media, JNU Delhi. He has experience of more than 11 years of teaching varied subjects related to Marketing at both Post Graduate and Undergraduate Level & having more than 5 years of Industry Experiences.

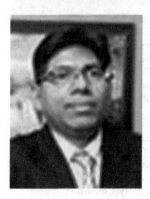

Dr. Mujibur Rahman is Ph.D, MBA, B.Tech from premier institute with 14 years of teaching experience. He has 8 publications in various journals. Area of interest is marketing and CRM.

Chapter 9
Socioeconomic Impacts and Opportunities of COVID-19 for Nepal

Deepak Chaudhary, Mahendra Sapkota, and Kabita Maharjan

1 Introduction

The COVID-19 has adversely affected Nepal's overall economy and health sector. It is speculated that it may take years to repair. Maintaining isolation and social distancing as a precautionary measure to contain the spread of COVID-19 altered social and economic life, eventually disrupting the business, trade, and mobility of people. Tourism, transport service, airspace, education, manufacturing, industrial sector, and hotel business have been seen suffering the most. Thus, millions of people have lost their jobs. The poor, marginalized people, and lower-class people who have been involved in informal employment sectors are seen mostly affected by COVID-19.

The pandemic greatly harmed the economic development in Nepal; the economic growth could be limited within 2.3% [1]. COVID-19 interrupted the supply chain of productions and goods and negatively impacted import–export. Serious concerns are being shown toward the proper management of quarantine and isolation centers in Nepal. Dozens of people died in quarantine itself. So, questions are raised about the pitfalls of the health system of Nepal. Quarantine is considered to cure corona patients. However, quarantines outside the capital have been portrayed as a hotbed of the Corona epidemic. Quarantines have been unsafe for women as some cases of sexual harassment were also reported there.

D. Chaudhary (✉) · M. Sapkota · K. Maharjan
Tribhuvan University, Kathmandu, Nepal
e-mail: dipak10@gmail.com

M. Sapkota
e-mail: sapkota.mahendra27@gmail.com

K. Maharjan
e-mail: kdkabs@gmail.com

© The Author(s), under exclusive license to Springer Nature Singapore Pte Ltd. 2021
P. K. Khosla et al. (eds.), *Predictive and Preventive Measures for Covid-19 Pandemic*,
Algorithms for Intelligent Systems, https://doi.org/10.1007/978-981-33-4236-1_9

Due to the lack of good governance, leadership, and coordination among inter-state machinery and financial constraints, the control of COVID-19 is not being effective. Poor management of quarantine and limited testing was the causes that contributed to a high number of COVID-19 cases in Nepal. These resulted in poor performance of the institutionalization of the public health system as well as the poor capacity of medical supplements in the country. Comparatively, Nepal faced a few fatalities (228 till 31 August 2020) but its consequences in socioeconomic and health sectors are unprecedented. The long-run effects of a sample of 12 major epidemics in Europe showed that the pandemics were followed by multiple decades of low natural interest rates, due to the depressed investment opportunities [2]. Nepal cannot be an exception.

The major objective of the paper is to examine the socioeconomic and health impacts of the COVID-19 and explore the opportunities in terms of the improvement in public health and socioeconomic life. The paper is prepared based on secondary data and discourse analysis.

2 Impacts of COVID-19 on Socioeconomic and Health Sectors

The World Bank has already made a forecast of its deteriorating situation in South Asia, including Nepal as it would linger up to 2021, with growth projected to hover between 3.1 and 4.0%, down from the previous 6.7% estimate [3]. The GDP growth of Nepal could shrink in 2.5 in 2020 compared to 7.1 in 2019 because of COVID-19 [4]. However, according to the International Monitoring Fund (IMF), Nepal's fiscal budget for the fiscal years of 2020/21 predicted that the economic growth would be shrunk within 1% [5]. The crisis created by COVID-19 is hitting on all of human development elements—income (low economic activity), health (causing a death toll over 300,000), and education (out-of-school) [6]. Furthermore, the world economic recession will reduce foreign investment within the country.

The consequences of COVID-19 can be seen in these sectors as follows:

2.1 Sectors of Gross Domestic Production (GDP) and Employment Situation

Figure 1 shows that the service sectors contribute 60% to the national GDP followed by agriculture (27%) and industry (13%) [7]. However, the service sector only contributes 22% of the employment sector in Nepal while the agricultural sector possesses the largest employer as it stands for 67% of total employment.

Fig. 1 Sectors to the GDP,
FY 2018/19

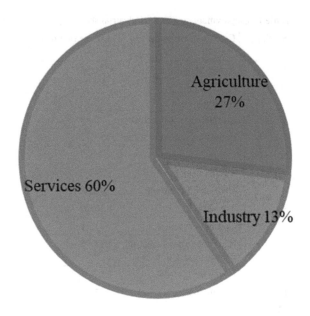

According to the Nepal Labor Force Survey, there are approximately 20.7 million people in the working-age in Nepal. Among, approximately 7.1 million are employed while 908 thousand is unemployed; the unemployment rate stands for 11.4% [8]. According to UNDP-Nepal [9], Nepal's economy largely depends on remittance (25% of GDP), tourism (8% of GDP), and agriculture (26% of GDP). However, the tourism, transportation, productive-industries, and construction field will shrink significantly.

According to a survey conducted in private industries by the Central Bank of Nepal, a total of 22.50% of workers lost their jobs during the lockdown [10]. 35% of businesses were partially closed during the four months lockdown (from March 24 till July 21, 2020). Hotel and restaurants were almost closed leading to 40% job loss. Small and medium enterprises lost 30.5% of their jobs. In the education sector, 22.5% of employment was cut. Most of the borrowing businesses made massive staff cuts. Of these, 70.59% were temporary and contract employees (see Table 1).

2.2 Workers in the Informal Sector

International Labor Organization defines that all jobs or employments in informal sector enterprises represent the informal sector. Informal sectors are not incorporated or registered with government authorities. Employment in formal and informal sectors collectively makes 7.1 million employed people in Nepal. Table 2 reveals that the informal employment sector in Nepal occupies 62.2%, while the formal

Table 1 Employment cuts to the industrial sectors (private) during the lockdown in percent

S. No.	Categories of industries	Share of employees cut	Share of temporary and contract employees (%)
1	Agriculture, forest, and fishing	21.35	80.19
2	Mining	16.67	75
3	Productive based industry	23.49	64.08
4	Electricity, gas, and water	39.71	44.09
5	Construction	26.67	78.5
6	Retail business	24.86	67.61
7	Hotel and restaurant	40.08	58.19
8	Transportation	18.29	91.67
9	Communication	21.31	64.2
10	Real state, room-rent and commercial activities	18.75	50
11	Education	5.6	88.33
12	Health and social works	15	97.43
13	Others	24.9	60.43
	Total	22.5	70.59

Table 2 Employment by sectors

Sectors of employment	Male	Female	Total
	Percent		
A. Formal	**40.3**	**33.5**	**37.8**
Agriculture	1.3	1.2	1.3
Non-agriculture	39	32.3	36.5
B. Informal	**59.7**	**66.5**	**62.2**
Agriculture	13.4	31.8	20.2
Non-agriculture	45.8	32.9	41
Private household	0.6	1.8	1
Total (A + B)	**100.00**	**100.00**	**100.00**

Bold signifies as per the legal provision of Nepal, the informal sector of employment is defined as a supplement to the national economy, and the enterprises are formally not registered with the government and do not have any tax liabilities. Similarly, the formal sector of employment comprises corporations (including quasi-corporate enterprises), owned either by the government or by the private sector or by both on the public-private partnerships, which are mandatory registered in the government and do have legal liabilities. This sector comprises semi-skilled and unskilled human resources, and labor-intensive enterprises, and most of the vulnerable, and peasantry people. However, the informal sector has a large contribution to employment in Nepal

sector occupies only 37.8% [11]. The agricultural sector shares 20.2%, and the non-agricultural sector shares 41% within the informal sector. Informal employment is higher among rural dwellers (90.9%) compared to urban residents (81.8%).

The poor and vulnerable people have been living in the informal sector for a long time, and this has encouraged them to move to the formal sector. Due to the lockdown to contain COVID-19, the closure of informal sectors and non-receipt of wages has negatively affected the livelihood of many poor people. Their condition is deplorable as they do not have proper savings, capital stocks, and physical assets. These workers have fewer chances of any immediate possibilities to search and engage with other sources of income-generating opportunities. The government lacks the proper database about the people working in the informal sector. So, numerous problems are seen arising while distributing relief packages. Many needy people are still seen yelling for relief packages.

2.3 Tourism

As of the Ministry of Culture, Tourism and Civil Aviation (2020), this sector has been supporting foreign exchange earnings, job creation, growth of economic activities, and overall economic development and prosperity [12]. Nepal's tourism sector is comprised of the partnership of government, private sector, households, professionals, and NGOs. A total of 1254 star and tourist standard hotels have operated with a bed capacity of 40,856 per day in 2018. Travel agencies, tour guides, tour operators, rafting agencies, trekking agencies, and guides are all associated with the tourism industry [13]. However, this sector has badly been hit by COVID-19 as a continuous lockdown strategy has been adopted in the country since March 24, 2020. All national and international transportation systems have been disrupted. According to the World Travel and Tourism Council (WTTC), Nepal's travel and tourism sector pumped Rs. 177 billion into the economy and supported more than 427,000 jobs last year [14]. It accounts for 7.5% of the national GDP. Nepal declared 'Visit Nepal' for 2020 expecting more than two million tourists from around the world, but it has been suspended amidst the COVID-19 pandemic. The small businesses, hotels and restaurants, lodges, and travel agencies have all been affected which are related to tourism. Consequently, thousands of people have lost their job. Both the domestic and international air movements are still uncertain.

2.4 Agriculture and Livestock Sector

Agriculture with livestock is the major means of livelihood for the majority of rural Nepalese people. This sector provides employment opportunities to around 65% of the total population and contributes to about 27% of the GDP in Nepal [15], and it is expected to reduce in the coming days. About 1.5 million people in this field will be directly affected. UN World Food Program (WFP) has predicted that there would be a significant reduction in the harvest of wheat and other winter crops. Ghanshyam Bhusal, a Minister of Agriculture and Livestock of Nepal, has warned all 753 local governments writing a letter to make aware of the food scarcity the country might face in the near future [16]. The total commodity productivity in Nepal's agriculture has steadily been increased since 1998. From 1992 to 2011, Nepal was seen ahead of Pakistan in total production, but much behind India and Bangladesh [17]. Nepal did export food grains before 1980, but now Nepal does import.

The disruption in the supply of agriculture-related goods like seeds, fertilizers, and herbicides to farmers is hindering agricultural production. Farmers were seen panicking during the lockdown since they could not reach to the market to sell their products (e.g., dairy products and vegetables). In the Udayapur District [18] alone, different vegetables worth 0.2 million rupees were wasted. A similar scenario could be seen across the country, which would badly affect the supply chains and distort the livelihood strategies in the villages. Moreover, the disturbance in the agricultural calendar, particularly of wheat and rice harvest, will have a severe socioeconomic impact among poor farmers.

2.5 Remittances

Remittance is largely contributing to the national GDP of developing countries like Nepal. It is the major source of foreign currency. Figure 2 reveals that remittances contributed less than 1% to Nepal's GDP until the late 1990s, lower than India and Bangladesh. But in 2008, it ascended to 21.7%, making Nepal the eighth largest remittance recipient in the world. Similarly, it significantly increased as it reached 31.4% in 2015 and Nepal became the second-largest recipient of remittances in the world. However, it dropped to 27.3% in 2019, making Nepal the sixth-largest recipient of remittances in the world.

Figure 3 shows that the flow of remittance increased by 1.7% in the first eight months of FY 2020 while the growth of the remittance was lower than 11.7% recorded in FY 2019. The flow of remittance increased nominally, but it is at a slower pace [19]. Because many workers who were destined to leave Nepal during the lockdown could not travel and some workers returned to Nepal due to COVID-19. Therefore, it is expected that remittances would be slow in the coming year. 7% of the total population are abroad for employment, and most of them are from rural areas. The proportion of all households that receive remittances is 56% in Nepal [20]. Remittances play a vital role in improving the socioeconomic condition, reducing poverty, and bringing social and political awareness in rural Nepal [21]. Meanwhile, millions of Nepali workers are facing uncertainty in migrant countries (Gulf, Malaysia, and South Asia, largely in India) because of prolonged lockdown due to COVID-19.

At least 700,000 migrant workers are expected to return from India after losing their employment [22] in the coming days. In the meantime, around 0.2 million migrant workers have already returned and most of them have been suffering from

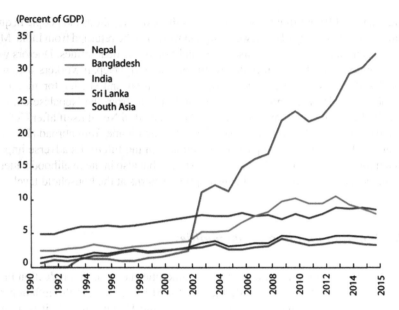

Fig. 2 Remittances as a share of GDP (*Source* WB, 2017). *Note* Data are for the first eight months of Fiscal Year

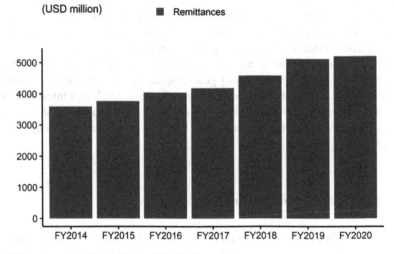

Fig. 3 Remittances in Nepal (*Source* WB, 2017)

COVID-19. Thousands of migrant workers are further expected to return. This may create several complexities and challenges in the employment sectors because of the high unemployment rate in Nepal which is 11.4%.

Remittance to Nepal is expected to drop by 14% this year, signaling economic distress stemming from the Covid-19 pandemic. In the mid of July, Nepal recorded

more than 15,000 confirmed cases with 35 deaths and thirty thousand people in quarantine [23], the majority of them were migrant workers who returned from India. Most
of them complained about the miserable condition of the quarantines. Doctors were
blamed not very professional in the treatment. Similarly, Nepali workers who were
unpaid and jobless were reported scrambled for food and shelter for months in
Sharjah, UAE. They did not receive any kind of help from the Nepalese embassy
[24]. On the one hand, many workers have been halted in Nepal itself after COVID-
19, and on the other hand, few workers have returned home from abroad [25]. This
scenario will have adverse impacts on remittance in the future. Its adverse impacts
will not limit up to national GDP growth next year, but also in the livelihood patterns,
income-generating activities, and consumption patterns at the household level.

2.6 Inflation and Food Commodities

COVID-19 also caused inflation in food commodities because of a reduction in the
movement of transportation. While the ADB [26] has estimated the inflation rate
in Nepal to be 7.5 in the post-COVID context, the UNDP predicts it to remain
6.3 as compared to 4.5 before COVID-19. Many farmers in Nepal wasted milk
(cow/buffalo) pouring on the ground due to the lockdown and lack of the market.
However, the rising food prices push up inflation to 6.87% [27]. The price of tomato
rose sharply to Nepalese Rupees (Rs) 95 per kg on Friday from 55 Nepalese Rupee
last week. Green vegetables jumped threefold to Rs.75 per kg from Rs. 25 a week
ago [28]. The vegetable consumption pattern is not changed so far.

Therefore, there is a risk of an immediate increase in the price of foodstuffs and
vegetables once the lockdown slightly gets loosened. Inadequate supply of chemical
fertilizers, seeds, and pesticides required for agriculture, and locust infestation, may
harm agriculture production and will result in inflation. Even so, the trend of inflation
in Nepal has been a fluctuation for a long time due to political unwillingness and
poor plans and policies.

2.7 Poor, Vulnerable Community and Women

About 31.2% of the population that is estimated to live between $1.9 (the international
poverty line adopted by Nepal) and $3.2 a day face significant risks of falling into
extreme poverty, primarily because of reduced remittances, job losses in the informal
sector, and rising prices for essential commodities as a result of COVID-19 [29].
According to the FAO [30], a total of 820 million people are expected to suffer from
hunger around the world and a largest number of undernourished people live in Asia,
mostly in South Asian countries.

According to NPC [31], the incidence of multidimensional poverty has reduced
from 39% in 2011 to 28.6% in 2018. Similarly, the poverty headcount incidence

in Nepal was 21.6% in 2015, and it has reduced to 18.7% in 2018/019. However, the literature suggests that the poverty rate may increase due to COVID-19. Mostly marginalized communities like rural Dalit, Muslims, Janajati/indigenous, and backward community represent the poorest community in Nepal in terms of income, consumption, and human development. This section of society will become more vulnerable as being curtailed from their job market and not having sufficient savings from their previous income to feed the family and sustain life. Besides, many poor people are unaware of COVID-19's impact on human health. They lack the precautionary knowledge like washing hands frequently with soap and water, usage of sanitizer, masks, and social distancing. Hence, they are more vulnerable than others. With the COVID-19 pandemic along with the negative outlook for the global economy, a significant share of vulnerable households faces the risk of falling back into poverty because of reduced remittances, agricultural production, and long vulnerability to natural disasters [32]. Lockdown has led to the loss of petty traders, salaried workers, and the poor, and they have been hit hard. In the rural areas, the marginalized farmers have limited access to health care facilities, quick financial support, food, and relief measures and they faced very hard during COVID-19.

Similarly, most of the migrant workers belong to this category. The illiteracy rate among them is high, and they have less access to the sustained job market.

Women

Women share 33.5% space in the formal sector of employment mostly in the non-agricultural sector. In the informal sector, women account for 66.5% (see Table 2). The lockdown resulted in the loss of jobs. Many women working in the hotel, travel agencies, and tourism businesses have lost their jobs because these businesses have been closed since the lockdown began. Besides, due to the closure of schools, children are staying at home, which has ultimately increased the workload of working women.

Likewise, during two months of lockdown, 293 cases of domestic violence and 39 cases of social violence were recorded [33]. Out of 39 social violence, 11 cases were self-initiated child marriage, 5 were forced child marriage by family members, and 11 were character assassination resulting in mental violence. In particular, the problems of violence and discrimination hit more of the women who belong to the so-called low caste/ethnic group, work in the informal sector, and who are already poor and unsecured in livelihood assets. If the pandemic continues likewise cases are expected to rocket. In essence, COVID-19 will increase the gender gap and inequalities.

2.8 Education

Lockdown is seriously affecting the education calendar. Examinations are either canceled or postponed due to the lockdown. Educational institutions have been closed since March. They do not seem to resume soon. Specific guidelines on online education and distance learning have been assured. Very recently in mid-April, some universities (e.g., Tribhuvan University) have endorsed the guideline. Yet, the online services are not reported to be effective and culturally less used. Low access to Internet services and poor technological know-how also matters in learning achievements. The online education system for young kids has been reported adding extra burden upon the parents while many teachers in many private schools have not received their salaries since lockdown started in April 2020 [34]. The new session of the education calendar does not seem to function as expected because of COVID-19. These scenarios imply mental and psychological stress among parents, teachers, and students.

2.9 Health Sector

According to the Economic Survey 2018/19 [35] of Nepal, there are altogether 4,517 health institutions. Among, 125 are government hospitals with 8,172 bed capacities, 2,640 doctors, and 14,347 nurses. Infectious and tropical disease hospital with 100 beds capacity is the only infectious disease hospital (STIDH) located in Kathmandu in Nepal that has a testing facility of coronavirus. In Nepal, COVID-19 cases are dealt with in government hospitals only. The limitations of health facilities in terms of numbers both hospital and health workers, infrastructure, quality, and lack of testing kits and mass testing have failed to control the spreading of COVID-19. For instance, many health workers were at risk without personal protective pieces of equipment, PPE. Initially, doctors involved in the treatment of COVID-19 affected patients were asked to stay in their respective hospitals, but the management of the hospitals could not manage such facilities, and doctors were forced to stay in their homes.

Similarly, many hospitals, patients with fever symptoms were not admitted. It was because of the fear and improper management of coronavirus treatment. Also, there are around 364 private hospitals and 14 private teaching hospitals in Nepal. However, only private teaching hospitals and few private hospitals were allocated for COVID-19 treatment after August, but most of them were reluctant to receive COVID-19 patients. The government could not mobilize those hospitals. Similarly, Nepal has less than 300 working ventilators for the entire population, which means on average one ventilator is available for 114,000 population [36]. Moreover, the highly-equipped hospitals with ICUs, CCUs, and ventilator services are located in urban centers; and two-third of them is in the capital city (Kathmandu). In essence, the poor health governance system is the reason for increasing affected cases and deaths too.

2.10 Social and Mental Stress

The migrants Nepalese who returned from foreign countries and India have been suggested to follow lockdown and stay in quarantine. However, there is no proper database and technological system to make effective surveillance. Thousands of Nepalese in India started walking home after India declared a complete lockdown on March 24 and stuck at the India border [37]. It is reported that they continuously travelled on foot even till 25 days and entered Nepal, but they stayed in quarantine in their villages as per the obligations adhered by the Government of Nepal. In a few cases, the migrants were also mistreated in the villages because some of them deliberately violated the isolation rules due to the fear.

Similarly, within the country, hundreds of workers returned to their birth village/place from Kathmandu on foot. It took them 4–7 days. In many places, security forces blocked them, but they walked through forest and farmland to reach their home-villages. Many were traveling in a miserable condition. Painful pictures of such migrants went viral with social media. Meanwhile, Nepal Human Rights and the Supreme Court ordered to allow them to go to their homes. More than 1200 suicidal cases were reported during the 74 days long lockdown; doctors say the pandemic's social-economic impacts have increased stressors, resulting in mental health problems [38]. Some studies have shown that when people start suffering from socioeconomic problems, stress increases, and eventually, this leads to suicide attempts.

Likewise, some health workers across the country faced social stigma as they were forcefully asked to leave their rooms fearing the spread of coronavirus. This has happened with many civilians. One incident is about a woman with her children who returned from her village Sindhupalchok District (mid-hill of the country). She was not allowed to enter the room in Kathmandu. Everyone was so scared. She managed to call the police, but the police failed to settle the dispute, and they were sent to the Teku Central Lab for a test. The medical team began interrogating them, asking about their travel history and symptoms. Those who rented the room were not allowed to enter the room until the house-owners received the testing report particularly [39] in Kathmandu.

3 Discussion for Opportunities in Terms of Rebuild and Reforms on Socioeconomic and Health Sectors

Despite the tremendous loss of human lives and the economy, COVID-19 has given some opportunities to follow several strategies and action plans to employ. Literature suggests that air pollution has drastically been reduced during the lockdown. In Kathmandu, people generally have been suffering from allergic cough and sneezing in the changing times of seasons (i.e., March and April) due to dust and air pollution for a decade. However, this year, very few people felt such problems, which is happily celebrated in social media as well. It seems that the health and environment are interrelated. The average concentration of PM 2.5 (pollutants that have a diameter of less than 2.5 μm) decreased by 34.9 μg per cubic meter (μg/m3) in Kathmandu from January 1 to April 24 during the lockdown [40].

Likewise, COVID-19 also created opportunities to enhance technologies to improve public service delivery, particularly for developing countries. It has been proved that technology can help to reduce pollution and corruption to a large extent. Schools and universities in many countries, including Nepal are trying to engage their students in online platforms. However, Nepal is still lacking behind in online education. Because Internet services are not well distributed across the country, it is still seen as a stake, and decision-makers are reluctant to use it. Cultural factor is connoted in this regard to some extent. Corruption has been rampant in public related offices in many developing countries including Nepal. The ordinary people heavily depend on the brokers, or mediators in many public-related offices to furnish their work, and it is institutionalizing corruption and dependency. E-services could break such malpractices and contribute to efficiency in the governmental institutions. Many developing countries like Nepal have been facing the poor delivery of public services. E-governance will provide better services without any prejudices and lingering.

In these circumstances, COVID-19 is a good opportunity to transform into the digitization that will strengthen decentralization and ensure transparency. The government of Nepal also realized this innovative context that COVID-19 has created opportunities in Nepal, especially in three fields: e-governance, e-commerce, and e-business [41]. It is a good opportunity to reform traditional bureaucracy equipping technology in fewer numbers considering efficiency and competency; e-governance-based bureaucracy will have more chances to tackle such challenges. It will further enhance public health governance. The role of technology in combating the pandemic can be significant [42]. The role of mega data in healthcare applications has been useful [43]. The only challenge is how technology like e-governance or e-services can be continued even after the COVID situation. Nepal's main challenge is, however, to strengthen good governance and institutional competencies in public services with digitization strategy. Nepal scores poor governance as it is 36 governance quality index only [44]. Nepal failed to provide a stimulating program to the targeted population and emergency response. It resulted in the movement led by youth against the government's ineffectiveness to respond to the COVID-19's impact in June. The government of Nepal had done little reducing the debt by 2% and added another three months to repay the loan for the business sector. It is said that all-accessible loans will be given for business in the affected areas, though there is no clear outline. There wasn't much discussion about employment.

To cope with the consequences of COVID-19, the country will need to adopt short-, mid-, and long-term strategies and policies. In short-term strategy, poor, small farmers, entrepreneurs, and private workers need to be protected for some time offering safety-net. In the mid-long-term recovery, resuming of transportation is crucial. Nepal's public transportation sector where private sectors have been dominating needs to be recommenced first taking various precautionary measures because its role in connectivity is essential. This sector is invested through bank loans mostly, and their concerns may be addressed through the relaxation in the interest of a loan. Meanwhile, the Nepal government has fewer resources for rebuilding post-COVID-19. For it, the unnecessary administrative expenditures and budgets allocated in unproductive fields must be cut down. The rebuild of agriculture, tourism, entrepreneurship, and public health and education should be placed in priority with a short-mid-long-term strategy because these are related to the majority of people's livelihood and the country's economy. The reforms in these fields will create employment and entrepreneurship.

3.1 The Rebuilding of Agriculture and Tourism Sectors

The long disruption in tourism, international trade and business, and lower remittances due to COVID-19 suggests that agriculture is the only sector that can likely contribute to national GDP and household economy in Nepal. Hence, it is a good opportunity for agricultural reform because it will avoid the risk of scarcity of food in the future and create employments. The agricultural sector needs to be rebuilt with both long- and short-term strategies targeting to create more jobs and surplus production. The majority of Nepalese depends on agriculture and its linkages. Agriculture with livestock is the major means of livelihood for the majority of Nepalese; however, agriculture in Nepal represents subsistence in nature and youths are reluctant to engage in it [45].

The agriculture sector is less attracted in terms of investment. In Nepal, this sector is still lacking modern technologies and tools. Food security has become a major issue after COVID-19. Encouragement to the agricultural sector is essential through special and subsidized loans and various discounts with technical supports. Subsidies and insurance in agriculture may help attract youths. The cash-generating agriculture system may be the option for a new generation. Other initiations like free education up to higher secondary schools to the poor farmer's children may also prompt them to engage in agriculture.

Agricultural development will enhance people to cope with future calamities and pandemic. Nepal does have fewer numbers of manufacturing industries for export purposes. So, agricultural development in terms of export could fill this gap that will boost the rural and national economy. In the post-COVID context, the returnee migrants from abroad can be engaged with different kinds of agricultural activities, including agro-based industries and entrepreneurial development. The linkage between agriculture and the market has been a major challenge in the path of modernization of agriculture in Nepal that needs to be seriously addressed. Hydroponic agriculture income may be a charm of youth. The farming is in water rather than soil; Nepal is rich in water resources. So, it can be a good opportunity to develop hydroponic agriculture. It will help to reduce micronutrient deficiency disease during COVID-19.

Similarly, tourism relates to income sources for a big number of people. Internal tourism should be prompted. It will support regional and national economies to some extent. Many tourism entrepreneurship like hotel business and travel agencies have largely been associated with tourism. Though Nepal has a high potential to develop the tourism sector, it lacks enough physical infrastructures.

3.2 Reforms of the Public Health System and Education

COVID-19 provides a lesson for the public health system worldwide. The public health service needs to be prioritized and developed with adequate technology, building, laboratories, and manpower which are inadequate in Nepal. For instance, Nepal has only one diagnostic center—National Public Health Laboratory, located in Kathmandu—testing for the coronavirus using real-time polymerase chain reaction (RT-PCR). Recently, each province is given such facilities, but not reliable because of the scarcity of skilled manpower and lacks infrastructural development. The role of private hospitals and laboratories in tackling such a pandemic could be a landmark, but they are not given such opportunities. The government's policy of public–private partnerships does not seem to work properly.

During the procurements of medical goods, scandal and irregularity were surfaced. While the private sector easily accessed these goods and provided to the government, poor governance has always been questioned in this regard. The lack of coordination between government and private health sectors is the major challenge as the government could not mobilize private laboratory and hospital for containing COVID-19.

However, the role of universities, health-related departments, and laboratories has played a key role in many developed countries, especially in the research field, the discovery of a ventilator, and drugs. For instance, Oxford University initiated the trial vaccine at the end of April. The Government of Nepal should take immediate action in making research institutions in Nepal to work to combat this pandemic. They should be identified and acknowledged through policies and incentive approaches. In Nepal, COVID-19 has been tested through rapid testing kits (RTK) and PCR method; PCR was recognized by WHO and its result is validated. However, the validation of RTK has been controversial. Such types of problems could be solved by laboratories, researchers, microbiologists, and doctors only.

At the same time, COVID-19 is accumulating stress on the people who are struggling with different kinds of physiological conditions, e.g. old age, illness, and poor immune systems, etc. People who already are patients with high blood pressure, sugar, and diabetes were seen as much panicking during the lockdown. Many cases of domestic violence and gender discrimination were also noticed. These incidents and circumstances are enough to predict psychological and stress impacts. Good public health governance can only tackle it and without prioritizing the health sector, this won't happen. Only below 5% of the total fiscal budget has been allocated for the health sector in Nepal. However, the budget for the fiscal year of 2020/21 increased by 2% compared to last year in health infrastructure. But looking at the implementation side so far, few believe it will yield the expected positive results; the expenditure capacity of the government has been poor. The private–public approach may be the best option in the reformation of the health sector.

COVID-19 in one way or another has become a reason for the educational transformation. It has opened up the minds to reform the value of education and educating methodology. Voices are being heard that online and student-oriented education system adopting technology should be encouraged. The centralized mentality (like board exam, which has been held by the federal government) and yearly exam-based education will not evaluate students as a whole. The school and universities should be modernized adopting recent technologies, learning methods, and evaluation systems. Basic education should be reliable, qualitative, and accessible for all. For it, the financial, as well as technical supports, should be allocated as per the needs assessment.

Basic education and health service must easily be available to everyone. The resilience of education and the health system ultimately help to empower people tackling epidemic and calamities that enhance inner strength to tackle challenges.

4 Conclusion and Implication

The literature suggests that the impact of COVID-19 in the socioeconomic and health sectors will be longer. Based on the above discussion, the Foreign Development Investment (FDI) may be slow due to global loss in economic growth. Similarly, inequality and poverty will be widened; the poor may face hardship. Covid-19 is sure to widen the gap between rich and poor. It could harm the goal of upgrading Nepal's economic condition by 2030 as projected by the Government of Nepal. Nepal has achieved incredible progress in poverty reduction over two decades, and its goal was to eradicate absolute poverty by 2030 as per the SDGs. COVID-19 pandemic will certainly have effects on Nepal's long-term development goals.

The creation of jobs within the country will be a major challenge for Nepal. The majority of migrants who returned home needs to engage in economic activities. A crisis created by COVID-19 may trigger inequality and have a disproportionate impact on the vulnerable population that needs to be addressed immediately. The reinforcement of social cohesion and peaceful coexistence is essential in preventing social tensions, inequality, and injustice. The gender violence was largely surfaced in Nepal during the pandemic and lockdown.

Moreover, the Nepal government does not have a scientific data of all the workers (including the absentee population), and thus the policy should be urged immediately to secure their job market and engage them in the productive fields. The recovery of economic losses may need to be fulfilled through sustainable approaches emphasizing policy reforms in health and education, agricultural development, e-governance, promotion of entrepreneurship equipping both short- and long-term strategies. Human resource management should be given priority for agricultural sectors, and hence, the policy needs to address such problems.

Similarly, the COVID-19 has stroke the layout of both public and private organizations in Nepal. The Ministry of Health and Population (MoHP) in Nepal is responsible for the overall policy formulation, planning, organization, and coordination of the health sector. In the future, this centralized layout will not work, and it should be reorganized enhancing local levels. The government needs to enhance the local level's capacity that has been responsible for delivering public services. However, the government of Nepal slightly increased budget in the health sector in terms of increment of bed and communicable hospital. Nepal will need debt for implementing such programs; therefore, it is necessary to come up with effective plans and strategies for proper utilization of debt. In the same way, the implementation part has always been difficult due to ineffective leadership and governance.

Hence, effective leadership and governance (especially e-governance) are crucial to create public health governance, making an effective public service delivery to a lower level of people who heavily depend on agriculture and remittances. Human resource management should be given priority for agricultural sectors, and hence, the policy needs to address such problems. The economic factors remain central because the crisis creates a recession, and recessions generally lead to higher death rates. The economy must consider the environment and must not forget public health issues. Therefore, Nepal must grab the opportunities created by COVID-19 to rebuild the socioeconomic and health sectors of Nepal.

References

1. MoF (Ministry of Finance). The Budget for the fiscal year of 2020/21 of Nepal. https://mof.gov.np/
2. Jordà O, Singh SR, Taylor AM (2020) Longer-run economic consequences of pandemics. Federal Reserve Bank of San Francisco Working Paper 2020-09. https://doi.org/10.24148/wp2020-09
3. World Bank (2020) Nepal must ramp up COVID-19 action to protect its people, revive economy. The World Bank. https://www.worldbank.org/en/news/press-release/2020/04/11/nepal-must-ramp-up-covid-19-action-to-protect-its-people-revive-economy
4. UNDP (2020) The social and economic impact of COVID-19 in the Asia-Pacific Region. Position Note prepared by UNDP Regional Bureau for Asia and the Pacific. Bangkok: United Nations Development Programme
5. NRB (Central Bank of Nepal) (2020) Monetary Policy of the fiscal year of 2019/20. https://www.nrb.org.np/contents/uploads/2020/04/Monetary_Policy_in_English-2019-20_Full_Text-new.pdf
6. UNDP, COVID-19 and human development: assessing the crisis, envisioning the recovery. https://hdr.undp.org/sites/default/files/covid-19_and_human_development_0.pdf
7. MoF (Ministry of Finance) (2020) Economic Survey 2018/19. https://mof.gov.np/uploads/document/file/compiled%20economic%20Survey%20english%207-25_20191111101758.pdf. Accessed on 15 June 2020
8. CBS (2019) Report on Nepal Labour Force Survey 2017/18. Central Bureau of Statistics (CBS), Kathmandu

9   Socioeconomic Impacts and Opportunities of COVID-19 for Nepal   165

9. UNDP-Nepal (2020) COVID-19 pandemic response; humanity needs leadership and solidarity to defeat the coronavirus. Retrieved from https://www.np.undp.org/content/nepal/en/home/cor onavirus.html

10. NRB (Central Bank of Nepal) (2020) Nearly a quarter of Nepal's workers lose jobs due to coronavirus—central bank. Retrieved from https://in.reuters.com/article/health-coronavirus-nepal/nearly-a-quarter-of-nepals-workers-lose-jobs-due-to-coronavirus-central-bank-idINKC N2591A8

11. NLFS (Nepal Labour Force Survey) 2017/18 (2019) Central Department of Statistics, Kathmandu. https://nepalindata.com/media/resources/items/20/bNLFS-III_Final-Report.pdf

12. MoCTCA (Ministry of Culture, Tourism and Civil Aviation). https://www.tourism.gov.np/ (2020, May 1)

13. MoCTCA (2019) Nepali Tourism Statistics 2018. Ministry of Culture, Tourism and Civil Aviation (MoCTCA), Kathmandu. Retrieved from https://tourism.gov.np/files/statistics/19.pdf

14. The Kathmandu Post (2017) Tourism pumped Rs177b into Nepal's economy. https://kathma ndupost.com/money/2017/03/31/tourism-pumped-rs177b-into-nepals-economy (2017 March 31)

15. MoALD (Ministry of Agriculture Livestock and Development) (2020) https://www.moald. gov.np/. Accessed on 14 June 2020

16. Onlinekhabar (2020) Danger of famine if the agricultural sector is not kept afloat. https://www. onlinekhabar.com/2020/04/856133 (2020, April 19)

17. World Bank (2017) CLIMBING higher: toward a middle-income Nepal (Nepal Country Economic Memorandum). Retrieved from https://www.worldbank.org/en/region/sar/public ation/climbing-higher-toward-a-middle-income-country

18. Annapurna Post (2020) Agriculture in trouble: chicken buried and decaying vegetables. Retrieved from https://annapurnapost.com/news/154361 (2020 April 27)

19. World Bank (2020) Nepal development update post-pandemic Nepal-charting a resilient recovery and future growth directions. file:///C:/Users/User/Downloads/Nepal-Development-Update-Post-Pandemic-Future-Growth-Directions%20(3).pdf (2020, July 23)

20. CBS. Nepal Living Standards Survey (NLSS-III) (2010/11) Vol. 2. Central Bureau of Statistics, Kathmandu

21. Chaudhary D (2020) Influence of remittances on socio-economic development in rural Nepal. Remittances Review 5(1):83–96. https://doi.org/10.33182/rr.v5i1.820

22. Ukyab Y (2020) From policy paradox to post-COVID resilience. UNDP Nepal. https://www. np.undp.org/content/nepal/en/home/blog/2020/From-policy-paradox-to-post-COVID-resili ence.html (2020 May 1)

23. MoHP (Ministry of Health and Population) (2020) https://covid19.mohp.gov.np/. 28 Aug 2020

24. The Kathmandu Post (2020) Jobless and without pay, migrant workers are returning home. But they have no recourse for compensation. https://tkpo.st/31JEE1y (2020, July 04)

25. The Kathmandu Post (2020) Remittance defies projections of a massive drop. https://tkpo.st/ 31qqmSN (2020, August 24)

26. Asian Development Bank (2020) Nepal Macroeconomic Update, 8(1). https://www.adb.org/ sites/default/files/institutional-document/577946/nepal-macroeconomic-update-202004.pdf

27. myRepublica (2020) Rising food prices push up inflation to 6.87 percent. https://myrepublica. nagariknetwork.com/news/rising-food-prices-push-up-inflation-to-6-87-percent/ (2020, April 19).

28. The Kathmandu Post (2020) Vegetables become scarce and costly as transporters stay away due to virus fears. https://tkpo.st/3bp3BRo (2020 April 27)

29. World Bank (2020) The World Bank in Nepal: overview. Retrieved from https://www.worldb ank.org/en/country/nepal/overview

30. FAO (2019) Global report on food crises 2019. Food and Agriculture Organization (FAO). sources/files/GRFC%202019_Full%20Report.pdf

31. NPC (National Planning Commission) (2018) Nepal's multidimensional poverty index: analysis towards action. National Planning Commission (NPC) & Oxford University, Kathmandu. https://www.npc.gov.np/images/category/Nepal_MPI.pdf

32. World Bank (2020) South Asia: poverty and equity. Retrieved from file:///C:/Users/USER/Desktop/Global_POVEQ_SAR%20PostCOVID-19.pdf
33. WORECNEPAL (2020) Risk and prevention of gender-based violence surveillance due to COVID-19 Epidemic. https://www.worecnepal.org/content/157/ (2020 June 12)
34. Onlinekhabar (2020) Demonstration of private school teachers demanding salary. https://www.onlinekhabar.com/ (2020 July 3)
35. Economic Survey 2018/19 of Nepal (2018/19) Ministry of Finance. https://mof.gov.np/uploads/document/file/compiled%20economic%20Survey%20english%207-25_201911111 01758.pdf
36. myRepublica (2020) Nepal has just one ventilator for 114,000 people. https://myrepublica.nagariknetwork.com/news/nepal-has-just-one-ventilator-for-114-000-people/ (2020, August 4)
37. Aljazeera (2020) Hundreds of Nepalese stuck at India border amid COVID-19 lockdown. Retrieved from https://www.aljazeera.com/news/2020/04/hundreds-nepalese-stuck-india-border-covid-19-lockdown-200401031905310.html (2020, April 1)
38. The Kathmandu Post (2020) Over 1,200 people killed themselves during 74 days of lockdown. https://tkpo.st/30G8m6N (2020, June 14)
39. The Kathmandu Post (2020) The housewife did not allow him to enter the room without testing the corona. https://ekantipur.com/feature/2020/04/29/158816532779897834.html (2020, April 17)
40. The Kathmandu Post (2020) Air quality improves in the world's major cities, including Kathmandu, under Covid-19 lockdowns. https://tkpo.st/3cXZKLM, https://tkpo.st/3cXZKLM (2020, January 5)
41. Onlinekhabar (2020) We also know that people die of hunger, let those who earn money buy and eat. https://www.onlinekhabar.com/2020/04/856223 (2020, April 19)
42. Chawla S, Mittal M, Chawla M, Goyal LM (2020) Corona virus–SARS-CoV-2: an insight to another way of natural disaster. EAI Endorsed Trans Pervasive Health Technol 6(22). https://doi.org/10.4108/eai.28-5-2020.164823
43. Kaur P, Sharma M, Mittal M (2018) Big data and machine learning based secure healthcare framework. Procedia Comput Sci 132:1049–1059. https://doi.org/10.1016/j.procs.2018.05.020
44. Shah A, Andrews M (2005) Assessing local government performance in developing countries. In: Shah A (ed), Public services delivery. The World Bank, Washinton, DC, pp 63–83
45. Chaudhary D (2018) Agriculture policy and rural Development in Nepal: an overview. Res Nepal J Dev Stud 1(2):34–46. https://doi.org/10.3126/rnjds.v1i2.22425

Chapter 10
Strategic Decision in Long and Short Run for Cross-Country Commodity Market in the Post-COVID 19 Era

Arya Kumar (ID)

1 Introduction

Trading between the cross countries is the only tool to boost up the economy number. A minor agreement with a developed country can set up in positioning the world trading and uplifting the domestic economy. However, the developed country, i.e., the United States recently refused India for duty-free trading in the US market till India unwraps exporting of the agricultural products in US markets. India is still considered as an agrarian country whose economy is developed only due to the demand for agro products worldwide, and US agri-business always keeps eye on developing its agricultural sector which is a non-starter for India.

Unlike India, China's economists experienced that the FDI mainly for the manufacturing sector will not boost up the economy in the long run. FDI is a means for exchanging technology, and US companies are highly advanced in locating its business units in developing countries that will make the US rich but not China. So instead of reinventing new technology at a cheaper price, it is better to enter a demanding area globally, i.e., agri-business.

As the world economy has stopped breathing and every sector has crashed down due to the pandemic issue Covid-19, it is observed that the food supply locally and globally has to fail down. As there is a strict restriction in the movement of goods and people within and outside the nation this brings to scarcity of foods and other amenities. The supreme commodities like fruits and vegetables have reduced their weightage in production and export due to the restriction of the value chain. Despite uncertainties due to Covid-19, Food and Agriculture Organization forecasted a comfortable rise of demand for cereals for the year 2020/21.

A. Kumar (✉)
Faculty of MBA, College of IT and Management Education, Biju Patnaik University of
Technology, Bhubaneswar, India
e-mail: arya4134@gmail.com

© The Author(s), under exclusive license to Springer Nature Singapore Pte Ltd. 2021   167
P. K. Khosla et al. (eds.), *Predictive and Preventive Measures for Covid-19 Pandemic*,
Algorithms for Intelligent Systems, https://doi.org/10.1007/978-981-33-4236-1_10

FAO is more concerned about the medium and long-term effects of pandemic, i.e., unemployment and national economy so the countries that are dependent on the food import are going to struggle badly to avail the resources to buy foods. However, some of the protectionists support the pandemic as an opportunity for an agro-based country like India or mainly who are willing to indulge them in agro-sector, i.e., USA and China by stating that the nation should focus less on local food prices as it weakens the national currencies so it is necessary to rely on the export of food products instead of trading domestically.

In the entire world, the most unpredictable price pattern is agro-based products. The reasons behind such are the climatic condition, export–import, quality of seeds, subsidy on agriculture, and many other economic variables. When such products are traded globally by some of the major producers, then it gets most important to have a track on the price forecasting in the long run. It is found that maize, rice, and wheat are some of the products that are widely consumed throughout the world result in which the prices of such products tend to be highly volatile. As a result, understanding the price dependencies and identifying the price movements get more important.

As farming-based countries like India and China, they completely rely on producing the agro products for consumption as well as exporting in the international market like soy, sugar, cotton, and cereal grains. Surprisingly, the most powerful and developed country, i.e., the USA fails to make a noticeable impact in the field of agriculture, so it always depends on these agro-based countries. But the issue lies as it is about price fixation. There are several reasons as discussed early that affect the prices.

Shahzad et al. [33], Kumar et al. [21], Bales et al. [7], Butt et al. [11] stated that the prices of the agricultural products are depended on various factors, few are the climatic condition, economic condition, EXIM policies or political hindrances. Taheripour and Tyner [34] opined that oil prices are the major reason behind the price hike of corn. Irwin and Good [17] conducted an empirical analysis along with theoretical concepts by considering the time series analysis that agricultural products follow the prices movement of its past prices, and this result also confirms long-run dependencies through (VECM) vector autoregressive and vector error correction models. Sekine and Tsuruga [32] analyzed empirically by considering the cross-country agro products and economic variables that state the macroeconomic variables of such countries affect the prices. Bentivoglio et al. [9] the study covers the empirical time series analysis considering the econometric tools, i.e., vector error correction model (VECM) and Granger causality tests on the ethanol prices and sugar prices that confirm the prices of agricultural products affect the ethanol prices but the opposite is not true. Zhang and Qu [35] the study considers the prices of oil on the agricultural commodities of China. It shows that there exists a volatility clustering and it also states that the oil price movement affects the agricultural products differently. It can be said that almost every agricultural products have asymmetric behavior. Except for natural rubber, other commodities like corn, soybean, bean pulp, strong wheat, cotton have a high influence on the change in oil price.

In past, many leading researchers contributed that the agricultural product's prices are more sensitive toward demands, supplies and of its prices [5, 10, 14, 19, 20, 25, 31]. Some of the researchers also suggested that change in oil prices affects the agricultural prices significantly in the international market [2, 4, 16, 24, 27, 28, 30, 12]. Few suggested that these price dependencies are also due to few substitute products and as per the availability of the products Abdulai and Rieder [1], Baek and Koo [6], Apergis and Rezitis [3], Rapsomanikis and Mugera [29] and Ozturk [26].

Out of several studies on identifying the price dependencies, one of the major impacts is the role of agro product prices of a country upon the ago product prices of another country. Clements et al. [13] investigated the association between agro products and countries. The resulting outcome confirms that the advanced country experiences cheaper pricing in comparison with advancing countries. Li et al. [22] an empirical analysis was conducted considering the USA and China as the key market player in the commodity segment. The study considered a wide range of agro products, i.e., cotton, sugar, corn, wheat, and soybeans. The result confirmed that China acts as the follower and the USA plays the role of the market leader in price fixation. Jiang et al. [18] considered the wheat, soy, sugar, and corn intra data prices of the USA and China. The resulting outcome depicts a potentially large profit on the flow of information from the different cross country for determining the prices.

Marini and McCorriston [23] experienced the price shock in the commodity market by using a vector autoregression model that shock produced as per country-specific cause the spillover in the commodity segment. Bekkers et al. [8] analyzed a study on food prices globally and locally. The outcome states that the per capita income of the nation has a significant impact on identifying food price behavior. Gale et al. [15] the study uses three different countries, i.e., China, USA, and Brazil for identifying the dependencies upon the prices of soybeans. The result states that China acts as the leader in exporting the soybeans followed with Brazil while it is found that the USA is the major importer of soybean throughout the world.

It is observed from that past studies that various elements and factors affect the price determination of the agro-based products. Based upon such many researchers proposed many tools and outcomes that are useful to deal with price fluctuation. But the major question arises is that will the same dependencies or factors will last for long if there is an unpredictable external global event, i.e., Covid-19 will help the same existing strategies? As per these research problems, the study will consider following objectives that are as follows:

- To identify the relation between the prices of the cross-country agro product.
- To measure the price association between the cross-country agro products.
- To confirm that the prices association established is for the short term or long term.

As per the above objective, the whole study considers various econometric models and interprets the result by revealing that whether the association will sustain long run or short run that the practitioners can implement right strategies in post-Covid-19 era.

2   Research Methodologies

Data Sources: The secondary data are collected from the commodity exchange of respective countries. The data include four major agro products that are traded locally and globally, i.e., corn, rice, soy, and wheat of three major countries in production and consumption, i.e., China, India, and the USA. The study considers the monthly return of all the agro products of all three countries from July 2013 to March 2020.

Data Tools:

(a) *Calculation of Adjusted Return*: The study considers the natural logarithm of closing prices.
    Mathematically: $R_t = \text{Log}(P_t/P_{t-1})$, where P_t and P_{t-1} are closing price of day t and $t - 1$, respectively.
(b) *Descriptive Statistics*: The study used the Jarque Berra test to understand for identifying the data distribution, i.e., mean, standard deviation, skewness, and kurtosis.
(c) *Test of Normality*: It states about the data characteristics that whether the data are normal or not normal, i.e., whether the data set follows a random or not a random walk.
(d) *Tests for Stationary*: It is a statistical analysis conducted to identify the statistical properties of a time series, i.e., mean, autocorrelation, variance are constant throughout the period. It can be measured through the unit root test.

$$\text{ADF} - \Delta Y_t = \alpha + \beta_t + \gamma Y_{t-1} + \partial_1 \Delta Y_{t-1} + \cdots + \partial_{p-1} \Delta Y_{t-p+1} + \epsilon_t$$

where $\alpha =$ constant, $\beta =$ coefficient of time trend and p-value is the autoregressive lag order, $\epsilon_t =$ error term for white noise.

$$\text{PP} - \Delta y_{t-1} = \alpha_0 + \gamma y_{t-1} + e_t$$

(e) *Granger Causality Test*: a test to measure the cause and effect relationship between the variables, i.e., whether x causes y or y causes x
(f) *Co-integration test*: The analysis uses the time series data, here its purpose is to identify whether the data set that are considered are moving parallel or not. Mathematically,

$$\lambda \max(r, r + 1) = -T \ln(1 - \hat{\lambda}_{r+1})$$

This is termed as the maximal eigenvalue statistics test, which can be defined as (λ**max**) as it is dependent on the value of maximum Eigen.

The next model used the trace statistics, as the trace of the matrix is based on likelihood ratio test. "It studies by adding more eigenvalue above (*i*th) eigenvalue to test whether it increases the trace" The equation can be calculated as

$$\lambda_{trace}(r) = -T \sum_{i=r+1}^{n} \ln(1 - \hat{\lambda}_{r-1})$$

As per the resulting outcome, the study will use.

(g) If the variable does not confirm co-integration, then test the short and long run through vector auto regression (VAR) or else run vector error correction model (VECM) in case of opposite.

Research Hypothesis

- H1: The cross-country agro products prices are not correlated to each other.
- H2: The cross-country agro products price does not have any causal effect.
- H3: The cross-country agro products prices are not co-integrated with each other.
- H4 There lays no short or long-run association between the cross-country agro products prices.

3 Data Analysis and Interpretation

The present paper considers a set of return series of the food crops that are traded globally to establish the directional relationship and price association between the food crops of the selected countries. But before implementing the research tools, the primary objectives are to identify the data normality through JB-test and understand the nature of the series through descriptive statistics. Table 1 shows the result of the JB-test for all the data series, i.e., the food crops corn, rice, soy, and wheat for three selected companies, i.e., China, India and USA.

The time series analysis includes the performances of the stock market for which the identification of data characteristics is mandatory. Table 1 depicts the output result of the data characteristics for all the variables for all the countries, i.e., China, India, and the USA and four different crops (corn, rice, soy, and wheat).

The output result of Jarque-Berra test is interpreted considering 5% level of significance to confirm the data behavior that states that out of twelve data series six are found to be normally distributed while rest is not normal in nature, i.e., rice (India and USA), soy (India and USA), and wheat (China and USA), it means all these prices follow a predictable pattern, i.e., there prices can be forecasted in near future; however, the remaining agro products for different countries like corn (China, India, and the USA), rice (China), soy (China), and wheat (India), all these series are not following a predictable pattern, i.e., it is required to identify how well the analysis can be made to support in price determination of this series. However, some of the

Table 1 Result of agro products test of normality

	Corn			Rice			Soy			Wheat		
	China	India	USA	China	India	USA	China	India	USA	China	India	USA
Observations	83	83	83	83	83	83	83	83	83	83	83	83
Probability	**0.000002**	**0.000003**	**0.000000**	**0.000000**	0.351642	0.381262	**0.000000**	0.103135	0.162522	0.093641	**0.017364**	0.101508
Jarque-Bera	25.99181	25.60662	34.22747	60.86573	2.090283	1.928536	226.1804	4.543425	3.633886	4.736566	8.106754	4.575232
Sum	-0.150189	1.040825	-0.695712	0.015353	0.192382	-0.056782	-0.010005	-0.035200	-0.455572	-0.063949	0.286425	-0.251706
Median	0.003783	0.007273	-0.005674	0.000000	0.000140	-0.002829	-0.004168	-0.004442	0.000839	0.000000	0.003841	0.001303
Mean	-0.001810	0.012540	-0.008382	0.000185	0.002318	-0.000684	-0.000121	-0.000424	-0.005489	-0.000770	0.003451	-0.003033
Std. dev	0.062636	0.073593	0.073143	0.072114	0.043261	0.061058	0.058070	0.066324	0.062824	0.060824	0.042523	0.079441
Kurtosis	5.576684	5.594927	5.953602	6.878769	3.673195	3.261471	10.50646	4.093147	3.460246	3.903183	4.342742	3.964657
Skewness	-0.468082	0.409475	-0.541602	0.799199	0.194440	0.349743	1.504547	0.172330	-0.457967	-0.372112	-0.367819	0.313207
Sum sq. dev	0.321706	0.444105	0.438695	0.426436	0.153461	0.305704	0.276519	0.360713	0.323642	0.303368	0.148272	0.517487
Minimum	-0.204421	-0.224591	-0.308383	-0.187469	-0.105424	-0.128350	-0.164631	-0.210756	-0.189689	-0.196001	-0.124053	-0.213408
Maximum	0.206734	0.294561	0.189608	0.308755	0.132638	0.198078	0.293376	0.184549	0.133925	0.145911	0.131389	0.254910

selected variables are found normal still these variables will be considered in subsequent analysis with an expectation of identifying the relationship or as a means to predict the series.

Apart from the Table 1 output, it also highlights few statistical results, i.e., about the data distribution which shows the result of kurtosis as more than the normal value, i.e., 3, it means the data are platykurtic in nature, it means the distribution follows a high peakedness while representing in graphical form, similarly the normal distribution for the data can be understood from its tail movement which is identified from the value of skewness when its result output is 0, and here, from the table output, it is clear that some of the values are either more than normal or less than normal, it means they are positively skewed, i.e., toward right-tailed, or negatively skewed, i.e., left tailed.

As the study of the Jarque Berra test is to understand the data characteristics, it is confirmed that the data are not normally distributed rather they follow a random walk. However, the deviations for all the data series are not too high. So, further study as per the research objective can be carried on.

The test of stationary highlights the data series maintains a uniform mean, variance, and covariance throughout the period. It means the resulting output will support the implication in the long run. Table 2 shows the result of a stationary test for all the agro products and the countries.

In time series analysis identifying the stationary of the data, series is just as it signifies the constant mean, variance, and covariance throughout the period. It is observed from Table 2 that the data series that consist of agro product corn with three different countries are statistically significant with 0.05 as the p-value, it means the test of stationery is true in this case that all the data series of corn, rice, soy, and wheat agro products of all three countries, i.e., China, India, and the USA are stationary in approach, i.e., the covariance, mean, and variance are constant throughout the period. So, it can be confirmed that the resulting outcome through this study can be accepted shortly and can be made to a generalized statement.

As per the research objective, the initial analysis that required confirming the degree of relationship between the variables, i.e., the countries as per the agro products needs to be made that is measured through correlation test and presented in Table 3.

Table 3 for the agro products corn confirms a weak but the highest degree of the relationships among all the variables, i.e., only 10.77% with China and the USA. The negative relation between each other is due to the availability of substitute products that are traded between each other. China is found to be the major producer of corn and export to various countries like the USA, but the USA depends on various substitute products and prefers to rely on other countries rather than China so there both prices move inversely from each other. Similarly, the major producer and consumers of rice worldwide are China and India. But surprisingly from the above output of price correlation, both of them show a positive but not a strong correlation with each other like China and the USA. These both countries show a medium but a strong correlation of prices of rice, it clears that the USA and China move parallel for the product rice as the USA hardly prefers to depend on rice as they are not the major

Table 2 Data stationary of agro products

Corn	China has a unit root							
			t-stat	$P*$			t-stat (adjusted)	$P*$
	Test statistic (ADF)		−12.76811	0.0001	Test statistics (PP)		−13.29427	0.0001
	Test critical values	Level (%)	10	−2.585861		Level (%)	10	−2.585861
			5	−2.897223			5	−2.897223
			1	−3.512290			1	−3.512290
	India has a unit root							
			t-stat	$P*$			t-stat (adjusted)	$P*$
	Test statistic (ADF)		−10.12275	0.0000	Test statistics (PP)		−10.12275	0.0001
	Test critical values	Level (%)	10	−2.585861		Level (%)	10	−2.585861
			5	−2.897223			5	−2.897223
			1	−3.512290			1	−3.512290
	USA has a unit root							
			t-stat	$P*$			t-stat (adjusted)	$P*$
	Test statistic (ADF)		−9.711980	0.0000	Test statistics (PP)		−9.829516	0.0001
	Test critical values	Level (%)	10	−2.585861		Level (%)	10	−2.585861
			5	−2.897223			5	−2.897223
			1	−3.512290			1	−3.512290
Rice	China has a unit root							
			t-stat	$P*$			t-stat (adjusted)	$P*$
	Test statistic (ADF)		−7.878421	0.0000	Test statistics (PP)		−24.2132	0.0001
	Test critical values	Level (%)	10	−2.586351		Level (%)	10	−2.58581
			5	−2.898145			5	−2.89723
			1	−3.514426			1	−3.51229
	India has a unit root							
			t-stat	$P*$			t-stat (adjusted)	$P*$
	Test statistic (ADF)		−6.693571	0.0000	Test statistics (PP)		−6.089907	0.0000
	Test critical values	Level (%)	10	−2.586103		Level (%)	10	−2.585861
			5	−2.897678			5	−2.897223
			1	−3.513344			1	−3.512290

(continued)

Table 2 (continued)

			USA has a unit root					
			t-stat	*P**			*t*-stat (adjusted)	*P**
Test statistic (ADF)			−10.37671	0.0000	Test statistics (PP)		−10.37671	0.0001
Test critical values	Level (%)	10	−2.585861		Level (%)	10	−2.585861	
		5	−2.897223			5	−2.897223	
		1	−3.512290			1	−3.512290	

Soy — **China has a unit root**

			t-stat	*P**			*t*-stat (adjusted)	*P**
Test statistic (ADF)			−7.323051	0.0000	Test statistics (PP)		−7.027869	0.0000
Test critical values	Level (%)	10	−2.585861		Level (%)	10	−2.585861	
		5	−2.897223			5	−2.897223	
		1	−3.512290			1	−3.512290	

India has a unit root

			t-stat	*P**			*t*-stat (adjusted)	*P**
Test statistic (ADF)			−8.136660	0.0000	Test statistics (PP)		−8.189249	0.0000
Test critical values	Level (%)	10	−2.585861		Level (%)	10	−2.585861	
		5	−2.897223			5	−2.897223	
		1	−3.512290			1	−3.512290	

USA has a unit root

			t-stat	*P**			*t*-stat (adjusted)	*P**
Test statistic (ADF)			−9.618676	0.0000	Test statistics (PP)		−9.610836	0.0001
Test critical values	Level (%)	10	−2.585861		Level (%)	10	−2.585861	
		5	−2.897223			5	−2.897223	
		1	−3.512290			1	−3.512290	

Wheat — **China has a unit root**

			t-stat	*P**			*t*-stat (adjusted)	*P**
Test statistic (ADF)			−8.255237	0.0000	Test statistics (PP)		−22.11859	0.0001
Test critical values	Level (%)	10	−2.586351		Level (%)	10	−2.585861	
		5	−2.898145			5	−2.897223	
		1	−3.514426			1	−3.512290	

(continued)

Table 2 (continued)

India has a unit root							
			t-stat	*P**		*t*-stat (adjusted)	*P**
Test statistic (ADF)			−8.041718	0.0000	Test statistics (PP)	−8.017230	0.0001
Test critical values	Level (%)	10	−2.585861		Level (%)	10	−2.585861
		5	−2.897223			5	−2.897223
		1	−3.512290			1	−3.512290
USA has a unit root							
			t-stat	*P**		*t*-stat (adjusted)	*P**
Test statistic (ADF)			−8.865153	0.0000	Test statistics (PP)	−12.25642	0.0001
Test critical values	Level (%)	10	−2.586103		Level (%)	10	−2.585861
		5	−2.897678			5	−2.897223
		1	−3.513344			1	−3.512290

*One sided-MacKinnon (1996)

Table 3 Result of agro products correlations

	CORN_CHINA	CORN_INDIA	CORN_USA
CORN_CHINA	1.000000	−0.073163	**−0.107776**
CORN_INDIA		1.000000	−0.023115
CORN_USA			1.000000
	RICE_CHINA	**RICE_INDIA**	**RICE_USA**
RICE_CHINA	1		
RICE_INDIA	0.114868	1	
RICE_USA	**0.219481**	0.023477	1
	SOY_CHINA	**SOY_INDIA**	**SOY_USA**
SOY_CHINA	1.000000	0.058468	0.079303
SOY_INDIA		1.000000	**0.433272**
SOY_USA			1.000000
	WHEAT_CHINA	**WHEAT_INDIA**	**WHEAT_USA**
WHEAT_CHINA	1.000000		
WHEAT_INDIA	0.030390	1.000000	
WHEAT_USA	−0.070778	**−0.078664**	1.000000

consumer they mainly produce it to trade, so if the international market tends to rise, they immediately prefer to raise its price to take the share in the international agro market.

Soy is a product that is not consumed in a daily habit but that is mainly used for various other activities mainly for feeding animals as organic food. A similar effect is found in the case of the USA that relies completely on purchasing soy to feed their cattle, sheep, and other animals. As a result, the USA prefers and depends on India as it supplies at the lowest price in comparison with others in the international market, due to such a reason if the price of the soy fluctuates in India, it will lead to a drastic price change for the USA. Unlike other agro commodities, wheat is also a product that is highly produced and consumed by all three countries. But wheat has never been a product that is to be accepted as major agro commodities for consumption like rice or soy. So when a correlation is made between the countries, the result was not too high rather it shows a weak and negative correlation between the prices of India and the USA.

Correlation analysis depicts the degree of relationship between the variables, but this analysis unable to explain the causal relationship between the variables i.e., which particular variable affects which particular variable significantly. In other words, to identify the cause and effect relationship between the variables, so it is required to test the causality by implementing the Granger causality test that is represented in Table 4.

Table 4 shows the result of Granger causality whose objective is to identify the cause and effect relationship. The resulting output considers lag 2 for identifying the price follow between the countries of an agro product, i.e., corn. The result shows that China follows the corn price of the USA, it means the relationship established between these two variables confirms a unidirectional flow where China fixes the prices of corn by following the USA, the reason is the USA is the major producer of corn globally that leads to trade in the international market. So as the China that produces for self-consumption so when the international market is found rising, they prefer to keep the price low, and when the price of the international market is less, then they raise the price and try to trade nationally; however, the prices fixed by China are always found to be lower in case of USA as they trade occasionally. As per the correlation matrix output, it is confirmed that USA and China hold a medium positive relation for the agro product rice, the reason is USA is completely depended on China for importing the rice as USA climate and land is not perfect for cultivating rice apart from that China is a country that keeps a wide range of various types of rice. These are the major reason for which the USA follows China's prices positively, i.e., a high price of China leads to a high price of the USA and vice versa.

As stated early the reason for the strong and positive correlation between the USA and India for the product Soy is due to the excess dependency of USA on the organic food to feed their cattle, sheep, and other animals. But there were no empirical support to approve. However, the reason behind such is confirmed after the resulting output of Granger causality that the price movement is from India to the USA, i.e., the USA market follows the price movement of the soy India that helps the USA in importing the commodity. The price movement is also observed for the

Table 4 Result of agro products granger causality

Hypothesis	Obs	F-statistic	Prob
Granger causality for agro products corn			
CORN_INDIA ## CORN_CHINA	81	1.34207	0.2674
CORN_CHINA ## CORN_INDIA		1.06165	0.3510
CORN_USA ## CORN_CHINA	**81**	**2.42294**	**0.0355**
CORN_CHINA ## CORN_USA		0.92949	0.3992
CORN_USA ## CORN_INDIA	81	1.16804	0.3165
CORN_INDIA ## CORN_USA		0.11676	0.8900
Granger causality for agro products rice			
RICE_INDIA ## RICE_CHINA	81	0.58371	0.5603
RICE_CHINA ## RICE_INDIA		1.07708	0.3457
RICE_USA ## RICE_CHINA	81	0.99153	0.7638
RICE_CHINA ## RICE_USA		**0.27035**	**0.0358**
RICE_USA ## RICE_INDIA	81	0.18601	0.8306
RICE_INDIA ## RICE_USA		1.00489	0.3709
Granger causality for agro products soy			
SOY_INDIA ## SOY_CHINA	81	0.03852	0.9622
SOY_CHINA ## SOY_INDIA		1.33720	0.2687
SOY_USA ## SOY_CHINA	81	0.73646	0.4822
SOY_CHINA ## SOY_USA		0.71391	0.4930
SOY_USA ## SOY_INDIA	81	0.49947	0.6088
SOY_INDIA ## SOY_USA		**2.41238**	**0.0264**
Granger causality for agro products wheat			
WHEAT_INDIA ## WHEAT_CHINA	81	1.34435	0.2668
WHEAT_CHINA ## WHEAT_INDIA		2.02720	0.1388
WHEAT_USA ## WHEAT_CHINA	81	2.00725	0.1414
WHEAT_CHINA ## WHEAT_USA		0.27384	0.7612
WHEAT_USA ## WHEAT_INDIA	**81**	**2.03018**	**0.0484**
WHEAT_INDIA ## WHEAT_USA		1.05626	0.3528

does not granger cause

agro product wheat where India depends on the price of the USA as the wheat is a product that is produced and consumed by all the three countries, but the USA is the market that supplies a major share in exporting the wheat globally. As it acts as the major market share, so the smaller producer like India depends on the price fixation or the movement of the USA.

The study holds the objective of identifying the association lies between the countries for price movement in the long run or short run. As the above analysis confirmed correlation as well as the directional relationship, but the price movement association is for the short or long run can be identified through the following test. But before analyzing such tests, the study should identify the co-integration between the variables. The purpose of identifying such is to confirm that the variables are moving parallel throughout the period.

The test of co-integration is one of the important analysis that is beneficial to establish the variables holds parallel moving characteristics, it means the variables considered confirm a similar kind of price movement in the long run. Table 5 confirms that the dependent and independent variables, i.e., corn China and the USA, respectively, act similarly in the long term as the probability value confirms at a 5% level of significance. Supporting to the objective of study the values of trace statistics, i.e., 78.16078 is found to be more than the critical value i.e. 15.495 and the max eigen value, i.e., 44.09114 also confirms the value more than the critical value 14.264 this result confirms that the variables are co-integrated with each other. A similar observation is also observed in case of rice, soy, and wheat agro products that confirms both the countries, i.e., USA and China, USA and India and the USA and China, respectively, are co-integrated with each other as the values of max-eigen and trace statistics are higher than that of the values of critical at the significance level 5%.

As the analysis of the co-integration test confirms the variables are co-integrated, so it is accepted that the variables move parallel in the future. But this analysis fails to confirm that this nature of behavior lies in the shortrun or long run, so the study will incorporate a vector error correction model (VECM) to confirm such kind of nature. It can be understood from Table 6 output.

The output result of the VECM model shows the value of the coefficient, i.e., $C(1)$ as negative, i.e., -1.566922 along with the subsequent p-values as 0.0000 which is considered as significant at 5% level of significance. This result output states that corn China and the USA both establish a long-run association with each other. To confirm that the analysis is true and holds the best result output, it can be further identified from the probability (F-statistics) which is significant in nature and the adjusted R-square values which are more than 60%. However, for other food crops, i.e., rice USA and China, soy India, and the USA and wheat USA and India does not confirm the presence of a long-run association between the variables as the probability value is not significant; however, they satisfy the other element that the coefficient value, i.e., $C(1)$ tends to be negative along with that the probability of (F-statistics) is significant and adjusted R-square is the result is good enough to confirm the testing model is true, but it does not provide a significant result so it can be concluded that there exists no significant long-run association between the above-said food crops.

As the result of VECM confirms the presence of long-run association, but several outcomes fail to confirm a long-run association. Perhaps there lies a short-run association between the series that can be measured and confirmed through the Wald test that is represented in the subsequent Table 7.

The analysis of the Wald test shows the resulting outcome of the short-run association between the variables, i.e., corn China and USA which depicts that the p-value of chi-square is significant at a 5% level that supports that the agro products corn holds a short-run price association between China and USA. But the similar result in the case of rice USA and China, soy USA and India, and wheat USA and India

Table 5 Agro products test of co-integration at level

Test of co-integration between corn USA and China

H0 No. of co-integrations	P**	Trace statistic	0.05 critical value	Max-Eigen statistic	0.05 critical value	Eigen value
None*	0.0000	78.16078	15.49471	44.09114	14.26460	0.423707
At the best 1*	0.0000	34.06964	3.841466	34.06964	3.841466	0.346799

Test of co-integration between rice China and USA

H0 No. of co-integrations	P**	Trace statistic	0.05 critical value	Max-Eigen statistic	0.05 critical value	Eigen value
None*	0.0000	70.98732	15.49471	48.08242	14.26460	0.451754
At the best 1*	0.0000	22.90490	3.841466	22.90490	3.841466	0.248971

Test of co-integration between soy India and USA

H0 No. of Co-integrations	P**	Trace statistic	0.05 critical value	Max-Eigen statistic	0.05 critical value	Eigen value
None*	0.0000	75.99756	15.49471	46.88703	14.26460	0.443500
At the best 1*	0.0000	29.11052	3.841466	29.11052	3.841466	0.305026

Test of co-integration between wheat USA and India

H0 No. of Co-integrations	P**	Trace statistic	0.05 critical value	Max-Eigen statistic	0.05 critical value	Eigen value
None*	0.0000	62.75029	15.49471	41.28701	14.26460	0.403149
At the best 1*	0.0000	21.46328	3.841466	21.46328	3.841466	0.235315

Table 6 Long-run association between agro products through VECM models

Depended variable: corn China; independent variable corn USA

	Coefficient	Std. error	t-statistic	Prob				
C(1)	−1.566922	0.244231	−6.415736	0.0000	S.E. of regression	0.059980	Akaike info criterion	−2.717565
C(2)	0.307854	0.195238	1.576816	0.1191	F-statistic	32.68282	Durbin–Watson stat	1.981769
C(3)	0.284102	0.114883	2.472969	0.0157	Log likelihood	114.7026	Hannan–Quinn criterion	−2.645938
C(4)	0.260281	0.076424	3.405761	0.0011	Adj. R^2	0.667248	S.D. dependent var	0.103980
C(5)	0.129753	0.077721	1.669482	0.0992	R^2	0.688308	Mean dependent var	0.000384
C(6)	0.000487	0.006706	0.072582	0.9423	Sum squared resid	0.266225	Schwarz criterion	−2.538913
					Prob(F-statistic)	0.000000		

Depended variable: rice USA; independent variable rice China

	Coefficient	Std. error	t-statistic	Prob				
C(1)	−0.071245	0.042408	−1.679974	0.0972	S.E. of regression	0.071736	Akaike info criterion	−2.359617
C(2)	−0.755251	0.119113	−6.340607	0.0000	F-statistic	12.35760	Durbin–Watson stat	2.150798
C(3)	−0.287671	0.114736	−2.507237	0.0144	Log likelihood	100.3847	Hannan–Quinn criterion	−2.287991
C(4)	0.346498	0.168448	2.057010	0.0432	Adj. R^2	0.418211	S.D. dependent var	0.094049
C(5)	0.192271	0.112000	1.716708	0.0902	R^2	0.455033	Mean dependent var	0.000405
C(6)	−0.000155	0.008022	−0.019317	0.9846	Sum squared resid	0.380805	Schwarz criterion	−2.180965
					Prob(F-statistic)	0.000000		

Depended variable: soy USA; independent variable soy India

	Coefficient	Std. error	t-statistic	Prob				
C(1)	−0.245767	0.172917	−1.421301	0.1594	S.E. of regression	0.072209	Akaike info criterion	−2.346476
C(2)	−0.618437	0.156261	−3.957723	0.0002	F-statistic	10.34445	Durbin–Watson stat	1.878819
C(3)	−0.219275	0.123842	−1.770599	0.0807	Log likelihood	99.85906	Hannan–Quinn criter	−2.274850
C(4)	−0.091785	0.202083	−0.454197	0.6510	Adj. R^2	0.371631	S.D. dependent var	0.091092
					R^2	0.411401	Mean dependent var	0.001597

(continued)

Table 6 (continued)

	Coefficient	Std. error	t-Statistic	Prob				
C(5)	0.024189	0.142606	0.169623	0.8658	Sum squared resid	0.385842	Schwarz criterion	-2.167824
C(6)	0.001720	0.008079	0.212902	0.8320	Prob(F-statistic)	0.000000		

Depended variable: wheat India; independent variable wheat USA

	Coefficient	Std. error	t-Statistic	Prob				
					S.E. of regression	0.047474	Akaike info criterion	-3.185227
C(1)	0.000338	0.038825	0.008693	0.9931	F-statistic	7.298170	Durbin–Watson stat	2.039837
C(2)	-0.592158	0.124923	-4.740166	0.0000	Log likelihood	133.4091	Hannan–Quinn criter	-3.113600
C(3)	-0.180526	0.117188	-1.540477	0.1277	Adj. R^2	0.285009	S.D. dependent var	0.056144
C(4)	0.014993	0.111184	0.134846	0.8931	R^2	0.330261	Mean dependent var	-0.001220
C(5)	0.102351	0.071060	1.440344	0.1540	Sum squared resid	0.166780	Schwarz criterion	-3.006575
C(6)	-0.001985	0.005312	-0.373776	0.7096	Prob(F-statistic)	0.000013		

Table 7 Short-run association between agro products through Wald test

Short-run causality between corn China and corn USA

Test stat	Value	df	P-value	Normalized Restriction (=0)	Value	Standard error
F-statistic	5.837466	(2, 74)	0.0044	C(4)	0.260281	0.076424
Chi-square	11.67493	2	0.0029	C(5)	0.129753	0.077721

Short-run causality between rice USA and rice China

Test stat	Value	df	P-value	Normalized Restriction (= 0)	Value	Standard error
F-statistic	2.165214	(2, 74)	0.1219	C(4)	0.346498	0.168448
Chi-square	4.330428	2	0.1147	C(5)	0.192271	0.112000

Short-run causality between soy USA and soy India

Test stat	Value	df	P-value	Normalized Restriction (= 0)	Value	Standard error
F-statistic	0.354905	(2, 74)	0.7024	C(4)	−0.091785	0.202083
Chi-square	0.709811	2	0.7012	C(5)	0.024189	0.142606

Short-run causality between wheat India and wheat USA

Test stat	Value	df	P-value	Normalized Restriction (= 0)	Value	Standard error
F-statistic	2.353994	(2, 74)	0.1021	C(4)	0.014993	0.111184
Chi-square	4.707988	2	0.0950	C(5)	0.102351	0.071060

for establishing of the short-run association is not sufficient to confirm the presence of short-run association as the p-value of chi-square is not significant, i.e., p-value is found more than 0.05. Hence, while understanding the price movement of the following crops concerning cross country will not reveal the accurate output, so fixing a price following the long-run association will put the price determiner a huge loss.

Here, as per the study objective, the analysis is carried on, and it is confirmed from the resulting outcome that how far the agro products are associated with the cross country. But before concluding and generalizing the study outcome, it is required to make a confirmation that all the analysis carried on supports the assumption for best fitting models.

The model of testing is accepted as true when the outcome of the p-value is more than 0.05. In general, it can be said when the residual of the data series established shows a non-serial correlation between the variables, then it can be accepted as the best model and helps in generalizing the output.

Here, from Table 8 output, it is confirmed that some of the residual outcomes confirm serial correlation, while some are not like in case of wheat India and USA

Table 8 Result of test of serial correlation between agro products

Agro products	F-statistic	Prob. F	Obs*R^2	P-value χ^2 (2)
Corn China and USA	0.029019	0.9714 (2, 72)	0.064434	**0.9683**
Rice USA and China	3.208765	0.0462 (2, 72)	6.547035	**0.0379**
Soy USA and India	4.845714	0.0106 (2, 72)	9.490765	**0.0087**
Wheat India and USA	1.276960	0.2851 (2, 72)	2.740481	**0.2540**

and corn China and USA have no serial correlation which is desirable to confirm the model is true, while rice China and the USA and soy USA and China have serial correlation as such outcome the further analysis for testing the assumption can be made.

Likewise the serial correlation, there is again testing to confirm that there is no heteroscedasticity in the residual outcome of the variables. Table 9 shows the compile result of such heteroscedasticity analysis.

The model of testing is further analyzed to identify the heteroscedasticity of the data series. Table 9 depicts that none of the data series are confirming the heteroscedasticity of the data series which is desirable for the model confirmation. The result of the p-value is more than 0.05, so the null hypothesis is accepted that the data series are not heteroscedasticity in nature. This outcome result is desirable to confirm that the model is the best fitting.

Table 10 reveals the outcome of normality test of the residual of all four agro products where the data series, i.e., corn China and the USA and soy India and the USA both have a non-normal distribution as the probability value is found significant at 5% level of significance apart from that the value of skewness and kurtosis are not normally distributed, i.e., the values are not exactly 0 and 3, respectively. Adding to it, the result confirms a negatively skewed for the series corn China and USA.

Table 9 Result of test of heteroscedasticity between agro products

Agro products	F-statistic	Prob. F	Obs*R^2	P-value χ^2 (6)	Scaled explained SS	P-value χ^2 (6)
Corn China and USA	1.037258	0.4084 (6, 73)	6.284544	**0.3921**	10.77955	0.0954
Rice USA and China	2.012121	0.0748 (6, 73)	11.65285	**0.0781**	12.65375	0.0489
Soy USA and India	1.770598	0.1171 (6, 73)	10.16325	**0.1179**	15.66254	0.0157
Wheat India and USA	0.709808	0.6427 (6, 73)	4.409954	**0.6214**	4.415073	0.6207

Table 10 Normality test of the residual of agro products

	Corn (China and USA)	Rice (USA and China)	Soy (USA and India)	Wheat (India and USA)
Probability	0.00000	0.119648	0.008563	0.756692
Kurtosis	5.009345	3.605317	4.602270	3.340186
Mean	−2.95e−18	−5.16e−18	0.000000	3.47e−19
Std. Dev	0.0058051	0.0069729	0.069886	0.045947
Skewness	−1.205791	0.476318	0.268765	−0.113526
Jarque Berra	32.84400	4.426409	9.520692	0.557598
Maximum	0.106882	0.199127	0.249506	0.120355
Median	0.0010643	−0.007425	0.005248	−0.001438

The above figure represents the data distribution for the rice agro products of two different countries, i.e., USA and China and wheat agro products of two different countries, i.e., the USA and India. The table outcome confirms that the residual of both the series are normally distributed adding to it by referring the skewness and kurtosis values are not accurate to normal but it is close to the normality, i.e., 0 and 3, respectively, so it can be said that the USA and China rice and the USA and India wheat prices are normally distributed which is desirable to confirm the model fitting.

As per the assumptions for accepting the model tested for the long-run and short-run association are true, we desire at that the assumptions need to be confirmed. As the study states that all the data series accepts assumptions, so it can be concluded that the models are best and the result outcomes are accurate.

4 Conclusion

The present study was to confirm the price associations between the variables, i.e., the agro products (corn, rice, soy, and wheat) with the three countries, i.e., China, India, and the USA to understand the price movement in normal practice that will support the practitioners, traders, policymakers, etc., to implement right strategies to take maximum benefit. As the economic condition is found to be disturbed due to uneventful and unpredictable event faced by the whole world, i.e., the pandemic event Covid-19 so it is utmost required to understand whether the past studies and outcomes are going to support in the long run or short run to deal with this pandemic event at present and in post-Covid-19 era. The result confirms that the prices of corn can be predicted by China by following the movement of the corn prices of the USA in both the long and short run, but the association is inversely proportional to each other. Likewise, for the rice product, the relationship establishment is simply the opposite of corn, i.e., the USA can identify the price of rice by referring to China. Similarly, in the case of soy and wheat, an opposite relation is confirmed between the USA and India where India helps USA in price determination of soy and USA support India in determining the price of wheat. In general, it can be said that this analysis of price association is worthy enough to fix the appropriate prices in advance to take the right strategies for local or international trading as well as the decision of importing or exporting after the Covid-19 era. However, this event might not last long as these events are experienced once in a century, but its impact may be felt for minimum a decade for the developing or under developing countries.

Managerial Implication

The present study considered the major three countries concerning the highest consumption and production of specific food crops. It is always challenging for food safety and maintaining price stability, as a result, the farmers or the practitioners unable to detect the future price movements and earning the desired return. In concise, this result outcome will support the policymakers and investors in adopting the right strategies in understanding the price movements and the pattern of association between the top producers and consumption that will reveal the trading price, volume and percentage of change in return in advance for maximizing their desired goal.

Limitations

The present study incorporated few food crops and only three countries based on the production and consumption which might be influenced by several other factors like climate, natural calamities, regional policies, and taxation that might affect the decisions of a practitioner. However, the present analysis considered a wide data set for the long-run association, and it is also observed that in the last two decades the mean value is not reverted as per the change in period. So, this result can be accepted widely for decision making.

Future Study

The present study is limited to few countries and crops, so to make the outcome as generalized statement, a further study is required considering more data set and including the macroeconomic variable, the climate and the rainfall of the particular region, understanding the psychology of the practitioners to measure the reality in an optimum manner.

References

1. Abdulai A, Rieder P (1995) The impacts of agricultural price policy on cocoa supply in Ghana: error correction estimation. J Afr Econ 4(3):315–335
2. Anderman TL, Remans R, Wood SA, DeRosa K, DeFries RS (2014) Synergies and tradeoffs between cash crop production and food security: a case study in rural Ghana. Food Secur 6(4):541–554
3. Apergis N, Rezitis A (2011) Food price volatility and macroeconomic factors: evidence from GARCH and GARCH-X estimates. J Agric Appl Econ 43(1):95–110
4. Avalos F (2014) Do oil prices drive food prices? The tale of a structural break. J Int Money Finan 42:253–271
5. Babula RA, Ruppel FJ, Bessler DA (1995) United States corn exports: the role of the exchange rate. J Agric Econ 13:75–88
6. Baek J, Koo WW (2010) Analyzing factors affecting US food price inflation. Can J Agric Econ/Rev Can D'agroeconomie 58(3):303–320
7. Bales C, Kovalsky P, Fletcher J, Waite TD (2019) Low cost desalination of brackish groundwaters by capacitive deionization (CDI)—implications for irrigated agriculture. Desalination 453:37–53
8. Bekkers E, Brockmeier M, Francois J, Yang F (2017) Local food prices and international price transmission. World Dev 96:216–230
9. Bentivoglio D, Finco A, Bacchi MRP (2016) Interdependencies between biofuel, fuel and food prices: the case of the Brazilian ethanol market. Energies 9(6):464
10. Bradshaw GW, Orden D (1990) Granger causality for the exchange rate to agricultural prices and export sales. West J Agric Econ 15:100–110
11. Butt S, Ramakrishnan S, Loganathan N, Chohan MA (2020) Evaluating the exchange rate and commodity price nexus in Malaysia: evidence from the threshold cointegration approach. Financ Innovation 6:1–19

12. Carro-Figueroa V (2002) Agricultural decline and food import dependency in Puerto Rico: a historical perspective on the outcomes of postwar farm and food policies. Caribbean Stud 77–107
13. Clements KW, Si J, Vo L (2017) Food and agricultural prices across countries and the law of one price. Available at SSRN 2968742
14. Denbaly M, Torgerson D (1992) Macroeconomic determinants of relative wheat prices: integrating the short run and the long run. Agric Econ Res 44:27–35
15. Gale F, Valdes C, Ash M (2019) Interdependence of China, United States, and Brazil in soybean trade. US Department of Agriculture's Economic Research Service (ERS) Report, New York, pp 1–48
16. Giraudo ME (2020) Dependent development in South America: China and the soybean nexus. J Agrarian Change 20(1):60–78
17. Irwin SH, Good DL (2009) Market instability in a new era of corn, soybean, and wheat prices. Choices (New York, N.Y.) 24(1):6–11
18. Jiang H, Todorova N, Roca E, Su JJ (2019) Agricultural commodity futures trading based on cross-country rolling quantile return signals. Quant Finance 19(8):1373–1390
19. Johnson PR, Grennes T, Thursby M (1977) Devaluation, foreign trade control, and domestic wheat prices. Am J Agr Econ 59:619–627
20. Kiptui M (2007) Does the exchange rate matter for Kenya's exports? A bounds testing approach. Prepared for presentation at the African Econometric Society 2007 conference, Cape Town, July 4 to 6 2007. Available at: https://www.africametrics.org/documents/conference07/Day%202/Session%205/KIPTUI%20Does%20the%20Exchange%20Rate%20Matter.pdf
21. Kumar A, Biswal SK, Swain PK (2019) A dynamic association between stock markets, Forex, gold and oil prices in Indian context. Revista ESPACIOSI 40(06)
22. Li N, Ker A, Rude J (2019) Modelling regime-dependent price volatility transmissions between China and US agricultural markets: a normal mixture bivariate GARCH approach (No. 1621-2019-2280)
23. Marini A, McCorriston S (2019) Price transmission in commodity networks (No. 1903).
24. Nellemann C (ed) (2009) The environmental food crisis: the environment's role in averting future food crises: a UNEP rapid response assessment. UNEP/Earthprint
25. Oyinlola MA (2008) Exchange rate and disaggregated import prices in Nigeria. J Econ Monetary Integr 9:89–126
26. Ozturk O (2020) Market integration and spatial price transmission in grain markets of Turkey. Appl Econ 52(18):1936–1948
27. Pham BT, Sala H (2020) The macroeconomic effects of oil price shocks on Vietnam: evidence from an over-identifying SVAR analysis. J Int Trade Econ Dev 1–27
28. Pokrivčák J, Rajčániová M (2011) The impact of biofuel policies on food prices in the European Union. Ekonomický Časopis 59(5):459–471
29. Rapsomanikis G, Mugera H (2011) Price transmission and volatility spillovers in food markets of developing countries. In: Methods to analyse agricultural commodity price volatility. Springer, New York, NY, pp 165–179
30. Rapsomanikis G, Hallam D, Conforti P (2006) Market integration and price transmission in selected food and cash crop markets of developing countries: review and applications. Agric Commod Markets Trade 187–217
31. Schwartz NE (1986) The consequences of a floating exchange rate for the U.S. wheat market. Am J Agr Econ 68:428–433
32. Sekine A, Tsuruga T (2018) Effects of commodity price shocks on inflation: a cross-country analysis. Oxford Econ Pap 70(4):1108–1135
33. Shahzad SJH, Hernandez JA, Al-Yahyaee KH, Jammazi R (2018) Asymmetric risk spillovers between oil and agricultural commodities. Energy Policy 118:182–198
34. Taheripour F, Tyner WE (2008) Ethanol policy analysis—what have we learned so far? Choices (New York, N.Y.) 23(3):6–11
35. Zhang C, Qu X (2015) The effect of global oil price shocks on China's agricultural commodities. Energy Econ 51:354–364

Chapter 11
Prediction of Novel Coronavirus (nCOVID-19) Propagation Based on SEIR, ARIMA and Prophet Model

G. Maria Jones and S. Godfrey Winster

1 Introduction

Coronavirus is an epidemic disease caused by SARS-CoV-2 (severe acute respiratory syndrome coronavirus2) which was first identified in Wuhan, China, in the year of 2019 and declared as a pandemic by World Health Organization (WHO) in March 2020. This kind of virus continues to threat the human life, and still, it is unclear about the origin of Corona. AIDS, HIV, Ebola, Zika, Spanish Flu, H1N1, H7N9 avian viruses affected millions of people across the globe. In twenty-first century two types of SARS originated from bats such as severe acute respiratory coronavirus (SARS-CoV) and Middle East respiratory Syndrome coronavirus (MERS-CoV) [1]. In late Dec 2019, unknown pandemic virus started to emerge from china which was quickly identified as Corona which is relatively similar as SARS occurred from 2002 to 2004 and MERS occurred in the year 2012. When SARS-CoV emerged, it quickly proliferates to 27 countries where 8100 people infected and 774 people were declared dead in twenty-first century. During MERS-CoV evolution, the infection reached about 1782 and death were about 640 in 2012 [1]. Corona has similar outbreak that has caused during 2002 and 2012. In 1918, around 500 and 17–50 [2] million people were affected and died due to Spanish flu which was considered as one of the deadliest epidemics in human history.

According to the statement declared by WHO, there are about 16,730,996 people affected by CoV2 and 658,991 people were died around the world [3, 4]. Initially, the outbreak of novel coronavirus were diagnosed as unknown pneumonia and also the source of nCoVid2019 have not yet determined. The other resources mentioned

G. Maria Jones (✉)
Department of Computer Science and Engineering, Saveetha Engineering College, Chennai, India
e-mail: joneofarc26@gmail.com

S. G. Winster
Department of Computer Science and Engineering, SRM Institute of Science and Technology, Kattankulathur, Chengalpattu, India

© The Author(s), under exclusive license to Springer Nature Singapore Pte Ltd. 2021 189
P. K. Khosla et al. (eds.), *Predictive and Preventive Measures for Covid-19 Pandemic*,
Algorithms for Intelligent Systems, https://doi.org/10.1007/978-981-33-4236-1_11

that infection has occurred from animals like bats. The virus has started to spread all parts of the world, especially, Asia, North America and Europe. Due to transmission factor, influence of geographical region and large population, virus propagation is uncontrollable. As of Jan 21, 2020, 276 were totally affected and 6 were died, by the time of March 15, the affected people were increased to 81,048 and 3204 died in China. At earlier stage of virus spread, it is important to control the propagation of virus from human to human in order to avoid huge disaster. About 30% of people used transportation to other places which resulted in difficulty to trace back the infected people. The virus has been spreading massively around the globe. Many countries declared a state of emergency, all events, and conferences have been canceled to reduce movement. All schools and universities are shut down to reduce the contact/interactions and also IT companies promoted work from home acts. These measures are effective to slow down the spread which referred as social distancing. Social distancing is one of the ways to reduce the interaction among people which will helps in reducing the transmission of virus.

Industry 4.0 is an upcoming technology which helps to tackle the viral infection in terms of wireless connectivity to service sector provides medical items and so on [5]. In many previous studies, only data-driven approaches are used and failed to use temporal analysis in the data. The prediction models like auto-regressive moving average (ARIMA), AR, MA are used to forecast the real-time series rates. Many research papers which include statistical and mathematical models for nCOVID-19 have been proposed for the dynamic model transmission range. Artificial intelligence, machine learning and deep learning are some of main factors in healthcare system and in many smart technologies. In this current paper, we introduced a novel method to modeling and analyzing the novel corona behavior. The work is classified into two segments. The first part deals with mathematical model which includes SEIR, and the second part works with ARIMA and prophet model which is based on prediction model. The following works are the main contribution of the paper.

1. To propose a novel method SEIR model to show how an nCoVid 2019 spreads among people.
2. To capture the interaction of coronavirus among people by a fractional equation for social distancing effort.
3. Extracting-related dataset from worldometer [3] and Our World in Data [6].
4. The time series prediction based on corona dataset for India with total affected rate till 17.07.2020 using ARIMA and Prophet algorithm.

The rest of the article is organized as follows: Sect. 2 presents the literature survey of coronavirus propagation and methods involved in SEIR and deep learning, Sect. 3 provides the SEIR mathematical model with the effect of social distancing, Sect. 4 gives the prediction model based on deep learning to find the propagation of corona, Sect. 5 provides the discussion on the inference of the models, and finally, the chapter concludes with conclusion of the work.

2 Related Work

In this section, a brief literature was done in terms of evolution of virus, virus propagation model using mathematics and time series prediction model in deep learning. Mathematical model is becoming an essential tool in modeling and analyzing the spread of virus with reproduction growth. The authors [7] used generalized Euler method and homotopy methods (HAM) to provide the solution for population dynamics in HIV virus, and also, they provided the numerical analysis of mathematical model. The traditional model susceptibility exposed infected recovered (SEIR) model showed the infection rate reached the peak when there were no counter measures were taken [8]. Machine learning methods are used to build corona formation, and also, prediction models like random forest showed the best result in terms of size, change of corona virus surface and change of formation and able to predict the corona protein formation in engineered nanomaterials [9]. The author has found that linear regression model is insufficient for analyzing time-dependent series. So, to predict the future values for pollution control within a time intervals, the SARIMA and prophet model are proposed [10]. The authors concluded that prophet forecasting models worked better in terms of log transmission with minimum value of RMSE and MSE values.

Another prediction model is ARIMA which predicts based on its historical data. The prediction model worked well for predicting the traffic flow. The authors used prophet models for analyzing and predicting the website traffic [11]. The novel idea is proposed by researchers [12] for analyzing the behavioral pattern of user smartphone by prophet algorithm to find out the continuous pattern and behavioral trend with the help of six daily behavioral patterns which are also used for training the model. The author [13] implemented prophet algorithm to analyze the result which was obtained by two different approaches. The variables were predicted in first approaches whereas the second approach used two variables like observed and forecasted values. Finally, the authors concluded the compared approaches are equally useful. The authors explored [14] the comparison model between BiLSTM and LSTM model by analyzing the performance and accuracy. The final result showed that adding extra layer during training, the accuracy gets improved by 38% for forecasting and also mentioned BiLSTM model gives good prediction when compared to ARIMA and LSTM prediction models. The spreading rate of COVID-19 has been increasing day by day. In order to slow down/control the virus propagation, social distancing plays an important role in society. The researchers [15] have used COVID-19 official data for analyzing the transmission model. Based on the existing data, the authors made prediction of virus outbreaks in future for South Korea, Iran and Italy.

3 SEIR Mathematical Modeling Based on Social Distancing

The outbreak of coronavirus is a kind of pandemic disease which brought a greater disturbance in all over the world. Even though China has been recovering, other countries are still suffering with increasing number of daily new cases which reach about $+16,730,990$ as on July 28. For analyzing the epidemic model, we have used SEIR model called compartmental model. SEIR represents the four segments, namely:

- Susceptible class
- Exposed class
- Infected class
- Recovered class.

Now, we are introducing three basic epidemiological quantities for modeling SEIR model. The first quantifier is infection rate denoted as β, where the number of people infected by single individual and probability of transmission rate. The second quantifier is recovery/death rate gamma γ which is the average ratio of the infected individuals which recover in the time unit and the final quantifier is sigma σ. The reproductive rate (R_0) of coronavirus can be defined as the ratio of infected rate and recovery rate which can be equated as in (1)

$$S' = -\beta S * \frac{I}{N}$$

$$E' = \beta S * \frac{I}{N} - \sigma E$$

$$I' = \sigma E - \gamma I$$

$$R' = \gamma I \tag{1}$$

where N = total population($S + E + I + R$), and this is a constant because $N' = S' + E' + I' + R' = 0$. We have considered ODE system with three parameters, namely β, γ and σ. For system (1), basic reproduction number is computed as below

$$R_0 = \frac{\beta}{\gamma}$$

Here we considered suitable positive real numbers for all vital parameters. The parameters values are $\beta = 0.3$, $\gamma = .09$ and $\sigma = 0.3$ where σ is termed as the rate at which an affected individual becomes infectious per unit time and also termed as symptoms development, γ is defined as the removal rate at which an infected person recovers per unit time, and β is termed as infection rate. The population size is N which is a constant and normalized to one. From Fig. 1, we can analyze the maximum infection occurs around 45th day and approaches zero after 100th day (i.e., the infection gets reduced by 100th day).

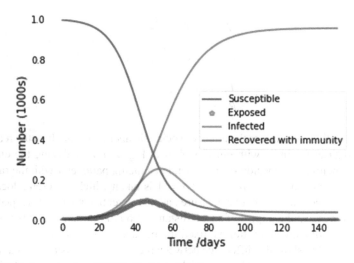

Fig. 1   SEIR dynamics for nCOVID-19

3.1   Social Distancing Applied for Coronavirus

One of the main characteristics of nCOVID-19 that makes spreading too fast to human beings where people would not have symptoms immediately but the infection keeps propagating to others without knowing them. There are only two methods to stop the pandemic such as vaccination/medicine and minimizing the contact with people which means reducing $R0$ value (i.e., reproduction number). Since there is no vaccination for nCOVID-19, we can control the spread of the pandemic by implementing social distancing/reducing the physical contact to each other. Social distancing refers avoiding contact huge gathering, minimum physical contact with everybody to reduce the spread of nCOVID-19. For our model, the term ρ(rho) is used to analyze the impact of social distancing for real-time population data. Here, the range is taken between 0 and 1, where 0 indicates fully isolated/quarantined and 1 indicates no one is locked down which is similar to the above model. In our study, we defined the terms for different levels of social distancing as mentioned below:

- No preventive measure: People are allowed to lead the normal life.
- Airport screening: Basic screening process has done only at airport.
- Self-isolation and quarantine: Infected people are quarantined.
- Schools and college closed: All schools and colleges are shut down on account of social distancing.
- Restrictions of travels.
- Full lockdown: Lockdown has been implemented around the globe.

To illustrate the effect of social distancing in controlling the spread, we introduce the parameter rho in the system (1) which is presented below.

$$S' = -\rho\beta S * \frac{I}{N}$$

$$E' = \rho\beta S * \frac{I}{N} - \sigma E$$

$$I' = \sigma E - \gamma I$$

$$R' = \gamma I \tag{2}$$

In this section, we discuss the effect of social distancing and analyze the real-time infected dataset for India with our model as in Fig. 2. For analyzing the effect of social distancing, ρ is considered as a social distancing parameter with the range of 0 to 1. As discussed before, $\rho = 0$ and $\rho = 1$ is taken which represents lockdown has implemented with preventive measure and no preventive measures, respectively. Figure 3 represents the impact of social distancing on the spread of nCOVID-19. In this case of India affected ratio, we fixed the parameters of ρ which varies as 0.9, 0.6, 0.4 and 0.2 to show the difference between the each social distancing parameter. From Fig. 3, we can analyze the peak of the infection if high when $\rho = 0.9$ whereas, the infection peak gets decreasing when ρ is reducing. Failing to adopt necessary measures of social distancing will turn out in high infection and death rate which will affect the whole healthcare system. As more and more measures are taken, infection is delayed, and the maximum peak is reduced considerably as represented in Fig. 3 so that medical care can be arranged and managed for all infective people.

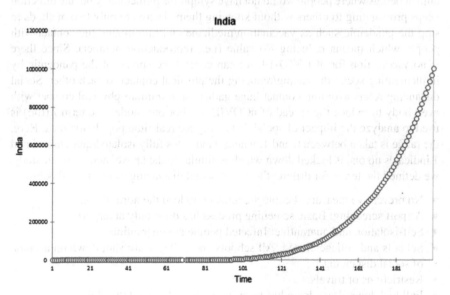

Fig. 2 Daily affected cases in India

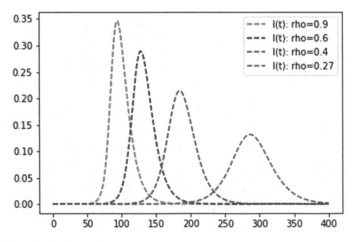

Fig. 3 Effect of social distancing

4   Time Series Analysis of Corona

A time series model is termed as a sequence of random points which is measured over successive times [16]. Mathematically, it is defined as a set of vectors $y(t)$, where t represents the time and $y(t)$ is treated as a random variable. The proper chronological order is arranged during the event. There are three kinds of time series variables which are used, such as univariate, bivariate and multivariate. A time series event containing only one variable is termed as univariate. An event containing two variables is termed as bivariate, whereas a time series event consisting of more than two variables is known as multivariate. According the worldwide affected data from Our World in Data website, the timeline analysis based on affected count around the globe is shown in Figs. 4 and 5. Time series is a collection of time intervals arranged in equal intervals and ordered chronologically. The collection of time interval is often referred as a time series frequency. A plot of time series often plotted as observed values will be placed on the y-axis and the time increment on the x-axis.

4.1   ARIMA

The term ARIMA stands for autoregressive integrated moving average which is a forecasting methodology based on the past events of time series comprised of date and time which is used to predict the future values. This model is categorized into three terms, and they are: P, D, Q
    where
    P is the order of autoregressive (AR).
    Q is the order of moving average (MA).

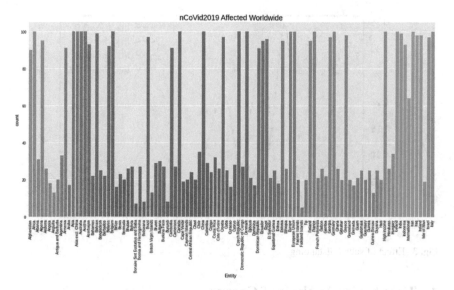

Fig. 4 Countries affected by coronavirus

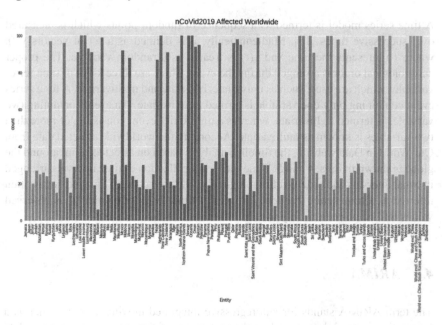

Fig. 5 Countries affected by coronavirus

D is the order of differencing.

ARIMA model is a linear regression model which uses its lag for predicting the future. The main approach in ARIMA model is to differencing which means subtracting the previous values from current values. Sometimes, more than one differencing is also needed based on the complexity of the problem. The term p refers to number of lags of Y used as predictors, and q refers to a lagged error present in this model. The AR model is represented in following equation.

$$X_t = \alpha + \beta_1 X_{t-1} + \beta_2 X_{t-2} + \cdots + \beta_n X_{t-n} + \in_1$$

$$X_t = \alpha + \sum_{m=1}^{n} \beta_m X_{t-m} + \in_1 \tag{3}$$

where X_{t-m} is the lag of the model, β_m is the coefficient of lag which estimates the model and α is the intercept term. Here, n represents the old value to forecast the value at the present observations. Like AR model, MA model is also developed where it depends on forecast error, and also, it is represented in the following equation,

$$X_t = \alpha + \varepsilon_t + \phi_1 \varepsilon_{t-1} + \phi_2 \varepsilon_{t-2} + \cdots + \phi_n \varepsilon_{t-n} \tag{4}$$

Here, ε_t is the error of autoregressive models and ε_{t-1} is represented in following equations.

$$X_t = \beta_1 X_{t-1} + \beta_2 X_{t-2} + \cdots + \beta_n X_n + \varepsilon_t$$
$$X_{t-1} = \beta_1 X_{t-2} + \beta_2 X_{t-3} + \cdots + \beta_n X_n + \varepsilon_{t-1} \tag{5}$$

From the above Eqs. (3), (4) and (5) of AR and MA model, we can combine the final equation of ARIMA model as below.

$$X_t = \alpha + \beta_1 X_{t-1} + \beta_2 Y_{t-2} + \beta_n X_{t-n} \varepsilon_t$$
$$+ \phi_1 \varepsilon_{t-1} + \phi_2 \varepsilon_{t-2} + \cdots + \phi_n \varepsilon_n \tag{6}$$

In this section, the author has discussed about the ARIMA modeling to forecast the future values of corona virus for next 30 days (i.e., from July 17, 2020).

The prediction model results are shown in Tables 1, 2 and 3 which show the fitness of the model, the standard error, upper bound, lower bound values which are set as 95%, and Table 3 represents the prediction values and residuals value, respectively.

In this section, we have analyzed the affected cases in India by using ARIMA model. The dataset comprised of total infected cases from Dec 31, 2019, to July 17, 2020. The prediction model shown in Fig. 6 shows the infection rate for next 30 days. Figure 7 represents the residual model with time step of infected cases.

Autocorrelation and partial autocorrelation plots are most widely used in all types of time series and prediction. This plot represents the relationship with an observation values in a time series with prior time vales of observation. The lags can be

Table 1 ARIMA fit statistics

Goodness of fit statistics	
Observations	174
DF	169
SSE	33,908,720.2
MSE	194,877.702
RMSE	441.449547
WN variance	194,877.702
MAPE(Diff)	379.4727
MAPE	352.726364
−2Log(Like.)	2628.18939
FPE	197,130.624
AIC	2638.18939
AICC	2638.54653
SBC	2653.98466
Iterations	13

Table 2 AR, MA and SMA bound values

Parameter	Value	Hessian standard error	Lower bound (95%)	Upper bound (95%)	Asympt. standard error	Lower bound (95%)	Upper bound (95%)
AR(1)	0.998	0.003	0.992	1.004	0.005	0.988	1.008
MA(1)	0.215	0.066	0.085	0.345	0.075	0.068	0.362
SMA(1)	−0.799	0.075	−0.946	−0.652	0.047	−0.891	−0.708

calculated by time series observation values with existing value (previous) time step. The correlation of the time series is calculated with a same series at previous times which is known as autocorrelation. Figures 8 and 9 show the autocorrelation and partial autocorrelation model for affected cases of nCOVID-19.

Descriptive Analysis India
   See Figs. 8 and 9.

Descriptive Analysis (Residuals)
   The autocorrelation of nCOVID-19 time series by lag is called Autocorrelation function (ACF) which is also termed as correlogram. Generally, the confidence level of upper and lower bound is set to 95%. The descriptive analysis of residuals for ACR and PACR is shown in Figs. 10 and 11.

Table 3 ARIMA prediction and residual values for nCOVID

Predictions and residuals					
Observations	India	ARIMA (India)	Residuals	Lower bound (95%)	Upper bound (95%)
1	0.000	0.000	0.000		
2	0.000	0.000	0.000		
3	0.000	0.000	0.000		
…	…	…	…		
23	0.000	70.109	−70.109		
24	0.000	72.062	−72.062		
25	0.000	74.128	−74.128		
26	0.000	68.497	−68.497		
⋮					
197	936,181.000	919,217.863	16,963.137	899,257.338	939,178.388
198	968,876.000	945,463.813	23,412.187	922,548.006	968,379.619
199	1,003,832.000	972,152.344	31,679.656	946,152.062	998,152.625
200		997,299.294		968,011.582	1,026,587.006
201		1,022,829.871		990,053.440	1,055,606.302
202		1,048,400.999		1,011,951.815	1,084,850.183
203		1,074,291.358		1,033,999.282	1,114,583.435
204		1,100,505.373		1,056,211.628	1,144,799.117
205		1,126,685.929		1,078,241.190	1,175,130.667
206		1,153,005.739		1,100,268.661	1,205,742.818
207		1,179,474.402		1,122,310.479	1,236,638.324
208		1,206,181.719		1,144,462.392	1,267,901.046
209		1,233,386.573		1,166,988.507	1,299,784.638
210		1,261,132.508		1,189,937.015	1,332,328.001
211		1,289,317.753		1,213,210.311	1,365,425.195
212		1,315,958.153		1,234,767.627	1,397,148.678
213		1,342,978.922		1,256,530.612	1,429,427.232
214		1,370,036.992		1,278,165.529	1,461,908.456
215		1,397,411.051		1,299,959.327	1,494,862.775
216		1,425,105.529		1,321,923.778	1,528,287.279
217		1,452,763.319		1,343,708.328	1,561,818.310
218		1,480,557.142		1,365,491.571	1,595,622.713
219		1,508,496.602		1,387,288.406	1,629,704.798
220		1,536,671.509		1,409,193.435	1,664,149.583
221		1,565,340.752		1,431,469.908	1,699,211.596

(continued)

Table 3 (continued)

Predictions and residuals					
Observations	India	ARIMA (India)	Residuals	Lower bound (95%)	Upper bound (95%)
222		1,594,547.882		1,454,165.360	1,734,930.405
223		1,624,191.136		1,477,181.683	1,771,200.589
224		1,652,286.364		1,498,487.103	1,806,085.624
225		1,680,758.789		1,520,002.601	1,841,514.976
226		1,709,265.348		1,541,391.895	1,877,138.800
227		1,738,084.737		1,562,939.907	1,913,229.567
228		1,767,221.392		1,584,656.793	1,949,785.991
229		1,796,318.215		1,606,190.724	1,986,445.706

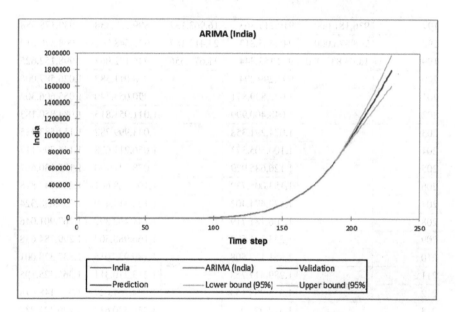

Fig. 6 Prediction model for India dataset

4.2 Prophet Time Series

Prophet is one of the time series algorithms, and it is an open-source software that can be implemented in Python and *R* for predicting the time series data. It was first published by Facebook data science team. When an LSTM algorithm gives lesser prediction than we expected, we used Prophet time series for forecasting the coronavirus infection for next 30 days. The prophet time series works with three main components, namely trend, seasonality and holidays. The following Eq. (4) is

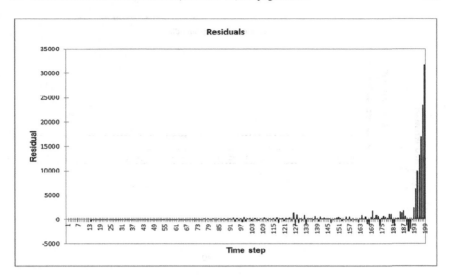

Fig. 7   Residuals model of nCOVID-19

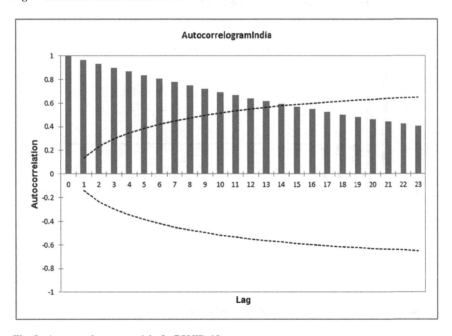

Fig. 8   Autocorrelogram model of nCOVID-19

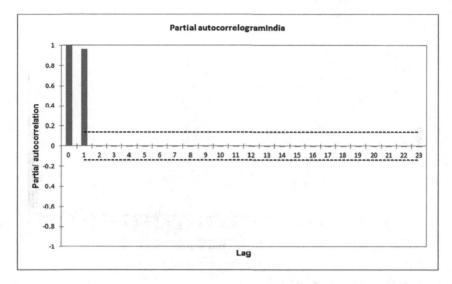

Fig. 9 Partial Autocorrelogram model of nCOVID-19

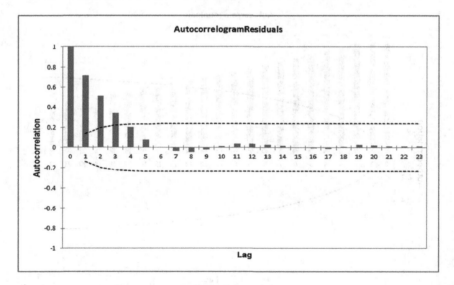

Fig. 10 Autocorrelogram residual model of nCOVID-19

used for a prophet time series prediction.

$$y(i) = g(i) + s(i) + h(i) + \in t \tag{7}$$

- $g(i)$—The time series with linear or logistic curve.
- $s(i)$—The occurrence of changes in terms of days, weeks, year or seasonality.

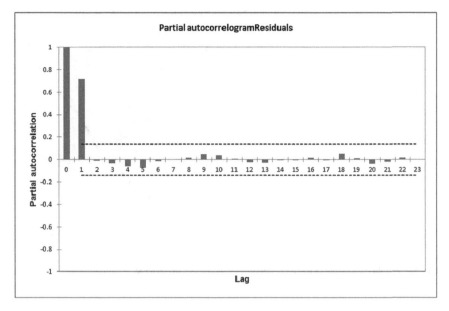

Fig. 11 Partial autocorrelogram residual model of nCOVID-19

- $h(i)$—The irregular data in effects of holidays.
- $\in (i)$—The error rate.

In this part, we analyzed forecasting for affected cases around India. The dataset comprised of total infected cases from Dec 31 2019 to July 17, 2020. The prediction model shown in Fig. 12 shows that infection will get increased till Aug 16 since prediction model is limited to 30 days. The prophet model analyzed the forecast components which includes trend, weekly and yearly components. In Fig. 13, there is an overall upward trend of coronavirus which forecasted till Aug 16, 2020.

Table 4 represents an extract result obtained from prophet prediction using nCOVID-19 dataset. In the prediction column, the India feature represents the daily affected cases with corresponding date. Based on it, the prophet forecasting was done for another 30 days (i.e. till Aug 16).

This type of time series allows us to predict the future based on past events. In prophet model, we can analyze the model effect according to weekly and yearly basis as shown in Fig. 14. Since our observations comprised of months and weeks, the output for yearly basis is not produced.

5   Discussion

Even though we have predicted the pandemic evolution of nCOVID-19, it is hard to evaluate the accuracy of prediction model. Due to the lack of reliable data from each

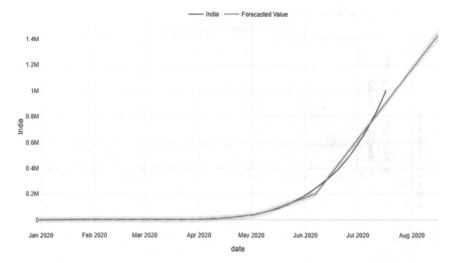

Fig. 12 Prophet forecasting for total infected case around worldwide

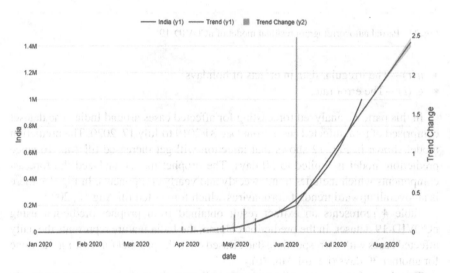

Fig. 13 Trend value analyses for total affected cases in India

website leads difficulty to trace the outbreak model. The mathematical and prediction modeling helped us in predicting and evaluating the evolution of pandemic outbreak through maintaining the social distancing also. From our study, we presented an earlier prediction of pandemic of nCOVID-19 based on SEIR model and time series analysis. The real-time epidemiological coronavirus data were initially analyzed to obtain the infection rate. In second section, the basic epidemic SEIR model without social distancing effort, whereas the next subsection includes the effort of social distancing which mitigates the effect of virus spreading. The author has used the

Table 4 Summary of prophet prediction from our study

Date	India	Forecasted_value	Forecasted_value_high	Forecasted_value_low
31-12-2019	0	−740.343178	20,573.06306	−24,644.44325
01-01-2020	0	−444.5891572	21,752.6354	−23,832.86577
02-01-2020	0	117.3582923	24,023.4588	−21,091.33523
03-01-2020	0	975.1128657	25,007.36878	−21,095.94388
⋮				
01-04-2020	1397	2129.439739	25,913.19147	−20,827.48429
02-04-2020	1965	3102.83033	26,803.89846	−20,794.00197
⋮				
15-07-2020	936,181	869,804.2182	893,132.1329	847,826.3304
16-07-2020	968,876	887,923.748	911,403.0247	863,110.4561
17-07-2020	1,003,832	906,339.0849	930,663.0998	882,644.3848
18-07-2020		920,929.3345	941,928.1191	897,223.7214
19-07-2020		939,298.394	964,470.1892	916,341.7961
20-07-2020		957,173.1083	979,790.5395	935,779.7143
21-07-2020		974,934.4001	997,788.3863	953,008.7155
22-07-2020		992,787.7364	1,017,066.702	969,695.7694
23-07-2020		1,010,907.266	1,032,975.49	988,643.6996
24-07-2020		1,029,322.603	1,053,282.121	1,005,260.261
25-07-2020		1,043,912.853	1,066,705.872	1,020,356.744
26-07-2020		1,062,281.912	1,085,386.879	1,037,651.511
27-07-2020		1,080,156.626	1,103,574.639	1,053,478.117
28-07-2020		1,097,917.918	1,123,039.78	1,071,994.354
29-07-2020		1,115,771.255	1,140,971.398	1,090,372.615
30-07-2020		1,133,890.784	1,159,673.154	1,107,202.949
31-07-2020		1,152,306.121	1,178,088.449	1,125,323.07
01-08-2020		1,166,896.371	1,194,225.811	1,139,250.291
02-08-2020		1,185,265.43	1,212,078.53	1,157,377.067
03-08-2020		1,203,140.145	1,231,420.781	1,172,936.2
04-08-2020		1,220,901.436	1,248,911.095	1,190,589.351
05-08-2020		1,238,754.773	1,268,478.449	1,205,653.581
06-08-2020		1,256,874.303	1,286,873.288	1,225,823.323
07-08-2020		1,275,289.639	1,308,040.81	1,240,272.637
08-08-2020		1,289,879.889	1,323,548.644	1,256,510.001
09-08-2020		1,308,248.949	1,342,088	1,272,561.635
10-08-2020		1,326,123.663	1,360,570.611	1,289,070.19

(continued)

Table 4 (continued)

Date	India	Forecasted_value	Forecasted_value_high	Forecasted_value_low
11-08-2020		1,343,884.955	1,377,669.411	1,303,590.368
12-08-2020		1,361,738.291	1,401,312.09	1,325,004.165
13-08-2020		1,379,857.821	1,420,269.411	1,337,229.28
14-08-2020		1,398,273.158	1,442,094.122	1,355,265.481
15-08-2020		1,412,863.407	1,455,886.844	1,366,931.799
16-08-2020		1,431,232.467	1,474,496.184	1,383,576.262

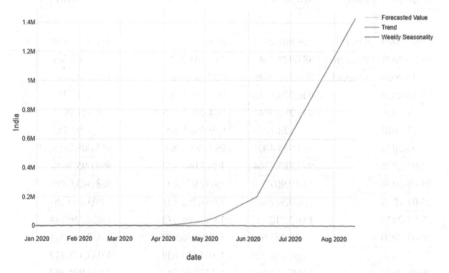

Fig. 14 Analysis of trend and weekly seasonality of predicted model

data from Our World in Data website for forecasting model which consists of real-time data about coronavirus for different ranges. Based on these data, the author has predicted for 30 more days which may lead to huge uncertainty outbreak in upcoming days. The spread of coronavirus is largely increasing due to physical contact, and this in turns infection and death rate are exponentially increasing. World Health Organization (WHO) and the Disease Control and Prevention Centers (CDC) have provided guidelines to control the spread of virus by social distancing, quarantine and self-isolation which are some best options to reduce the spread of nCOVID-19. One of the major problems is lack of medical equipment's which includes masks, ventilators, medical personals and also proper drug for treating infected patients. According to the source [17] reporting, doctors in New York are facing apocalyptic scenarios of infection, death and lack of medical equipment to protect the people and healthcare takers from deadly infection.

6 Conclusion

Our mathematical modeling based on SEIR was more effective in analyzing and modeling the nCOVID-19 pandemic propagation. Furthermore, the effect of social distancing works well for flattening the curve of real-time data for India affected cases in order to reduce the spread of disease and also we implemented deep learning model based on time series for forecasting the epidemic. Prophet time series model represents the early prediction of nCOVID-19 which helps us to take preventive measure and take necessary steps like social distancing to stop the spread of virus.

References

1. Anthony SJ et al (2017) Global patterns in coronavirus diversity, vol 3, no 1, pp 1–15
2. Spreeuwenberg P, Kroneman M, Paget J (2018) Reassessing the global mortality burden of the 1918 influenza pandemic. Am J Epidemiol 187(12) https://doi.org/10.1093/aje/kwy191
3. https://www.worldometers.info/coronavirus/
4. Torgan C (2015) Lymphatic vessels discovered in central nervous system. Office of Communications and Public Liaison. National Institutes of Health (U.S.) [Online]. Available: https://www.nih.gov/news-events/nih-research-matters/lymphatic-vessels-discovered-central-nervous-system. Accessed: 17 Mar 2020
5. Javaid M, Haleem A, Vaishya R, Bahl S, Suman R (2020) Diabetes & metabolic syndrome: clinical research & reviews industry 4.0 technologies and their applications in fighting COVID-19 pandemic. Diab Metab Syndr Clin Res Rev 14(4):419–422
6. Roser M, Ritchie H, Ortiz-Ospina E, Hasell J (2020) Coronavirus pandemic (COVID-19). Published online at OurWorldInData.org. Retrieved from https://ourworldindata.org/coronavirus
7. Arafa AAM, Rida SZ, Khalil M (2013) The effect of anti-viral drug treatment of human immunodeficiency virus type 1 (HIV-1) described by a fractional order model. Appl Math Model 37(4):2189–2196
8. Zhou Tang, Xianbin Li, Houqiang Li (2020) Prediction of New Coronavirus Infection Based on a Modified SEIR Model. medRxiv. https://doi.org/10.1101/2020.03.03.20030858
9. Duan Y et al (2020) Prediction of protein corona on nanomaterials by machine learning using novel descriptors. NanoImpact 17:100207
10. Samal KKR, Babu KS, Das SK, Acharaya A (2019) Time series based air pollution forecasting using SARIMA and prophet model. In: ACM international conference proceeding series, pp 80–85
11. Subashini A, Sandhiya K, Saranya S, Harsha U (2019) Forecasting website traffic using prophet time series model. Int Res J Multidiscip Technovation 1(1):56–63
12. Chunmin M, Runjie X, Lin C (2019) Real-time recognition of smartphone user behavior based on prophet algorithms, pp 4–6
13. Tyralis H, Papacharalampous GA (2018) Large-scale assessment of prophet for multi-step ahead forecasting of monthly streamflow. Adv Geosci 45(2017):147–153
14. Siami-namini S, Tavakoli N, Namin AS (2019) A comparative analysis of forecasting financial time series using ARIMA, LSTM, and BiLSTM

15. Li L, Yang Z, Dang Z, Meng C, Huang J, Meng HT (2020) Propagation analysis and prediction of the COVID-19 main results, vol 12
16. Adhikari R, Agrawal RK (2013) An introductory study on time series modeling and forecasting. arXiv Prepr. arXiv 1302.6613
17. Mary V. https://www.cidrap.umn.edu/news-perspective/2020/03/what-can-hospitals-still-do-prep-covid-19

Chapter 12
Innovative Strategies to Understand and Control COVID-19 Disease

Sadia Qamar, Amna Syeda, and M. Irfan Qureshi

1 Introduction

The disease coronavirus known as COVID-19 was first reported in 2019, mid-December in China (Wuhan) with the causative agent of the disease Severe Acute Respiratory Syndrome Coronavirus-2 (SARS-CoV-2). The health specialist of Wuhan claims that they noticed a few cases of unusual pneumonia and consecutively researched till discovered that the causal agent was coronavirus, published genome sequence of the same. It was discovered that the causal agent of this disease was the RNA virus relative to a similar group of coronavirus that has caused the Middle East Respiratory Syndrome (MERS) pandemic in 2012 and Severe Acute Respiratory Syndrome pandemic (SARS) in 2003 [1]. In total, 215 countries have been reported with cases of COVID-19, and the total number touched above 26.66 million as of September 04, 2020; the USA is the most (about 6.3 million), followed by Brazil (4.0 million), India (4.5 million) and Russia (1.0 million). India is reporting the largest number of daily cases (87,115 on Sep 04, 2020). In total, 876,203 deaths and around 18.8 million recovered cases so far. Earlier, the Emergency Committee of WHO on January 30, 2020 declared SARS-CoV-2-borne disease a worldwide health emergency and gave the disease an official name on Feb 11, 2020 as COVID-19. The disease has raised worldwide concern due to its very high rate of transmission, infectivity, and a high number of deaths.

Coronaviruses belong to the family Coronaviridae, and they were termed subsequently for their crown-shaped spikes present on the surface of the virus. Coronaviruses are sub-divided into alpha, beta, and gamma and also delta to date (Fig. 1).

S. Qamar · A. Syeda · M. Irfan Qureshi (✉)
Proteomics and Bioinformatics Lab, Department of Biotechnology, Jamia Millia Islamia, Delhi, India
e-mail: mirfanq@gmail.com

S. Qamar
e-mail: zadiaqamar11@gmail.com

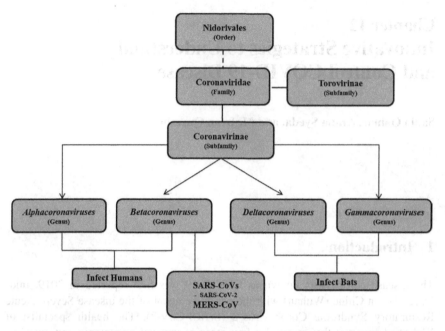

Fig. 1 A member of order Nidorivales, family Coronavirinae has four genera including *Betacoronaviruses*; SARS-CoVs (e.g., SARS-CoV-2), MERS-CoV, etc.

The genome of SARS-CoV-2 ranges from 27 to 32 Kb, and it belongs to the RNA virus family. Coronavirus is an enveloped, single-stranded positive-sense RNA virus having a poly-A tail at 3′ and cap structure at 5′ [2]. The virus has four structural proteins which are the spike protein (S), a viral envelope protein (E), membrane protein (M), and inner nucleocapsid protein (N) which are essential for the proper assembly, maintaining its structure, and also required to regulate its function [3]. The most important structural proteins among these four are the S protein and N protein.

The N protein helps the virus for capsid development and the structure of the virus properly, and S protein helps the virus in the attachment to the host cells [4]. The spike protein is composed of three sections consisting of the anchor domain, large ectodomain, and an intracellular tail. These play the foremost role in attaching to the cells of the host. Furthermore, ectodomain is divided into two subunits S1 and S2, where the former is the receptor binding and the S2 subunit is the membrane fusion subunit. And since these subunits possess a crown-shaped structure or clove trimeric form, so that is why coronavirus is named (crown = corona) [5]. It has also been found that both SARS-CoV-2 and the SARS-CoV have a similar type of receptors mainly the receptor-binding motif (RBM) and the receptor-binding domain (RBD) [6]. During the SARS infection, the receptor-binding motif of the spike protein gets attached directly to the ACE2 in the host or human cells [7]. The protein angiotensin-converting enzyme-2 is known to be expressed in several organs chiefly in the lungs, intestine, and kidney which are the major targets of the unique SARS-CoV-2 [8].

Moreover, coronavirus infects the human or host cell through the receptor of ACE2 leading to pneumonia, damage to the cardiovascular system, and acute myocardial damage [9].

Mode of Transmission

The transmission of SARS-CoV-2, according to current reports, started from the human seafood market in Wuhan, China, where selling wild animals might be the cause of the zoonotic infection. It is claimed that bats are the likely reservoir of the virus before spreading to humans from pangolins [10]. Numerous studies have recorded the transmission of SARS-CoV-2 from humans to humans via direct contact between humans or the virus-containing droplets coming as a result of talking, coughing, or sneezing from an infected person [11]. Nearby contamination of the virus occurs via large droplets, while small droplets containing the virus tend to be air-borne and thus lead to transmission of the viral particles across long distances [12]. Traveling between cities and nations has been so frequent and convenient in today's time which has added to spreading the viral infection at a much higher rate [13]. A major reason for the marked increase in the infected cases across the globe is the rapid rate of spreading the infection and the asymptomatic carriers which led to the escalation of the disease, thus becoming a pandemic. Some recent reports have suggested the possible transmission of the SAR-CoV-2 virus from humans to their pets such as dogs and cats [14]. The detail of how the transmission occurred is still been studied. The most susceptible to rapid transmission is the elderly people and those already suffering from underlying medical conditions such as cancer, lung infections, heart disease, and hypertension; hence, utmost care is required for such a group of people.

2 Potential Strategies for Study and Diagnosis of Disease

The COVID-19 disease has originated unique human health and also a financial crisis. The extent of the crisis has called an urgent response worldwide from the scientists, medical specialists, and the governing officials. This crisis demands some immediate innovative solutions. To meet the increasing demands, the use of innovative technologies has been proposed. This chapter is the description of the novel emergent technologies to limit the threat of disease development and treatment for the prevention and cure of COVID-19. The potential strategies used in the study and also in the diagnosis of the diseases are described.

2.1 Bioelectronics and Biosensors

Biosensing is a tool that detects biochemical or biological agents by using a biomimetic or biologically derived element while either binding the target molecule called analyte or undergoing a biochemical reaction (such as the use of enzyme-based biosensors). This binding result can thus transduce a signal directly (surface plasmon resonance or impedance measurements) or by using other signaling molecules (such as optically active compounds, fluorophores, and enzymes) as labels [15]. Recently, two biosensing unamplified systems utilizing CRISPR technology have been introduced. One is used for analyses of microRNA (electrochemical CRISPR) biosensor, and the other is used for the detection of the genetic mutation (CRISPR chip) employing Cas9 [16]. Moreover, CRISPR-based biosensor would also target the two distinctive genomic sequence of SARS-CoV-2 (RdRP gene and E gene) simultaneously. Also, CRISPR-biosensors technology can address mutations in the genome of SARS-CoV-2 in a specific way. Another approach that is recently demonstrated is an optical biosensor combing localized surface plasmon resonance and plasmonic photothermal effect to distinguish a similar sequence of genes with high diagnostic sensitivity [17]. An alternative appropriate way is the use of sensor material (substrate) that can be functionalized with the recombinant antigens of the virus and further can be used for binding the immunoglobulins. Through this method, it becomes feasible to detect a history of past-COVID-19 infection (through IgG) and also used to identify the presence of coronavirus infection (through IgM) [18]. These devices are a necessary tool for monitoring the SARS-CoV-2 infection using plasma, blood, or even a drop of human serum.

2.2 Artificial Intelligence

Artificial intelligence has a wide range of applications and features that can be applied to help our response to coronavirus disease. Researchers have used various models like deep and machine learning models to identify and to study COVID-19 treatment. The machine learning permits the viral genomes datasets study and hence can upsurge our basic information of the coronavirus disease. To identify the probable origin and also to provide a precise taxonomic classification of the novel COVID-19, scientists have employed models of machine learning [19]. Control of the pandemic usually relies on the accurate and early diagnosis of the disease. Artificial intelligence based on deep learning and machine learning models was proposed by Mei et al. that combines clinical information (such as history of exposure, laboratory test results, and reported systems) with the demographic information (such as sex, age) with results of chest imaging for speedy identification of the COVID-19 patients [20]. Also, imaging modalities have worked as a tool for COVID-19 detection, observing the disease course, and evaluating the complications. To meet the challenges, artificial intelligence has empowered various imaging approaches such as X-rays and CT scans by providing reliability and accuracy [21]. Deep learning models have also been used recently to develop a CT scan system which can identify patients of COVID-19 and also measure the infection burden [22]. Application of artificial intelligence software usually decreases the need for annotations of the radiologist, thereby lifting a major burden from the medical staff [23]. An artificial intelligence model also predicts high mortality problems development such as acute respiratory distress syndrome. This property could be utilized to identify the features of the disease presentation at the initial stage; these features are the occurrence of myalgias, elevated level of hemoglobin, mildly raised alanine aminotransferase [24]. The principles based on machine learning can also be useful in predicting whether commercially available drugs can be used for the cure of disease.

2.3   Mathematical Modeling

For the prediction of the transmission rate of COVID-19, the mathematical modeling tool has been at lead nowadays. Mathematical models include a set of differential equations that are known to mimic the actuality and can further be refined to get novel information about the virus. To discover probable scenarios of the spread of the epidemic, this interplay is very essential. Scientists everywhere in the domain are giving their best to capture the interaction among various factors that are ranging from individuals or micro-pathogens or interplay between populations, interaction with the environment, demographic conditions, and socio-economic conditions. Models which have been used generally for various infectious disease are susceptible–infected–recovered (SIR), individual-based models (IBM), and susceptible–exposed–infected–recovered (SEIR). The new models that have been developed during the pandemic COVID-19 are the stereographic Brownian diffusion epidemiology model used to explain the spread of the virus [25, 26]. Substantial facts about the spread of the virus remain unidentified, hence limiting the accuracy of predictions.

2.4   3D Printing

3D printing is emerging quickly and could help design medical equipment and can provide desirable materials more readily at a cheaper cost. This disease has caused a global scarcity of significant medical supplies, which also includes protective equipment (face shields, facemasks, and also goggles) [27]. The 3D laser allows scanning and measurement of the parameters of the face, thus enabling the fabrication of personalized masks [28]. To avoid efficiently the droplets and air from entering the edges, face masks should be fitted properly. Protective face shields can also be made using the open-source data with suitable material, i.e., biodegradable, and hence allowing on-demand production at home [29]. The 3D technology utilization would further increase access to these medical supplies. This technology can also help in the making of oropharyngeal and nasopharyngeal swab tests. The 3D printing aid in the fabrication of these materials would permit populating testing. Furthermore, this technology can also be used for ventilators splitters production with flexible flow control valves which enable two patients to use the same ventilator at the same time with different requirements of oxygen. Application of 3D printing can also revolutionize the production of equipment in terms of their efficiency, cost, and quantity.

2.5 Big Data

With the design of the big data for the analytics of important information from all over the domain can be made easily available to the doctors, scientists, the epidemiologists, and also to the policymakers. Big data has been demonstrated to be a suitable device for rapid real-time assessments [30]. Big data could play a significant role in checking coronavirus-related hospital outbreaks. The provision and storage of contact history and individual travel history permit the screening and tracing to be done for all visitors and patients before they come to the medical facility. The government in Taiwan has included and also examined various big data from Taiwan centers for disease control, the National Immigration Agency, and the National Health Insurance Administration. This has delivered the actual evidence for the quarantine station of each clinic and hospital in the state. Thereby, all the visitors are separated through personal documentation and any doubted carriers are examined before entering [31]. This type of model might assist a way to limit the spread of disease. This type of framework could be applied to permit quicker immigration allowance at sea borders and at airports. For instance, in Taiwan, the NIA and NHIA launched the entry quarantine method, and this method also uses the past fourteen-day travel history along with their ID card data for the screening of coronavirus. The date from this travel history is made at the phase of arrival or departure at the Taiwan airport. Travelers at this time are necessary to complete a health declaration form.

2.6 Robotics

Robotics can be used to decrease the risk of coronavirus in both patient and provider. As compared to the open surgery and conventional laparoscopy robotics surgery affords safer alternate in terms of COVID-19. Robotics can reduce direct exposure of medical staff and perform various procedures. Remote controlled or autonomous robots can execute ultraviolet surface sterilization through intelligent navigation and also through the identification of high-touch/high-risk zones [32]. Robotics can collect the daily measurements of temperature in patients suffering from coronavirus independently. Furthermore, robotics can also conduct independently the nasopharyngeal swab tests [31]. Robotics used to carry these functions would decrease the direct contact of staff with novel coronavirus infected patients and would also let the staff distribute their time toward the other patients [33]. Drones and unmanned aerial vehicle (UAV) can also recognize the carriers of the COVID-19. Unmanned aerial vehicles can detect the temperature of the ground surface at certain heights and send the optical images thermal images captured, measured data, and also the GPS map location to the server. UAVs can also be used to take the body temperature and thus enable us to identify COVID-19 patients at a very early stage. Additionally, this technology reduces mortality by enabling the distribution of test kits equipment and medical supplies in areas hard to reach [34].

2.7 Theranostic Nanoparticles

The size, charge, low toxicity, and chemical modification abilities of the NPs help them to overcome several barriers. For the delivery of numerous therapeutic moieties such as drug, antibodies, vaccine, and peptides, various efforts have been made for the development of nanoparticles based intranasal delivery systems as a safe and effective tool. The nanoparticles used in the medical field are known to hold great potential in diagnostic solutions and the development of novel theranostic for treating COVID-19. Since SARS-CoV-2 has a diameter of about 125 nm, and thus, fitting in the nanoscale range and thus biocompatible NP can be very favorable to detect and simultaneously to neutralize the novel coronavirus by various approaches as investigated previously against several viral infections such as MERS and SARS coronavirus. These theranostic NPs can increase the delivery of various therapeutic drugs, delivery of peptide inhibitors, specific and selective delivery of siRNA, stimulate the immune system, and prevent the entry of coronavirus into the cell. Hence, NP could be a promising method to combat coronavirus.

3 Current Strategies Used for the Treatment of COVID-19

3.1 Immunological Approaches

Convalescent plasma: Convalescent plasma is chosen usually when there is no particular drug or vaccine available for the emerging infectious disease. It can be employed for passive immunotherapy. A favorable result has been reported by Yeh et al. for using convalescent plasma for the cure of healthcare workers infected with the SARS-CoV [35]. The possibility, safety, and also clinical efficacy of the convalescent plasma in ill patients suffering from the infection of MERS-CoV was tested by Chen et al. [36]. Convalescent plasma, if obtainable could be considered for the cure of patients infected with the SARS-CoV2.

Monoclonal antibodies (mAbs): Biological drugs that are composed of the mAbs have been produced for the cure of several illnesses. This method is also being considered for SARS-CoV treatment and shows promising results. A human IgG1 monoclonal antibody known as CR3022 that is known to bind S protein of SARS-CoV has been developed [37]. The mAbs could neutralize SARS-CoV efficiently and also inhibit the formation of syncytia in between the cells expressing the ACE2 receptor of the SARS-CoV and those expressing the spike protein [38]. Another human IgG1 monoclonal antibody called CR3014 has been produced and found that it can impede the infection of coronavirus in ferrets and also neutralize the SARS-CoV [39]. Recently, Ju et al. described isolation followed by characterization of the 206 RBD-specific monoclonal antibodies which is derived from the single B-cells of individuals infected with the SARS-CoV-2 [40]. These mAbs can be used for prevention as well as for the cure of SARS-CoV-2. Those agents which block the S protein binding of the ACE2 receptor might also have the potential to be used for COVID-19 treatment.

Blockers of cytokine: Production of cytokines is the underlying disease process in COVID-19 severe cases, and thus, neutralization of certain cytokines may be considered as an innovative method for the treatment of such disease and also decreasing the rate of mortality and morbidity. It was reported by Huang et al. that in coronavirus infection increased level of IP-10, IFN-γ, IL-1ß, and MCP-1 and greater concentration of TNF-α, G-CSF, MCP-1A, and MCP-1 were found in those patients needing cure at ICU than those who are not treated at the ICU [41]. Also, it was reported by Conti P et al. that the pro-inflammatory cytokines such as IL-6 and (IL)-1β are associated with lung fibrosis development in COVID-19 [42]. And the suppression of these pro-inflammatory cytokines might have a significant therapeutic effect. One immunosuppressive cytokine known as IL-37 acts on mTOR and further increases adenosine monophosphate kinase activity which suppresses the production of numerous cytokines including TNF, IL-6, and IL-1β and thus inhibits inflammation. IL-37 cytokine could be a possible therapeutic agent for inhibiting the inflammation [42]. In future, cytokine blocker targeting the receptor of IL-6 in COVID-19 may be developed as a therapeutic agent. FDA approved mAbs against interleukin-6 receptors which are available for the cure of rheumatoid arthritis. This is promising that the pharmaceutical corporations have initiated the clinical trials of the anti-interleukin-6 receptor for coronavirus treatment. Various immunological approaches used in the treatment of COVID-19 have been with shown in Fig. 2 their mechanism of action (Table 1).

Interferons (IFNs): Interferons are produced as a result of the innate immune response against the viral infection, and they are capable of inhibiting viral replication. Recombinant interferon-α which is given three days before the infection might decrease the replication of the virus and also lung injury, as compared with the clinical trial and with control in monkeys [43]. Inhalation of interferon-α can also be considered. IFN-α-2a in combination with ribavirin drug was used in the cure of MERS-CoV-infected patients, and the survival rate of patients was found to be

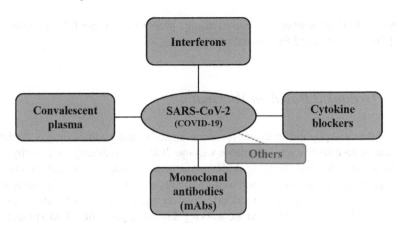

Fig. 2 Various immunological approaches used for the COVID-19 treatment

Table 1 Various therapeutic agents and their mechanism of action

Therapeutic agent	Evidence level	Mechanism of action	References
Immunotherapeutic potential convalescent plasma	Cell and clinical use	Neutralization of viral infectivity	[36]
Monoclonal antibody CR3014	Cell	Neutralization of viral infectivity	[39]
Monoclonal antibody CR3022	Cell and clinical use	Binds potentially to the receptor-binding area of Spike protein	[37]
mAbs single-chain variable region fragments, scFv, 80R	Cell	Potentially acts against the S protein (S1 domain)	[38]
Cytokine blocker cytokine IL-37	Cell	Impedes the inflammation, by acting on the mTOR and thus the activity of adenosine monophosphate kinase enzyme is increased	[42]
Cytokine blocker Lianhuaqingwen	Cell	Hinders IL-6 receptor and anti-inflammation	[45]
Cytokine blocker antibody against IL-6 receptor	Clinical use	Anti-inflammation and inhibits the IL-6 receptor	
TMPRSS2 Serine protease	Cell	Binds the spike protein of virus, leading to the spike protein priming by host the cell protease through receptor ACE2	[46]

improved [44]. Moreover, the above findings propose that these IFNs permitted by the FDA could be used for coronavirus treatment.

3.2 Treatment Based on Vaccination

One of the most popular strategies for reducing and treating coronavirus is the development of an effective and affordable vaccine. It aims at reducing the severity level of the disease, the viral shedding, and its transmission. Although several targets have been identified for the production of the vaccine, extensive work, and clinical trials are still required for developing an effective vaccine for the COVID-19. Scientists and researchers across the world are working day and night to help find a potentially effective vaccine against COVID-19 (Table 2).

The DNA vaccine: DNA vaccines are based on nucleic acid that is made up of plasmid-DNA encoding antigens that would be expressed in the cells of the host.

Table 2 Some vaccines under clinical trials (ClinicalTrials.gov; Apr. 30, 2020) [50]

Platform	Vaccine candidate	Immunogen	Subject	Study location	Phase
DNA-based	INO-4800	S protein	18–50 years	United States	NCT04336410 Phase I
mRNA based	mRNA1273 vaccine	S protein	18–55 years	USA	NCT04283461 Phase I
Adenovirus viral vector	Ad5-nCoV	S protein	18–60 years	China	NCT04341389 Phase II
	ChAdOx1 nCoV-19	S protein	18–55 years	United Kingdom	NCT04324606 Phase I/II
Live-attenuated vaccines	BCG	Danish strain 1331	Healthcare workers (>18 years	Australia	NCT04327206 Phase III
		Tice strain	Healthcare workers (18–74 years)	USA	NCT04348370 Phase IV
Lentivirus vector	LV-SMENP-DC (modified DCs) Covid-19/aAPC (modified aAPCs)	Polyprotein protease and Structural proteins	6 months to 80 years	China	NCT04276896 Phase I/II NCT04299724 Phase I
Bifidobacterium vector	bacTRL-Spike	S protein	19–45 years	Canada	NCT04334980 Phase I
Inactivated whole virus vaccine	inactivated SARS-CoV-2 vaccine	Whole virus	18–59 years	China	NCT04352608 Phase I/II

These vaccines can be made at very low cost and are produced rapidly. However, the need for a particular delivery system for persistence in the host cells and probable genomic integration and to attain good immunogenicity is a remaining concern [47]. DNA vaccines that encode S protein of MERS-CoV and also SARS-CoV have been shown to provide protective immunity by neutralizing the antibody response and stimulate T cell in human studies and also in the mouse model [48].DNA vaccine known as INO-4800 targets the SARS-CoV-2 spike protein.

The mRNA vaccine: Vaccines based on the mRNA usually encodes the antigen of interest and usually contains 50 and 30 UTR, whereas the self-amplifying RNAs that are derived from the virus not only encode antigen but also encodes the replication system of the virus that allows amplification of intracellular RNA and the abundant protein [49]. The mRNA-based vaccine delivery has been upgraded by the use of nanoparticles made up of lipids for intradermal and also intramuscular injection [47]. Additionally, mRNA vaccines have an advantage over the conventional vaccines since they are free from infectious pathogens. Hence testing is rapidly efficient, relatively safe, and cost-effective. In the USA, the mRNA vaccine against COVID-19 was mRNA-1273 which was the first to be advance to clinical trial phase I, currently which is employing the healthy volunteers of age from 18 to 55 years to evaluate the immunogenicity, reactogenic response, and safety.

Viral vector vaccine: Viral vector can also be used as a potential tool for the development of the vaccine. Viral vector vaccines deliver the genes to the target cells specifically and without adjuvant can increase immunogenicity and also induce a vigorous T cell response to remove the cells infected with the virus. Though the results of such vaccines have been promising in various animal models, but still before use in humans some obstacles need to be overcome. These obstacles mainly include genotoxicity, the ability to evade preexisting immunity, and genetic stability. The most commonly used vector is the (Ad5) adenovirus serotype-5 since this vector can be produced easily and has a wide range of viral tropism and a high level of expression [51].The ability of the Ad5 viral vector to increase mucosal immunity by affecting the epithelial cells of the gut and the respiratory tract where ACE2 receptors are expressed at higher levels makes it a valuable vaccine against the COVID-19. A vaccine candidate, AD5-nCoV, that encodes the S protein of COVID-19 is the first proved and confirmed vaccine to be safe for human use and also to process to the clinical trial phase II in China. Another vaccine is known as ChAdOx1 nCoV-19 which is made of non-replicating adenovirus vector of chimpanzee along with the S protein genetic sequence. The vector signifies the substitute to the human adenovirus vector owing to its good safety and also lack of the preexisting immunity among the population of humans [52].

BCG vaccine: The most usually administered vaccine globally is the BCG vaccine (Bacillus Calmette-Guerin) that contains the live-attenuated strain of the bacteria *Mycobacterium bovis* for protecting against tuberculosis. In many countries such as China, Japan, and Taiwan where TB is very prevalent or where there is a high possibility of exposure to tuberculosis, worldwide vaccination is recommended at birth with a single dose of Bacillus Calmette-Guerin, whereas other countries like Switzerland, France, and Spain have withdrawn their vaccine policies since the incidence of the infection of tuberculosis has declined. Some countries like Italy, the USA, and Netherland have yet to accept vaccine policies [53]. The vaccination of BCG has been shown to induce non-specific or heterologous effects against the non-mycobacterial pathogens, and this property is termed as trained immunity (which is the capability of the innate immunity memory to provide an enhanced response against diverse microbes) [54]. The significant potential of BCG has been detected in human and mouse studies for diverse viral pathogens [55]. Various epidemiological studies found that BCG vaccination is also linked with the reduction of mortality rate in neonates and the reduction of respiratory diseases in elderly people. Recent studies proposed the important relation of BCG immunization with the occurrence, development of the disease, and also mortality due to coronavirus [56]. Many researchers suggested that countries without the global programs for vaccination of BCG have been affected very severely as compared with the countries with the use of the BCG vaccines in neonates. Clinical trials have been started in healthcare workers who are exposed to the COVID-19 pandemic to ensure the safety of the BCG vaccination. Before any evidence, BCG vaccination is not expected to be recommended by the WHO for the prevention of the coronavirus [57].

For the development of potential vaccine, lentivirus vector systems also represents an attractive technology. Two vaccine candidates such as LV-SMENP-DC and COVID-19/aAPC which were made by dendritic cells and artificial APCs with lentivirus expressing immune-modulatory genes and multiple viral genes act as a Trojan horse against the infection of coronavirus. To evaluate the immune reactivity and safety of the vaccine, clinical trials are ongoing. *Bifidobacterium* is a non-pathogenic, domestic, and anaerobic bacteria that is found in the human intestine. They offer numerous advantages such as high safety levels, low cost, noninvasive administration, and low antibiotic resistance. The most interesting characteristic is that the *bifidobacterium* tends to stimulate mucosal antibodies against foreign antigens [58]. Moreover, some strains have been used for enterovirus and Hepatitis C virus vaccine development [59]. The vaccine candidate is known as bacTRL-Spike which has live-attenuated *Bifidobacterium longum*, and it usually has the synthetic plasmid-DNA that encodes the novel SARS-CoV-2 spike protein.

The clinical trial is underway which is planned to estimate the tolerability of the orally delivered vaccines in the healthy adults and also to assess the safety of the vaccine. Inactivated whole virus (IWV) preparation is the fastest method for the production of vaccines, and these vaccines have been made successfully for enterovirus and influenza virus. These vaccines are made generally by the exposure of the contagious virus to physical and also chemical agents, e.g., gamma irradiation or formaldehyde, to kill the infectivity and retaining the immunogenicity. The major concern for the IWV vaccines is the need to use antigen in a larger amount to elicit antibody response and the possibility of producing Th2 hypersensitivity [60].

3.3 Antiviral Drugs

Currently, no therapies or drugs are approved by the US FDA for the treatment of COVID-19. No antiviral drugs have adequate proof that they have the potential to treat coronavirus. Steroid dexamethasone has however been found effective in the recovery of critical patients. Various drugs have been carefully chosen to treat coronavirus patients; most of these drugs were usually considered for other illnesses such as HIV infections, influenza, Ebola, parasitic infection, inflammatory disease, and immune therapy for autoimmune disease. One of the most sought-after strategies for reducing and treating the COVID-19 is the development of SARS-CoV-2-based vaccine. It aims at reducing the severity level of the disease, the viral shedding, and its transmission. Although several targets have been identified for the production of the vaccine, extensive work and clinical trials are still required for developing an effective vaccine for the novel COVID-19. Scientists and researchers throughout the world are working day and night to help find a potentially effective vaccine against COVID-19. Few commonly used drugs are described, and a list of the drug against the COVID-19 is given in Table 3.

Ribavirin: It is a drug having a wide range of activities and whose curative property was discovered in 1972. Ribavirin is an antiviral medicine for hepatitis C treatment, and it is used usually in combination with the interferon–α. Ribavirin competes for the RdRp active site, and it is approved by the FDA.

Lopinavir/Ritonavir: Lopinavir targets HIV, and it is a protease inhibitor which was recognized in 2000 by the FDA. Lopinavir inhibits viral proteins formation by

Table 3 Drug available commercially for the cure of COVID-19

S. No.	Drug	Disease treated	References
1	Ribavirin	RSV pneumonia and RSV	[71]
2	Lopinavir and Ritonavir	MERS and SARS	[72]
3	Chloroquine	SARS, HCoV-OC43	[73]
4	Ruxolitinib	COVID-19	[67]
5	Indinavir	COVID-19, SARS	[42]
6	Acyclovir	COVID-19, SARS, MERS	[74]
7	Baricitinib	COVID-19	[75]
8	Tocilizumab	COVID-19	[76]
9	Favipiravir	COVID-19	[63]
10	Remdesivir	COVID-19, SARS, MERS	[63]
11	Darunavir	COVID-19	[64]
12	Carfilzomib	COVID-19	[63]
13	Baloxavir marboxil	COVID-19	[77]
14	Umifenovir	SARS and Feline Coronavirus	[78]

mimicking its structure [61]. Lopinavir along with the drug oseltamivir was further reported to result in the complete recovery after novel COVID-19 infection.

Remidesivir: Remidesivir is an analog of adenosine nucleotide, and it was also used in the treatment of SARS-CoV, Ebola, and MERS-CoV. It is a potential and promising drug that pauses the replication of the viral genetic makeup by premature termination of nascent viral RNA. Remdesivir has shown therapeutic and prophylactic activity in nonclinical models. Also, in vitro results have revealed that it has potential against the novel SARS-CoV-2 [62].

Hydroxychloroquine and chloroquine: Hydroxychloroquine and chloroquine both drugs are directed against malaria and used in the cure of avian influenza chronic inflammatory disease, e.g., rheumatoid arthritis, erythematosus, and systemic lupus [63]. Hydroxychloroquine and chloroquine are known to block the entry of the virus into the cells by impeding glycosylation of receptors of the host, endosomal acidification, and proteolytic processing. Immunomodulatory effects by inhibition of lysosomal activity and autophagy in host cells and also through attenuation of production of cytokine [64]. The experiences of Europe, the USA, and also China have shown the clinical effects of these drugs in the initial phase, but inadequate effects have been shown in the later phases [65]. A previous study show that hydroxychloroquine drug was associated with the decrease or disappearance of viral load in the patients suffering from COVID-19 infection and this effect was further strengthened by the drug azithromycin [66].

Baricitinib: Various anti-inflammatory drugs, particularly JAK and STAT inhibitors, may be useful against viral infections and also effective against the cytokines elevated levels. For instance, a recent study has shown that baricitinib drugs used in remidesivir combination elevate the activity of the drug against infection of the virus [67].

Favipiravir: Favipiravir is an antiviral drug, and it has got its approval from the Shenzhen Health Commission for the cure of patients infected with the COVID-19 [68]. Favipiravir is known to compete with the purine nucleosides and also impedes the replication of the virus by incorporating into the viral RNA, thereby inhibiting RdRp.

Umifenovir: Umifenovir targets the interaction of ACE2/S protein and further inhibits the viral envelope membrane fusion [69]. Umifenovir is presently approved in China as well as in Russia for the prevention and cure of influenza and also being tested in COVID-19 clinical trials based on the in vitro data against the infection of SARS [70].

3.4   Indian Medicinal Plants Against SARS-CoV-2

Indian herbs since prehistoric times have been used for the prevention and cure of numerous diseases including viral infections and respiratory infections. AYUSH's holistic approach of medicine emphasizes prevention via variation of lifestyle, preventive mediations for immunity improvement, dietary management, and simple therapies based on symptoms [79]. Medicinal plant *Sphaeranthus indicus* and *Vitex trifolia* have been known to decrease the inflammatory cytokines via a pathway of NF-kB (a pathway that is associated with the SARS-CoV respiratory diseases) [80]. The plants, *Allium sativum* and *Glycyrrhiza glabra* [81, 82] are known to target SARS-CoV replication and thus arising as the promising candidate for the treatment of the SARS-CoV-2. Another herb *Clerodendrum* has been found to have the activity to deactivate the ribosome of the virus, and thus, this can be explored for its efficacy in targeting novel SARS-CoV-2. Likewise, *Strobilanthes Cusia* also blocked the RNAgenome of the virus thus targeting HCoV [83]. A study has recognized the antiviral properties of some ethnomedicinal plants against bronchitis, and it showed that *Verbascum Thapsus*, *Justicia adhatoda*, and *Hyoscyamus niger* have reduced the infections caused by the influenza viruses. Furthermore, several plants have also shown the inhibitory effects against the ACE such as *Punicagranatum*, *Embeliaribes*, *Cynara scolymus*, *Coriandrum sativum*, and *Boerhaavia diffusa* [84]. Among these, all plants except *Punicagranatum* were non-specific inhibitors [85] while *Punicagranatum* usually showed a competitive effect. Moreover, these herbs need to be explored further to observe their activity on the SARS-CoV-2 entry into the cell of the host. Another species of plant *Andrographis paniculata* has the potential against viral respiratory infections, and it also suppressed caspase-1 and interleukin-1β and NLRP3 molecules which are involved widely in the pathogenesis of both SARS-CoV-2 as well as the SARS-CoV [86]. Some plants like *Vitex negundo*, *Solanumnigrum*, and *Ocimum sanctum* have been known to target the HIV reverse transcriptase property and thus can be further studied for the cure of SARS-CoV-2 infection. Hence, these medicinal plants might have the potential to ameliorate the COVID-19 symptoms. Research has to be carried out to explore the efficacy of these medicinal plants against the SARS-CoV-2. Several therapeutic plants that have been used broadly for respiratory illness are described below in Table 4.

4   Conclusion and Future Recommendations

Scientists across the globe are working tirelessly in characterizing and understanding the mechanism behind SARS-CoV-2 to be able to come up with effective therapies and vaccines against it. Several vaccines have been designed and are been tested for their effectiveness through animal and human trial testing across the world: 321 vaccine candidates and of which 32 candidate vaccines are in clinical trials as on September 02, 2020 [96]. With current supporting therapies and treatments, more research needs to be done toward understanding the underlying mechanism of viral entry, cellular replication, transmission, and pathogenicity to enable the formation of an effective intervention such as antiviral drug/s or vaccine/s. A study has suggested the role of serine–proline–arginine–arginine (SPRR) residues present in the surface proteins in higher infectivity and pathogenicity of lethal human viruses including

Table 4 List of few Indian medicinal herbs that might have the potential to inhibit the SARS-CoV-2 and other viruses

S. No.	Plant	Target	Mechanism	Virus	References
1	*Acacia nilotica*	–	Inhibition	HIV-PR	[87]
2	*Allium sativum*	–	Hemagglutinating and proteolytic activity	SARS	[81]
3	*Andrographis paniculata*	Capase-1, NLRP3, and IL-1β	Suppression	SARS-COV and likely on SARS-CoV-2 as well	[86]
4	*Boerhaavia diffusa*	ACE	Inhibition	–	[85]
5	*Clerodendrum inerme Gaertn*	Ribosome	Inactivation	SARS-CoV-2	[88]]
6	*Coriandrum sativum*	ACE	Inhibition	–	[89]
7	*Cynara scolymus*	ACE	Inhibition	–	[85]
8	*Embelia ribes*	ACE	Inhibition	–	[85]
9	*Glycyrrhiza glabra*	–	Inhibition of replication of the virus	SARS; HIV-1	[90]
10	*Hyoscyamus niger*	Ca^{2+}	Inhibition and Bronchodilator	–	[91]
11	*Ocimum sanctum*	–	Inhibition	HIV-1	[92]
12	*Punica granatum*	ACE	Inhibition	–	[85]
13	*Solanum nigrum*	–	–	HIV-1	[59]
14	*Sphaeranthus indicus*	–	Inhibition	Herpes virus and mouse coronavirus	[93]
15	*Strobilanthes cusia*	–	Blocking	HCoV-NL63	[83]
16	*Vitex negundo*	–	Inhibition	HIV-1	[94]
17	*Vitex trifolia*	–	Reduction	SARS-COV	[95]

SARS-CoV-2 [97] that could serve as a point of treatment. More studies need to be conducted to curb its transmission to animals and ways to effectively prevent its spread, especially among elderly people, children, and healthcare workers without hampering much of the economic condition of the nations. Proper travel screenings and public precautionary guidelines need to be incorporated. Also, the variations observed in the epidemiology of the SARS-CoV-2 across various countries depicting probable mutations in the virus need to be studied as well. More accurate, cost-effective, and less time-consuming diagnostic methods need to be developed which can differentiate patients infected with SAR-CoV-2 from those infected with other similar diseases such as influenza and allergies. Such an approach will help in avoiding any confusion and depression among patients with similar respiratory symptoms as of COVID-19.

References

1. Lu R, Zhao X, Li J, Niu P, Yang B, Wu H et al (2020) Genomic characterization and epidemiology of 2019 novel coronavirus: implications for virus origins and receptor binding. Lancet 395:565–574
2. Chen J (2020) Pathogenicity and transmissibility of 2019-nCoV—a quick overview and comparison with other emerging viruses. Microbes Infect 22:69–71
3. Schoeman D, Fielding BC (2019) Coronavirus envelope protein: current knowledge. Virol J 16:69
4. Walls AC, Park YJ, Tortorici MA, Wall A, McGuire AT, Veesler D (2020) Structure, function, and antigenicity of the SARS-CoV-2 spike glycoprotein. Cell 181:281–292
5. Zumla A, Chan JF, Azhar EI, Hui DS, Yuen KY (2016) Coronaviruses—drug discovery and therapeutic options. Nat Rev Drug Discov 15:327
6. Tai W, He L, Zhang X, Pu J, Voronin D, Jiang S, Zhou Y, Du L (2020) Characterization of the receptor-binding domain (RBD) of 2019 novel coronavirus: implication for development of RBD protein as a viral attachment inhibitor and vaccine. Cell Mol Immunol 1–8
7. Phan T (2020) Novel coronavirus: from discovery to clinical diagnostics. Infect Genet Evol 79:104211
8. Zhao Y, Zhao Z, Wang Y, Zhou Y, Ma Y, Zuo W (2020) Single-cell RNA expression profiling of ACE2, the receptor of SARS-CoV-2. Am J Resp Crit Care Med 5:756–759
9. Zheng M, Song L (2020) Novel antibody epitopes dominate the antigenicity of spike glycoprotein in SARS-CoV-2 compared to SARS-CoV. Cell Mol Immunol 17:1–3
10. Zhou D, Dai SM, Tong Q (2020) COVID-19: a recommendation to examine the effect of hydroxychloroquine in preventing infection and progression. J Antimicrob Chemother 75:2016–2017
11. Zhou P et al (2020) A pneumonia outbreak associated with a new coronavirus of probable bat origin. Nature 579:270–273
12. Morawska L, Cao J (2020) Airborne transmission of SARS-CoV-2: the world should face the reality. Environ Int 139
13. Biscayart PA, Lloveras S, Chaves T, Schlagenhauf P, Rodriguez-Morales AJ (2020) The next big threat to global health? 2019 novel coronavirus (2019-nCoV): what advice can we give to travellers? Interim recommendations January 2020, from the Latin-American Society for travel medicine (SLAMVI). Travel Med Infect Dis 33:101567
14. Leroy EM, Ar Gouilh M, Brugere-Picoux J (2020) The risk of SARS-CoV-2 transmission to pets and other wild and domestic animals strongly mandates a one-health strategy to control the COVID-19 pandemic. One Health 100133. hhttp://doi.org/10.1016/j.onehlt.2020.100133
15. Dincer C, Bruch R, Costa-Rama E, Fernandez-Abedul MT, Merkoçi A, Manz A, Urban GA, Güder F (2019) Disposable sensors in diagnostics, Food, and environmental monitoring. Adv Mater 31:1806739

16. Bruch R, Urban GA, Dincer C (2019) Unamplified gene sensing via Cas9 on graphene. Nat Biomed Eng 3:419–420
17. Qiu G, Gai Z, Tao Y, Schmitt J, Kullak-Ublick GA, Wang J (2020) Dual-functional plasmonic photothermal biosensors for highly accurate severe acute respiratory syndrome coronavirus 2 detection. ACS Nano 14:5268–5277
18. Vogel G (2020) New blood tests for antibodies could show true scale of coronavirus. https://doi.org/10.1126/science.abb8028
19. Randhawa GS, Soltysiak MPM, El Roz H, de Souza CPE, Hill KA, Kari L (2020) Machine learning using intrinsic genomic signatures for rapid classification of novel pathogens: COVID-19 case study. PLoS ONE 15(4):e0232391
20. Mei X, Lee H-C, Diao K, Huang M, Lin B, Liu C et al (2020) Artificial intelligence-enabled rapid diagnosis of patients with COVID-19. Nat Med 26:124–1228
21. Hosny A, Parmar C, Quackenbush J, Schwartz LH, Aerts H (2018) Artificial intelligence in radiology. Nat Rev Cancer 18(8):500–510
22. Gozes O, Frid-Adar M, Greenspan H, Browning PD, Zhang H, Ji W et al (2020) Rapid AI development cycle for the coronavirus (COVID-19) pandemic: initial results for automated detection & patient monitoring using deep learning CT image analysis. arXiv e-prints [Internet], 1 Mar 2020
23. Zheng C, Deng X, Fu Q, Zhou Q, Feng J, Ma H et al (2020) Deep learning-based detection for COVID-19 from chest CT using weak label. MedRxiv. https://doi.org/10.1101/2020.03.12.20027185
24. Jiang X, Coffee M, Bari A, Wang J, Jiang X, Huang J et al (2020) Towards an artificial intelligence framework for datadrive prediction of coronavirus clinical severity. Comput Mater Contin 62:537–551
25. Bekiros S, Kouloumpou D (2020) SBDiEM: a new mathematical model of infectious disease dynamics. Chaos Solitons Fractals 136:109828
26. Peirlinck M, Sahli Costabal F, Linka K, Kuhl E (2020) Outbreak dynamics of COVID-19 in China and the United States. Biomech Model Mechanobiol 1–15. https://doi.org/10.1007/s10237-020-01332-5
27. WHO: Clinical management of severe acute respiratory infection when novel coronavirus (nCoV) infection is suspected. https://www.who.int/publicationsdetail/clinical-management-of-severe-acute-respiratory-infection-when-novelcoronavirus-(ncov)-infection-is-suspected
28. Swennen GRJ, Pottel L, Haers PE (2020) Custommade 3D-printed face masks in case of pandemic crisis situations with a lack of commercially available FFP2/3 masks. Int J Oral Maxillofac Surg 49(5):673–677
29. Wesemann C, Pieralli S, Fretwurst T, Nold J, Nelson K, Schmelzeisen R et al (2020) 3-D printed protective equipment during COVID-19 pandemic. Materials (Basel) 13(8):1997
30. Wang CJ, Ng CY, Brook RH (2020) Response to COVID-19 in Taiwan: big data analytics, new technology, and proactive testing. JAMA 323:1341–1342
31. Chen FM, Feng MC, Chen TC, Hsieh MH, Kuo SH, Chang HL et al (2020) Big data integration and analytics to prevent a potential hospital outbreak of COVID-19 in Taiwan. J Microbiol Immunol Infect. https://doi.org/10.1016/j.jmii.2020.04.010
32. Yang G-Z, Nelson B, Murphy RR, Choset H, Christensen H, Collins S et al (2020) Combating COVID-19—the role of robotics in managing public health and infectious diseases. Sci Robot 5(40):5589
33. Robert-Guroff M (2007) Replicating and non-replicating viral vectors for vaccine development. Curr Opin Biotechnol 18(6):546–556
34. Anggraeni S, Maulidina A, Dewi MW, Rahmadianti S, Rizky YPC, Arinalhaq ZF et al (2020) The deployment of drones in sending drugs and patient blood samples COVID-19. BioRxiv 5(2):8
35. Yeh KM, Chiueh TS, Siu LK, Lin JC, Chan PK, Peng MY, Wan HL, Chen JH, Hu BS, Perng CL, Lu JJ, Chang FY (2005) Experience of using convalescent plasma for severe acute respiratory syndrome among healthcare workers in a Taiwan hospital. J Antimicrob Chemother 56(5):919–922

36. Chen L, Xiong J, Bao L, Shi Y (2020) Convalescent plasma as a potential therapy for COVID-19. Lancet Infect Dis 20:398–400
37. Tian Y, Rong L, Nian W, He Y (2020) Review article: gastrointestinal features in COVID-19 and the possibility of faecal transmission. Aliment Pharmacol Ther 51:843–851
38. Sui J, Li W, Murakami A, Tamin A, Matthews LJ, Wong SK, Moore MJ, Tallarico AS, Olurinde M, Choe H, Anderson LJ, Bellini WJ, Farzan M, Marasco WA (2004) Potent neutralization of severe acute respiratory syndrome (SARS) coronavirus by a human mAb to S1 protein that blocks receptor association. Proc Natl Acad Sci USA 101(8): 2536–2541
39. Ter Meulen J, van den Brink EN, Poon LL, Marissen WE, Leung CS, Cox F, Cheung CY, Bakker AQ, Bogaards JA, van Deventer E, Preiser W, Doerr HW, Chow VT, de Kruif J, Peiris JS, Goudsmit J (2006) Human monoclonal antibody combination against SARS coronavirus: synergy and coverage of escape mutants. PLoS Med 3(7):e237
40. Ju B, Zhang Q, Ge X, Wang R, Yu J, Shan S, Zhou B, Song S, Tang X, Yu J, Ge J, Lan J, Yuan J, Wang H, Zhao J, Zhang S, Wang Y, Shi X, Liu L, Wang X, Zhang Z, Zhang L (2020) Potent human neutralizing antibodies elicited by SARSCoV-2 infection. bioRxiv
41. Huang C et al (2020) Clinical features of patients infected with 2019 novel coronavirus in Wuhan, China. Lancet 395:497–506
42. Conti P, Ronconi G, Caraffa A, Gallenga CE, Ross R, Frydas I, Kritas SK (2020) Induction of pro-inflammatory cytokines (IL-1 and IL-6) and lung inflammation by coronavirus-19 (COVI-19 or SARS-CoV-2): anti-inflammatory strategies. J Biol Regul Homeost Agents 34:2
43. Loutfy MR, Blatt LM, Siminovitch KA, Ward S, Wolff B, Lho H, Pham DH, Deif H, LaMere EA., Chang M, Kain KC, Farcas GA, Ferguson P, Latchford M, Levy G, Dennis JW, Lai EK, Fish EN (2003) Interferon alfacon-1 plus corticosteroids in severe acute respiratory syndrome: a preliminary study. JAMA 290(24):3222–3228
44. Lee JY, Bae S, Myoung J (2019) Middle East respiratory syndrome coronavirus encoded ORF8b strongly antagonizes IFN-beta promoter activation: its implication for vaccine design. J Microbiol 57(9):803–811
45. Runfeng L, Yunlong H, Jicheng H, Weiqi P, Qinhai M, Yongxia S, Chufang L, Jin Z, Zhenhua J, Haiming J, Kui Z, Shuxiang H, Jun D, Xiaobo L, Xiaotao H, Lin W, Nanshan Z, Zifeng Y (2020) Lianhuaqingwen exerts anti-viral and anti-inflammatory activity against novel coronavirus (SARS-CoV-2). Pharmacol Res 156:104761
46. Hoffmann M, Kleine-Weber H, Krueger N, Mueller MA, Drosten C, Pöhlmann S (2020) The novel coronavirus 2019 (2019-nCoV) uses the SARS-coronavirus receptor ACE2 and the cellular protease TMPRSS2 for entry into target cells. https://doi.org/10.1101/2020.01.31.929042
47. Rauch S, Jasny E, Schmidt KE, Petsch B (2018) New vaccine technologies to combat outbreak situations. Front Immunol 9:1963
48. Modjarrad K, Roberts CC, Mills KT, Castellano AR, Paolino K, Muthumani K et al (2019) Safety and immunogenicity of an anti-Middle East respiratory syndrome coronavirus DNA vaccine: a phase 1, open-label, single-arm, dose-escalation trial. Lancet Infect Dis 19:1013e22
49. Pardi N, Hogan MJ, Porter FW, Weissman D (2018) mRNA vaccines—a new era in vaccinology. Nat Rev Drug Discov 17:261e79
50. Shih H-I, Wu C-J, Tu Y-F, Chi C-Y (2020) Fighting COVID-19: a quick review of diagnoses, therapies, and vaccines. Biomed J
51. Ura T, Okuda K, Shimada M (2014) Developments in viral vector based vaccines. Vaccine 2:624e41
52. Dicks MD, Spencer AJ, Edwards NJ, Wadell G, Bojang K, Gilbert SC et al (2012) A novel chimpanzee adenovirus vector with low human seroprevalence: improved systems for vector derivation and comparative immunogenicity. PLoS ONE 7:e40385
53. Zwerling A, Behr MA, Verma A, Brewer TF, Menzies D, Pai M (2011) The BCG world atlas: a database of global BCG vaccination policies and practices. PLoS Med 8:e1001012
54. Netea MG, Joosten LA, Latz E, Mills KH, Natoli G, Stunnenberg HG et al (2016) Trained immunity: a program of innate immune memory in health and disease. Science 352:aaf1098

55. Moorlag S, Arts RJW, van Crevel R, Netea MG (2019) Non-specific effects of BCG vaccine on viral infections. Clin Microbiol Infect 25:1473e8

56. Miller A, Reandelar MJ, Fasciglione K, Roumenova V, Li Y, Otazu GH (2020) Correlation between universal BCG vaccination policy and reduced morbidity and mortality for COVID-19: an epidemiological study. medRxiv. https://doi.org/10.1101/2020.03.24.20042937

57. Kam YW, Kien F, Roberts A, Cheung YC, Lamirande EW, Vogel L et al (2007) Antibodies against trimeric S glycoprotein protect hamsters against SARS-CoV challenge despite their capacity to mediate FcgammaRII-dependent entry into B cells in vitro. Vaccine 25:729e40

58. Kandasamy S, Chattha KS, Vlasova AN, Rajashekara G, Saif LJ (2014) *Lactobacilli* and *Bifidobacteria* enhance mucosal B cell responses and differentially modulate systemic antibody responses to an oral human rotavirus vaccine in a neonatal gnotobiotic pig disease model. Gut Microb 5:639e51

59. Yu Y-B (2004) The extracts of *Solanum nigrum* L. for inhibitory effects on HIV-1 and its essential enzymes. Korean J Orient Med 10:119–126

60. Agrawal AS, Tao X, Algaissi A, Garron T, Narayanan K, Peng BH et al (2016) Immunization with inactivated Middle East respiratory syndrome coronavirus vaccine leads to lung immunopathology on challenge with live virus. Hum Vaccines Immunother 12:2351e6

61. Wu A et al (2020) Genome composition and divergence of the novel coronavirus (2019-nCoV) originating in China. Cell Host Microbe 27:325–328

62. Sheahan TP, Sims AC, Leist SR, Schafer A, Won J, Brown AJ et al (2020) Comparative therapeutic efficacy of remdesivir and combination lopinavir, ritonavir, and interferon beta against MERS-CoV. Nat Commun 11:222

63. Wang J (2020) Fast identification of possible drug treatment of coronavirus disease-19 (COVID-19) through computational drug repurposing study. ChemRxiv

64. Zhou D, Dai SM, Tong Q (2020) COVID-19: a recommendation to examine the effect of hydroxychloroquine in preventing infection and progression. J Antimicrob Chemother 75:1667–1670

65. Tan L, Wang Q, Zhang D, Ding J, Huang Q, Tang YQ et al (2020) Lymphopenia predicts disease severity of COVID-19: a descriptive and predictive study. Signal Transduct Targeted Ther 5:33

66. Gautret P, Lagier JC, Parola P, Hoang VT, Meddeb L, Mailhe M et al (2010) Hydroxychloroquine and azithromycin as a treatment of COVID-19: results of an open-label nonrandomized clinical trial. Int J Antimicrob Agents 105949

67. Stebbing J, Phelan A, Griffin I, Tucker C, Oechsle O, Smith D, Richardson P (2020) COVID-19: combining antiviral and anti-inflammatory treatments. Lancet Infect Dis 20:400–402

68. Wu C, Liu Y, Yang Y, Zhang P, Zhong W, Wang Y, Wang Q, Xu Y, Li M, Li X (2020) Analysis of therapeutic targets for SARS-CoV-2 and discovery of potential drugs by computational methods. Acta Pharm Sin B 10:766–788

69. Kadam RU, Wilson IA (2017) Structural basis of influenza virus fusion inhibition by the antiviral drug Arbidol. Proc Natl Acad Sci USA 114:206e14

70. Khamitov RA, Loginova S, Shchukina VN, Borisevich SV, Maksimov VA, Shuster AM (2008) Antiviral activity of arbidol and its derivatives against the pathogen of severe acute respiratory syndrome in the cell cultures. Vopr Virusol 53:9–13

71. McIntosh K, Kurachek SC, Cairns LM, Burns JC, Goodspeed B (1984) Treatment of respiratory viral infection in an immunodeficient infant with ribavirin aerosol. Am J Dis Child 138:305–308

72. Chu C, Cheng V, Hung I, Wong M, Chan KH, Chan KS, Kao R, Poon L, Wong C, Guan Y (2004) Role of lopinavir/ritonavir in the treatment of SARS: initial virological and clinical findings. Thorax 59:252–256

73. Vincent MJ, Bergeron E, Benjannet S, Erickson BR, Rollin PE, Ksiazek TG, Seidah NG, Nichol ST (2005) Chloroquine is a potent inhibitor of SARS coronavirus infection and spread. Virol J 2:69

74. Peters HL, Jochmans D, de Wilde AH, Posthuma CC, Snijder EJ, Neyts J, Seley-Radtke KL (2015) Design, synthesis and evaluation of a series of acyclic fleximer nucleoside analogues with anti-coronavirus activity. Bioorg Med Chem Lett 25:2923–2926

75. Richardson P, Griffin I, Tucker C, Smith D, Oechsle O, Phelan A, Stebbing J (2020) Baricitinib as potential treatment for 2019-nCoV acute respiratory disease. Lancet 395:30–31
76. Diao B, Wang C, Tan Y, Chen X, Ying L, Ning L, Chen L, Li M, Yueping L, Wang G (2019) Reduction and functional exhaustion of T cells in patients with coronavirus disease (COVID-19). medRxiv
77. Li G, Clercq E (2020) Therapeutic options for the 2019 novel coronavirus (2019-nCoV)
78. Hsieh LE, Lin CN, Su BL, Jan TR, Chen CM, Wang CH, Lin DS, Lin CT, Chueh LL (2010) Synergistic antiviral effect of *Galanthus nivalis* agglutinin and *nelfinavir* against feline coronavirus. Antiviral Res 88:25–30
79. Ministry of Ayush (2020) Government of India: homeopathy for prevention of coronavirus infections. https://www.covidhomeo.com/2020/05/ayush-ministry-govt-of-india-issues.html
80. Srivastava RAK, Mistry S, Sharma S (2015) A novel anti-inflammatory natural product from *Sphaeranthus indicus* inhibits expression of VCAM1 and ICAM1, and slows atherosclerosis progression independent of lipid changes. Nutr Metab 12:20
81. Keyaerts E, Vijgen L, Pannecouque C, Van Damme E, Peumans W, Egberink H, Balzarini J, Van Ranst M (2007) Plant lectins are potent inhibitors of coronaviruses by interfering with two targets in the viral replication cycle. Antiviral Res 75:179–187
82. Nourazarian A (2011) Effect of root extracts of medicinal herb *Glycyrrhiza glabra* on HSP90 gene expression and apoptosis in the HT-29 colon cancer cell line. Asian Pac J Cancer Prev 1–16
83. Tsai YC, Lee CL, Yen HR, Chang YS, Lin YP, Huang SH, Lin CW (2020) Antiviral action of Tryptanthrin isolated from *Strobilanthes cusia* leaf against human coronavirus NL63. Biomolecules 10:366
84. Hussain F, Jahan N, Rahman K, Sultana B, Jamil S (2018) Identification of hypotensive biofunctional compounds of *Coriandrum sativum* and evaluation of their angiotensin-converting enzyme (ACE) inhibition potential. Oxidative Med Cell Longevity 3:1–11
85. Khan MY, Kumar V (2019) Mechanism & inhibition kinetics of bioassay-guided fractions of Indian medicinal plants and foods as ACE inhibitors. J Tradit Complement Med 9:73–84
86. Liu YT, Chen HW, Lii CK, Jhuang JH, Huang CS, Li ML, Yao HT (2020) A diterpenoid, 14-deoxy-11, 12-didehydroandrographolide, in *Andrographis paniculata* reduces steatohepatitis and liver injury in mice fed a high-fat and high cholesterol diet 12:523
87. Mishra S, Aeri V, Gaur PK, Jachak SM (2014) Phytochemical, therapeutic, and ethnopharmacological overview for a traditionally important herb: *Boerhavia diffusa* Linn. Biomed Res Int 808302
88. Olivieri F, Prasad V, Valbonesi P, Srivastava S, Ghosal-Chowdhury P, Barbieri L, Bolognesi A, Stirpe F (1996) A systemic antiviral resistance-inducing protein isolate from *Clerodendrum inerme Gaertn*. Is a polynucleotide: adenosine glycosidase (ribosome-inactivating protein). FEBS Lett 396:132–134
89. Pandey A, Bigoniya P, Raj V, Patel KK (2011) Pharmacological screening of *Coriandrum sativum* Linn. for hepatoprotective activity. J Pharm Bioallied Sci 3(3):435
90. Cinatl J, Morgenstern B, Bauer G, Chandra P, Rabenau H, Doerr H (2003) Treatment of SARS with human interferons. Lancet 362:293–294
91. Gilani AH, Khan A, Raoof M, Ghayur MN, Siddiqui BS, Vohra W, Begum SP (2008) Gastrointestinal, selective airways and urinary bladder relaxant effects of *Hyoscyamus niger* are mediated through dual blockade of muscarinic receptors and Ca2+ channels. Fundam Clin Pharmacol 22:87–99
92. Rege A, Chowdhary AS (2014) Evaluation of *Ocimum sanctum* and *Tinospora cordifolia* as probable HIV protease inhibitors. Int J Pharm Sci Rev Res 25:315–318
93. Galani VJ, Patel BG, Rana DG (2010) *Sphaeranthus indicus* Linn.: a phytopharmacological review. Int J Ayurveda Res 1:247–253
94. Nair R (2012) HIV-1 reverse transcriptase inhibition by *Vitex negundo* L. leaf extract and quantification of flavonoids in relation to anti-HIV activity. J Cell Mol Biol 10:53–59
95. Liou CJ, Cheng CY, Yeh KW, Wu YH, Huang WC (2018) Protective effects of casticin from *vitex trifolia* alleviate eosinophilic airway inflammation and oxidative stress in a murine asthma model. Front Pharma Col 9:635

96. Le TT, Cramer JP, Chen R, Mayhew S (2020) Evolution of the COVID-19 vaccine development landscape. Nat Rev Drug Discov. https://www.nature.com/articles/d41573-020-00151-8
97. Qureshi MI, Asim M. Probing occurrence and probable roles of new insert in spike glycoprotein of SARS-CoV-2. SSRN. https://doi.org/10.2139/ssrn.3605888

Chapter 13
An Investigation on COVID 19 Using Big Data Analytics and Artificial Intelligence

G. Rajesh, S. Karthika, J. Ashwinth, R. Shanmugapriya, and X. Mercilin Raajini

1 Introduction

Artificial intelligence (AI) in medical applications helps to optimise the hospital, patient and disease management efficiently. These techniques assist the doctors in decision making effectively and efficiently by analysing the patient's time critical data. The pandemic situation arrived globally due to COVID-19, and its implications are one of the unintended consequences which affected the mankind. The AI with big data helps the world to fight against the COVID-19. This chapter investigates how big data and AI are used in the monitoring and mitigation and management of COVID-19.

G. Rajesh (✉) · S. Karthika · J. Ashwinth · R. Shanmugapriya
Department of Information Technology, MIT Campus, Anna University, Chennai, India
e-mail: raajiimegce@gmail.com

S. Karthika
e-mail: karthisubbu.92@gmail.com

J. Ashwinth
e-mail: ashwinthj@gmail.com

R. Shanmugapriya
e-mail: shanmurajendran2@gmail.com

X. Mercilin Raajini
Department of ECE, Prince Shri Venkateshwara Padmavathy Engineering College, Chennai, India
e-mail: raajii.mercy@gmail.com

P. K. Khosla et al. (eds.), *Predictive and Preventive Measures for Covid-19 Pandemic*,
Algorithms for Intelligent Systems, https://doi.org/10.1007/978-981-33-4236-1_13

1.1   Big Data

Big data, the name itself describes that it deals with a large volume of data. The information can be any of the following form: structured, unstructured or semi-structured. A huge variety and volume of data is dealt with. With the help of big data, smart decision making is handled. It also gives a systematic prediction for the data. Big data involves a sequence of steps by which the data is captured from source; sequentially, it analyses, visualises, updates secure and stores the data. Its usage is needed in a variety of domains like marketing, banking, e-commerce, health care, secure zones, government organisations and so on. In health care, big data collects the data, analyses and makes predictions with the patient's data. On using the patient's data with traditional data, it was unhelpful, since healthcare data is highly complex and tough to understand. As big data can deal with all volumes of data, it plays a significant role in the health care of today's world. Big data has also made its role in the pandemic COVID-19. Section III describes how big data functions on COVID-19.

1.2   Data Analytics

Data analytics aims at an optimal solution in the business world. It involves preloading the existing data and provides the most exceptional solution for any complex problems. The resultant entirely relies on analysing the data. For instance, in a hospital, the patient's data is collected, and risk factors of each patient can be analysed using data analytics. For proper planning, data analytics is pertained in the healthcare sector. Another instance explains about a country taking the census, and each citizen's bio-data is stored and gathered as data requirements (data mining) in data analytics initially. Every citizen's information is carried out either through online, personal appearance, through a third party or agents, etc., which allows collecting information (data warehousing) of each individual. It becomes the second phase in data analytics. The third phase of data analytics involves by maintaining a database or spreadsheet, which results in a statistical data (statistical analysis) and can give the summary for the data has been collected. On the end of summarisation, duplicates and errors are validated and also clean up the NA values appeared in the data. Final stage of data analytics is carried out by an analyst (Data presentation or visualization stage). Finally, it can be shared as a visual presentation to the stakeholders. For this presentation, data visualisation tools are needed, which may cognisance in a better way.

Data analytics shows most favourable results for business models previously, but it can also be favourable for health care, cyber sectors, governmental organisations, banking and so on. In healthcare applications, data analytics aggregates a large number of patient's data and keeps track of each patient, which helps in identifying the risks and recoveries of patients. Performance factors remained much better than the traditional analysis of using data analytics. Survival analytics plays a significant role in healthcare data analytics. For each persistent the survival rate and the health condition is foreseen. In COVID-19, some concepts of data analytics are also involved. Section IV describes the role of data analytics on COVID-19.

1.3   Covid-19

A shrimp seller from the seafood market of Wuhan city of Hubei province was found to be the first positive case on novel coronavirus (2019-nCOV) in December 2019. The 2019-nCOV virus has the capability of spreading through human–human interaction [1], i.e., a person who is tested positive, is in contact with others, then the virus will infect them. Initially, a few individuals from the market were infected. People, who were in contact with the market area started to suffer and after that individuals who were in contact with those infected cases and so on it spreads exponentially. Within a few days, thousands were tested with 2019-nCOV. China government announced to lock down the city of Wuhan on 23 January 2020. People who were travelling outside the city became a carrier of 2019-nCOV. It started to spread across China. After that, it started to spread across countries. A lady who travelled from Wuhan to Thailand was the first outside country to get affected on 2019-nCOV.

Similarly, USA, Nepal, France, Malaysia, Australia, Singapore, South Korea, Vietnam, Taiwan, Italy, Philippines, India, UK, Canada, Germany and Japan started to confirm new cases on 2019-nCOV. Italy started to affect more than China, and also, mortality rate in Italy started to increase. World Health Organization (WHO) announced officially "COVID-19" as the name of the disease caused by 2019-nCOV on 11 February 2020. Following this report, on 11 March 2020, WHO has reported COVID-19 disease as a pandemic. As of now dated on 21 May 2020, 5.1 Million of world's population are affected by COVID-19. Around 2.1 Million were recovered, and 0.3 Million were dead due to COVID-19. The situation is explained in Fig. 1; the blue coloured line depicts the overall active cases on COVID-19 across the world.

For curing this disease, no medicine has found yet. The only solution is lockdown to control the spread of disease. If anyone is found to be affected by COVID-19, then the person who was in contact was quarantined for a few days to identify whether they are infected or not. WHO has also announced to wear a mask, not to touch face, nose, eyes, mouth and also to wash hands to avoid the spread of disease frequently. Figure 2 depicts how COVID-19 spreading over the globe, and the exponential growth of the infection is portrayed.

Out of 195 countries, 172 countries were affected by this pandemic disease. In India, initially, COVID-19 was only countable, and later, when people started arriving from various countries, the patient's count started to increase gradually. Till today's survey in India, over 112,442 total cases were affected, and 3438 deaths were confirmed on COVID-19 cases. The following graph (Fig. 3) explains the symbolic view of confirmed, recoveries and death of COVID-19 patients in India.

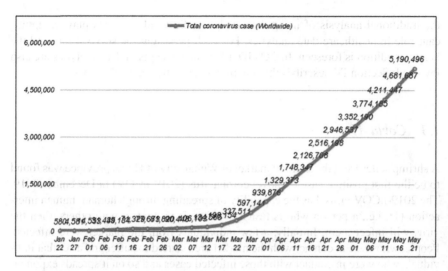

Fig. 1 Total cumulative count of COVID-19 patients all around the world (excluding death rate)

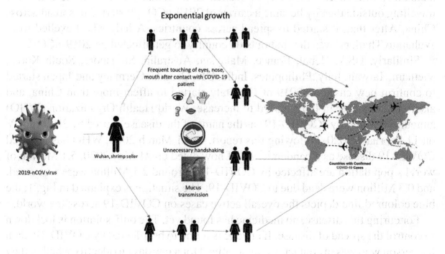

Fig. 2 COVID-19 transmission across the world

One of the solutions for COVID-19 was identified that plasma from people who have recovered from this infection can donate their plasma which is to be dripped into the infected patients [2]. The plasma contains the antibodies which might kill the virus and cures the person. However, this should be an effective treatment, since the cases are rapidly increasing, and it should be controlled as much. Convalescent plasma showed a positive result in many cases. Even though plasma therapy may recover a patient, harm may underlie. Transfusion-related reactions like unknown pathogens may also combine along with plasma, and it might get transfused to the

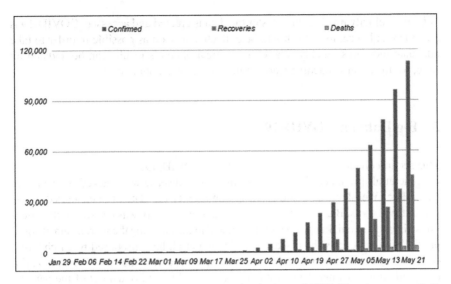

Fig. 3 Daily cumulative of confirmed, recoveries and deaths on COVID-19 patients across India from January–May 2020

patient. For instance, under the research of dengue, plasma therapy ultimately failed since it made a replication of the virus in the plasma [3]. Nevertheless, there are no studies to prove that COVID-19 can be wholly cured using plasma therapy. Countries like China, USA, Italy and Canada were involved in the research [4].

Various tests like swab test, nasal aspirate, tracheal aspirate, sputum test, blood test, viral test, antibody test are few tests handled for measuring the positive and negative results on COVID-19. Even though the healthcare domain works much on COVID-19, big data and data analytics increases the efficiencies and helps the better way of practice on this disease. Necessitate of big data and data analytics on COVID-19 is elucidated in Sects. 3 and 4.

2 Characteristics of Big Data

Volume: Volume of the data is increased exponentially since it is updated regularly. For COVID-19, large volume of patient's data, laboratory records, doctor's advice, medical claims, genetic data, image data on diseases, the structure of disease and so on are maintained as big data.

Variety: Variety of data involves different types of sources available throughout the healthcare sector. As discussed in our paper, myocardial injury data was taken on COVID-19.

Velocity: Velocity involves how faster the data is created and accessed. COVID-19 is a pandemic; hence, its data should be collected as soon as possible in order to take adequate measures quickly. Therefore, critical patient's results can be updated on time; for this, many machine learning techniques were applied.

3 Big Data on COVID-19

This section elucidates the role of big data on COVID-19.

Chae et al. [5] stated that in Korea, infectious disease was tracked by using big data. Here, Web look data and Internet community big data are considered as the surveillance tools. Based on the surveillance tools, a study was carried on the infectious disease like chickenpox, scarlet fever and malaria. Using the search data, it could predict how infectious the disease was. Huang et al. have proposed research based on temperature and humidity; dengue fever spreads across the city of Australia. For this prediction, weather data with temperature and humidity dataset of the patients in Australia was used [6]. Ganasekaran and Abdulrehman [7] have stated that the clinical and non-clinical datasets can predict with two weeks of history to find how the outbreak of the disease would be. When the infections were small, it is not much necessary for involving big data. When the infection started to rise, then big data will play its role by predicting. In many relevant data, machine learning and deep learning algorithms were used for learning about the diseases. Based on the previous studies, data is collected for an infectious disease like Ebola, influenza, pneumonia and H1N1, which gave the details of the risk factors [8] including the survival rate of the patient. These studies made a footpath on COVID-19 outbreak. The following diagram explains the prominent data involvement in COVID-19 (Fig. 4).

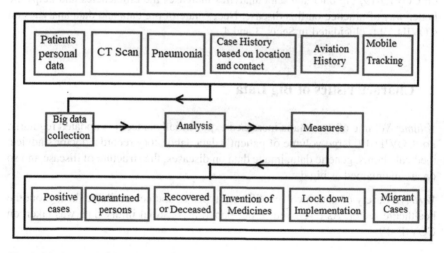

Fig. 4 Big data analysis on COVID-19

Numerous biological dataset was referred for finalising the structure of coronavirus. The trial test was done with Wuhan data, which supported on identifying the people who have migrated from Wuhan city. With the help of this data, Peng, et al. found an easy way for quarantining the people who were in contact with the migrated people [9]. China government has prepared data on the outbreak of COVID-19 results. The data explains the details of the patient's record and who were in contact with patient, X-ray and CT scans of the patient, case history of the infected person and where the patient resides. Based upon the source, it gave a favourable output for China on identifying the number of infected people and who are the persons should be quarantined [10]. It was also identified that big data was used in the tracking of the symptoms earlier by matching the symptoms of pneumonia [11]. With the help of these comparisons, it tested either positive or negative case.

Aviation data identified the air passengers who had fled from China which was explained by Zhao et al. [12], In their work, it has mentioned that from Wuhan airport, around 90,000 passengers fled all over the world. With the help of the multi-linear model, the data was identified. Spearman correlation method was used for tracking based on the Web users who gone away from Wuhan. For this, Zhao, et al. have employed GIS technology which gave successfulness for China government on identifying the patient's record. Big data is analysed for hidden populations too. With the assistance of this, it can predict that who else will be affected by the disease. Two weeks of data from Wuhan hospitals were recorded. The data was classified into active cases, recovered and deceased. On this surveillance, big data made a forecast [13] that at the end of February, the COVID-19 cases would reach around 1 million all over the world. After considering China, the other countries like Thailand, Italy and Korea also started employing big data on COVID-19. With the help of the combined dataset of all these countries, Castorina et al. analysed the velocity of the virus spread using macroscopic growth law [14].

The assistance of CT scan images [15] of chest data gave an analysis on COVID-19. The CT scanner made a study and gave a decision that isolation of patients is must since it can have human–human transmission [16]. For this, a separate COVID-19 classifier was found which covered lung and chest CT scan data across many hospitals in China. Centred on, this model was trained, validated and tested [17]. Based on the increasing results, China officially made Wuhan city to shut down. Following this, many countries started to put their country in lockdown [18].

The Facebook dataset was used for implementing social distancing by big data [19]. Yi-Cheng Chan and Ping-En Lu stated that minimum distance should be maintained between people and massive gathering of people which should be avoided in order to prevent the spread of coronavirus. On applying this, many countries found useful on minimising the spread of the virus [16]. The above studies show the effectiveness of significant data role on COVID-19. Even a proper dataset was not provided; initially, big data found a challenge; later through help of many government organisations, hospital data and aviation data paved the way for big data taking part in COVID-19.

4   Data Analytics on COVID-19

Predictive analytics is a type of data analytics which has made its role by predicting the target. Prediction analytics is mainly focused on business models. Applying data analytics, the risk of a company can be found of ease by predicting the target. Depending on engineering, in health care, it has described how predictive analytics is applied which is explained. Predictive analysis is classified into two strategies: regression and classification. Regression is applied for continuous target values, and classification is applied for discrete target values. The following model explains logistic regression model based on regression [20].

4.1   *Logistic Regression Analysis*

Logistic regression is applied for continuous as well as discrete outcomes. The outcome will be true/false, 0/1, yes/no, low/high from a given set of independent variables. Based on the response variable, logistic regression is classified into simple logistic regression (for nominal response variable) and ordinal logistic regression (for ordinal response variable) [17].

The logistic regression formulation is as follows:

$$P(Y = 1|X_1, \ldots X_n) = \frac{1}{1 + e^{(\beta_0 + \beta_1 x_1 + \ldots \beta_n x_n)}} \quad (1)$$

Here, $P(Y = 1|X_1,\ldots, X_n)$ always lies between 0 and 1.

From the above equation, we can infer that the output will be in the form of logistic sigmoid, from the inputs $P(Y = 1|X_1,\ldots, X_n)$. Since the sigmoid function is useful for predicting the probability value, it is applied in the logistic regression technique. Hence, it remains easy to calculate since the outcome always lies between 0 and 1, which helps understand each feature [21].

Using this logistic regression technique, COVID-19 predicted the recovery rate of patients. Data is collected based on positive patients, demographic data, clinical notes, laboratory records and blood test samples. After collecting these data, the mean and standard deviation were calculated. Using the mean and standard deviation, Fishers test and Student t-test were calculated. On applying these results in Eq. (1) of logistic regression, it predicted that the patient is at risk or not. Both univariate and multivariate characteristics of logistic regression were used to calculate the factors.

Several studies made that COVID-19 patients are also having symptoms of pneumonia. A study [18] was made that >65 years and <14 years are the main infectors of COVID-19. In 500 patients, who experienced the symptoms of pneumonia, around 367 members were recovered from the disease. Here, logistic regression was applied, and the probability value was calculated. If the P-value is less than 0.001, then it is supposed to have high risk, and if the P-value is greater than 0.001, then it is

Table 1 Clinical strategy on COVID-19 for myocardial injuries

Disease	Total number of cases = 500	Survival group (n = 367)	Death group (n = 133)	Comparison value	P value
Myocardial injury	59 (25.6)	30 (16.80)	38 (101.5)	60.285	<0.001
Cardiac insufficiency	90(15.11)	40 (7.12)	17 (83.8)	85.187	<0.001
Time from admission to detection of hs-cTnI [d, M (Q_1, Q_3)]	1 (1,1)	1 (1,1)	1 (0,1)	−1.215	0.224

supposed to have high recovery. Table 1 explains the clinical strategy of COVID-19 for myocardial injuries which made calculation [22]. The P-value column describes the value of P and predicts less and significant risks of patients. This dataset was taken from Wuhan Pulmonary Hospital between December 2019 and May 2020 [23].

where d refers to the detection of myocardial injury and cardiac insufficiency in the first and third quartiles.

On applying the dataset, the P-value is calculated as 0.001 as the least value for myocardial patients who are under significant risk.

The graph (Fig. 5) shows the exponential increase of patients affected through COVID-19. The lesser probability of myocardial injury has less survival rate, and the greater probability of myocardial injury has a high rate of survival. This was calculated on an average of 120 days, i.e. in the month of January–May 2020.

This made the forecast on how COVID-19 will be risky between age group factors [24]. It predicted that within a few days, how the growth of COVID-19 patients will be. Based on this prediction, China government took measures by providing a new hospital for COVID-19 patients and control measures like lockdown was handled. Following China, Italy, Singapore, Thailand, Australia, USA, India and several other countries started to follow the same rules.

4.2 Kaplan–Meier Analysis

Another method of data analytics was applied to COVID-19 which was survival analysis. Kaplan–Meier analysis of survival analysis was used to find the survival rate of the patients from COVID-19 [25].

Kaplan–Meier analysis is used to estimate survival value and hazard function form the given data. The survival function is denoted by:

$$S_t = \frac{\text{number of individuals surviving longer than } t}{\text{total number of individuals studied}} \tag{2}$$

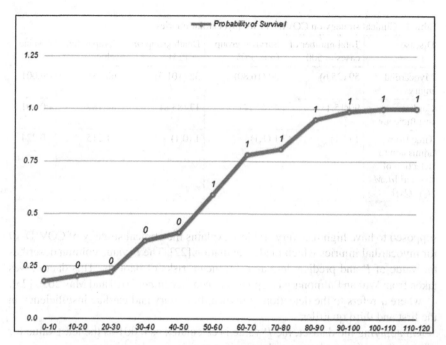

Fig. 5 Plot diagram for logistic regression calculated for patients on 120 days interval on COVID-19

Here, t denotes survival period. It also shows that before t, no event takes place. In Kaplan–Meier analysis, product limit method is used. It is given as:

$$S_t = \prod_{t_i \leq t}\left[1 - \frac{d_i}{n_i}\right] \tag{3}$$

The above equation is used to calculate S (survival probability), t_i is the duration of study made at the point i, d_i is the number of death at i, and n_i is the number of individuals in risk.

Kaplan–Meier analysis made a study on 500 patients of COVID-19. The data was collected from various hospitals based on the recovery and deceased results [26]. This study made that person who is having a myocardial injury is having high risk when infected with COVID-19 [11]. It also considered the age factors to determine the resultant. It gave a result for 500 patients, and 25.6 per cent of patients had myocardial injuries, and their survival rate (S) is only 16.80% [27]. From Table 1, it describes the study of myocardial injury patients on surviving rate.

The above plot was taken for 500 patients on COVID-19 (Fig. 6). It shows that in 125 days of history, myocardial patients found to have a higher risk of COVID-19. The green line shows COVID-19 patients without myocardial injury, and they have low risk on death rate, and the red line shows COVID-19 patients with myocardial

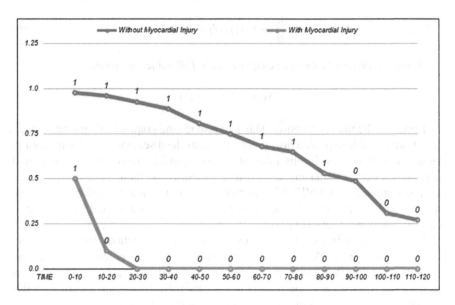

Fig. 6 Risk analysis for myocardial patients

injuries who have a high risk on death rate. This result made the hospitals to give more attention to myocardial injury patients [28].

4.3   Compartmental Models

Another research was done with compartmental models. SIR model is one of the useful mathematical models used for predicting infectious disease. SIR model was implemented to predict the outbreak of COVID-19 in China [29]. SIR model [25] has three compartments—susceptible, infectious, recovered or deceased. Each prediction is made more accessible with the help of this SIR model. The susceptible equation is given as

$$\frac{\mathrm{d}s}{\mathrm{d}t} = -bs(t)I(t) \tag{4}$$

The infectious equation is given as,

$$\frac{\mathrm{d}r}{\mathrm{d}t} = kI(t) \tag{5}$$

The recovered or deceased equation is given as,

$$\frac{di}{dt} = bs(t)I(t) - kI(t) \tag{6}$$

Based on the resultant of these equations, S, I, R values are found.

$$S(t) + I(t) + r(t) \tag{7}$$

Here, n is the total population. This will provide the graph of SIR model through which we can able to predict how much infectious the disease was. Ridge regression technique [30] was used to find the rate of susceptibility, infectious and recovered patients who come under myocardial injuries. Based on these calculations, it was similarly applied for COVID-19. Due to the SIR, it was able to predict the average rate of the disease. The following diagram explains the plot of the total number of cases rise within 50 days (Fig. 7).

Here, the curve in the plot explains the number of infectious cases all around the country of China. The plot describes that blue lines are indicated as infectious patients, green lines are indicated as susceptible, and pink lines are indicated as recovered cases. It describes how many myocardial patients were affected by COVID-19 and what is the infectious and recovery rate of those persons.

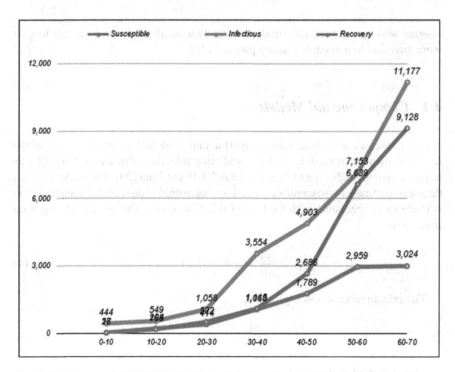

Fig. 7 Plot diagram of COVID-19 infection in China based on the SIR model

4.4   Other Applications of Big Data on COVID-19

The following section explains the other application of big data in the monitoring and mitigation to prevent COVID pandemic.

4.4.1   Spotting the Hotspot Areas

In most populated countries, the hotspot identification played a significant role by spotting which zone is profoundly affected by COVID-19. On the basis, people may stop visiting those places. Big data collected the person's living place and filtered that particular place. It also grouped them as clusters to show how far that place is infected. For example, places that have been deeply affected in India, were marked as dark red zone (Fig. 9), the next level of affected places was marked as the red zone if the moderate number of infection then it was marked as pink, if a few cases then will be marked as yellow and if it is a free zone it is marked as green. This colour method for the zones was decided using big data. The same method was followed globally (Fig. 8). Big data was also employed for predicting the percentage of infection to the total population of the country, which can give a result of how far the country is affected.

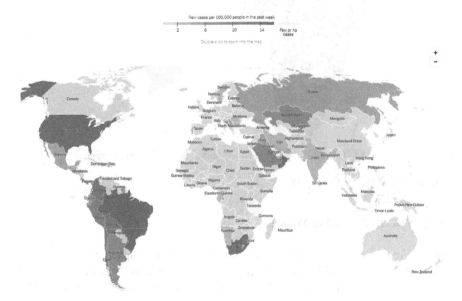

Fig. 8   Global tracker on COVID-19

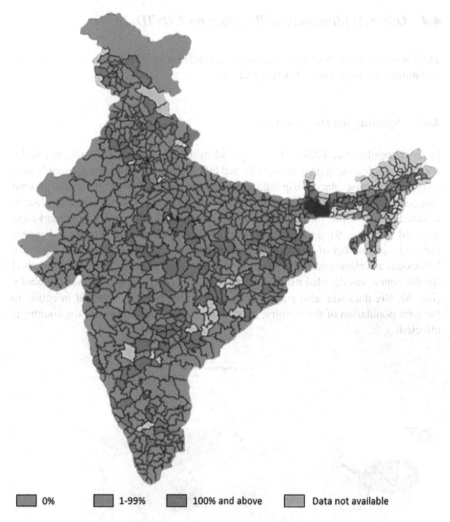

0%   1-99%   100% and above   Data not available

Fig. 9 India tracker on COVID-19

4.4.2 Death Prediction Models

Death prediction model used big data for analysing the impact, and it predicted COVID-19 cases resulting in how the death rate would be by using the model researchers identified that the death rate on COVID-19 cases can be minimised. This model was developed at the University of Washington, USA. Since, in the USA, lockdown was not employed, over 90,000 people died due to COVID-19 disease. On making a study from the other countries, social distancing was the only measure which was identified. After this, USA stated to maintain social distancing. Within two days, the rate of new cases started to decrease, which also paved the way for less death rate. This study was made entirely using big data and data analytics. Global economic growth mainly depends on the USA; hence, the lockdown was still a question mark.

4.4.3 Testing on COVID-19

For a few people, it is possible to take COVID-19 test in hospitals. However, if there is a significant population, only critical and life-risking patients can be admitted in the hospital. Because many will have a common cold, they might suspect and go for treatment. To overcome this, a decision was taken to take the test before identifying the condition of the patient. Big data analysed symptoms of COVID-19 cases, and it gave a rapid result on how to treat the patient. If a person has a mild infection, they were asked to self-isolate in their home itself. As COVID-19 is a communal transmission, for a thousand positive cases, they could have spread for ten thousand people as a hospital cannot provide much space for all the positive cases. Applying big data not only plays a significant role, but also it needs a medical assistant in order to decide on how critical the patient is.

4.4.4 Mobile Applications

In many countries, mobile applications were developed since it can give the accurate location of a person. Countries like India, China, UK, Australia, Singapore and many other countries have developed their app. These apps are useful by giving a notification on which zone a person is from and how far their zone is affected. Each country developed these apps on their regional languages. It also collects the user's name, phone number, identification number, age, address, postal code, profession, etc. This will collect the information, and the health department of each country does the monitoring. For every 20 days, the data of a person is erased, and again, the data is collected from the person. However, the government server will have all the data which is controlled by big data. Some applications in countries are listed below in Table 2.

5 Comparative Summary

All three models showed outsmart results. Through logistic regression model, it showed the survival rate alone. Kaplan–Meier analysis showed results of myocardial injuries and without myocardial injuries. SIR model showed results on how much persons will get infected and recovered, and hence, it proves to be more useful than the other two models. Since it shows results on compartments, it holds good.

Table 2 Countries and their applications on COVID-19

Country	Application
India	Arogya Setu
	Test Yourself Goa
	Mahakavach
	Corona Kavach
	COVA Punjab
	Test Yourself Puducherry
	COVID-19 Quarantine Monitor-Tamil Nadu
	Quarantine watch
	Corona watch
	GoK-Direct Kerala
	COVID-19 feedback
China	Close contact detector
Israel	Hamagen
Australia	COVIDSAFE
United Kingdom	NHS COVID-19
Singapore	Trace together

6 Challenges Faced

On using big data and data analytics, it found great results like predicting the outbreak of COVID-19, vaccines to be used, precautional measures to be taken, tracking the virus spread, comparing with the results of pneumonia, and many other techniques like logistic regression, Kaplan–Meier analysis and SIR models were implemented to predict the COVID-19 cases. These analyses can predict accurate values only but not approximately. It was majorly successful in many hospitals by utilising big data and data analytics on COVID-19. In an analysis of 30 hospitals in China, it was found that 90% of prediction was accurate [31]. However, these are made successful in facing many challenges. The proper dataset was not ready within a few days of the coronavirus spread. Even though the technologies were used, still it is a challenge for controlling the spread of the virus. A proper medicine was unable to discover using several medicinal datasets. Including this privacy, challenges were also faced [32]. In order to control the virus spread, GPS location, travel reports, daily reports, medical reports and personal history of patients must be shared. These are stored as data to identify that patient might not be the carrier of the virus. Hence, the personal data of each patient is managed by big data. However, it was a tough challenge to maintain privacy for these data.

The big data and data analytics should be recommended to use overall the world for fighting against the pandemic COVID-19 since it may help in flattening the curves of rising by applying many technological solutions on the healthcare industry.

6.1 Big Data and Economic Challenges

Even a person is under self-isolation, there is a possibility on positive cases of COVID-19. So far, it was not made a point that the virus can transmit through air. Also, coronavirus tends to live on environmental surfaces for a while. Immunity power of a human decides on fighting with this deadly virus.

Without considering big data and data analytics, COVID-19 has made an impact in economic position, health care, education, business, pharmaceuticals, IT sector, automobiles manufacturing division and so on. According to the International Monetary Fund (IMF), a medium scale of unemployment of 8.4% has now increased to 10.5% due to the COVID-19 lockdown in many countries. A study was made that unemployment in the USA has an average of 2–3%, but now, it has increased to 10%. Many workers furloughed. COVID-19 has also made a fall in stock markets. It created a situation to slash the interest rates in many banks, in order to provide ease, but this will make a fall in the economic growth of a country. If this tends to continue, then there will be a 4% fall in the global economy, which may lead to recession. This has mainly affected countries like India and China, which are the largest manufacturing countries.

Due to the pandemic, airways were also banned in many countries, which may hold good for many, but it may also create much unemployment by without giving them a chance for immigration. On banning the transports, oil and gas industries are facing hurdles. The crude oil prices started to shrink due to less demand for it. It also reached a 5.2% loss globally. The automobile industry also faced the impact. Since these industries have a massive number of workers, the production unit will be completely halted. Export and import of these industries will also see a drawback. Only when there is a zero possibility of COVID-19 cases, economic life can return.

7 Conclusion

Overall review of big data and data analytics role on COVID-19 was discussed in this paper. The brief introduction of how big data and data analytics were applied in healthcare was reported. Role of predictive analytics and survival analytics of data analytics stream on COVID-19 was explained with accurate results. Pneumonia, CT scan data, myocardial infection data and several infectious diseases played a significant role in COVID-19 big data [33]. Aviation and mobile tracking data were very helpful in identifying the migration of people from one place to another. Some other real-time applications on COVID-19 were also discussed as a part. It also elaborated the comparative study on three different models of big data analytics applied to myocardial injury. A view on challenges so far faced using this big data and data analytics was explained. COVID-19 has no medicine yet, but it can be controlled only by social distancing and maintaining cleanliness around the city.

References

1. Phan LT, Nguyen TV, Luong QC et al (2020) Importation and human-to-human transmission of a novel coronavirus in Vietnam. N Engl J Med
2. Xu Z, Shi L, Wang Y et al. Pathological findings of COVID-19 associated with acute respiratory distress syndrome. Lancet, pp 420–422
3. Gao GF (2020) From A to Z: attacks from emerging and re-emerging pathogens. Cell 1157–1159
4. Stahl K, Bode C, David S (2020) First do no harm-beware the risk of therapeutic plasma exchange in severe COVID-19. Critical Care
5. Chae S, Kwon S, Lee D (2018) Predicting Infectious disease using deep learning and big data. Int J Environ Res Public Health 15(8)
6. Huang X, Clements ACA, Williams G, Milinovich G, Hu W (2013) A threshold analysis of dengue transmission in terms of weather variables and imported dengue cases in Australia. Emerg Microbes Amp Infect 2:e87
7. Gansekaran K, Abdulrehman SA (2020) Artificial intelligence applications in tracking health behaviours during disease epidemics. Springer International Publishing, pp 141–155
8. Lew TWK, Kwek TK, Tai D et al (2003) Acute respiratory distress syndrome in critically ill patients with severe acute respiratory syndrome. JAMA 374–380
9. Peng L, Yang W, Zhang D, Zhuge C, Hong L (2020) Epidemic analysis of COVID-19 in China by dynamic modelling. arXiv preprint:2002.06563
10. https://www.researchgate.net/deref/http%3A%2F%2F, www.nhc.gov.cn%2F
11. Ouidit GY, Kassiri Z, Jiang C et al (2009) SARS-coronavirus modulation of myocardial ACE2 expression and inflammation in patients with SARS. Eur J Clin Invest
12. Zhao X, Liu X, Li X (2020) Tracking the speed of novel coronavirus (2019-ncov) based on big data. medRxiv
13. Hu Z, Ge Q, Jin L, Xiong M (2020) Artificial intelligence forecasting of COVID-19 in China. arXiv preprint arXiv:2002.07112
14. Castorina P, Iorio A, Lanteri D (2020) Data analysis on coronavirus spreading by macroscopic growth laws. arXiv: 2003.00507
15. Wang S, Kang B, Ma J, Zeng X, Xiao M, Guo J, Cai M, Yang J, Li Y, Meng X et al (2020) A deep learning algorithm using CT images to screen for coronavirus disease (COVID-19). medRxiv
16. Yi-Cheng C, Ping-En L (2020) A time-dependent SIR model for COVID-19 with undetectable infected persons, April
17. Hastie T, Tibshirani R, Friedman J (2001) Elements of statistical learning: data mining, inference and prediction. Springer, Berlin
18. Rong-Hui D, Li-Rong L, Cheng-Qing Y, Wen W, Ming L et al (2020) Predictors of mortality for patients with COVID-19 pneumonia caused by SARS-CoV-2: a prospective cohort study. Eur Respiratory J
19. Mittal M, Kaur I, Pandey SC, Verma A, Goyal LM (2019) Opinion mining for the Tweets in healthcare sector using fuzzy association rule. EAI Endorsed Trans Pervasive Health Technol 4(16)
20. Jiang S, Li Q (2020) Mathematical models for devising the optimal SARS-COV-2 eradication in China, South Korea, Iran and Italy, Lancet
21. Baesens B et al (2005) Neural network analysis for personal loan data. J Oper Res Soc 1089–1098
22. Bauch CT, Lloyd-Smith JO, Coffee JO, Galvani AP (2005) Dynamically modelling SARS and other newly emerging respiratory illnesses: past present and future. In: Epidemiology, pp 791–801, Nov 2005
23. Huang C, Wang Y, Li X et al (2020) Clinical features of patients infected with 2019 novel coronavirus in Wuhan, China. Lancet 395:497–506
24. Dong Y, Mo X et al (2020) Epidemiology of COVID-19 among children in China. Pediatrics

25. Chawla S, Mittal M, Chawla M, Goyal LM (2020) Corona virus—SARS-CoV-2: an insight to another way of natural disaster. EAI Endorsed Trans Pervasive Health Technol 6(22)
26. Chen C-J (1999) Epidemiology: principles and methods. Linking Publishing Company
27. Wang L, He W, Yu X, Liu H, Zhou W, Jiang H (2020) Effect of myocardial injury on the clinical prognosis of patients with new coronavirus pneumonia. Chin J Cardiovascular Dis 48
28. Ruan Q, Yang K, Wang W, Jiang L, Song J (2020) Clinical predictors of mortality due to COVID-19 based on an analysis of data of 150 patients from Wuhan, China. Intensive Care Med 641–643
29. Report of the WHO-China Joint Mission on Coronavirus Disease [EB/OL] [2020–03–05] (2019)
30. Majumder M, Mandl KD (2020) Early transmissibility assessment of a novel coronavirus in Wuhan, China. SSRN J
31. Mittal M, Balas VE, Goyal LM, Kumar R (eds) (2019) Big data processing using spark in cloud. Springer, Heidelberg
32. Dayal BS, MacGregor JF (1996) Identification of finite impulse response models: methods and robustness issues. Ind Eng Chem Res 35(11):4078–4090
33. Gao H, Liu CH, Wang W, Zhao J, Song Z, Su X, Crowcroft J, Leung KK. A survey of incentive mechanisms for participatory sensing. IEEE Commun Surv Tutorials 17:2

Chapter 14
Rise of Online Teaching and Learning Processes During COVID-19 Pandemic

Koushal Kumar and Bhagwati Prasad Pande

1 Introduction

Since December 2019, the world has been witnessing the rapid spread of the novel *Corona Virus Disease 2019 (COVID-19)* from Wuhan, China, to the entire globe. This highly contagious virus was declared a pandemic by the World Health Organization (WHO) on March 11, 2020. This widely transmittable disease has affected all the spheres of our lives such as economy, business, manufacturing, health sector, education, and livelihood [1]. The pandemic has deeply affected the educational systems all around the globe, and they have been derailed from their normal operations. The outbreak of the pandemic caused schools, colleges, and universities to remain closed for an indefinite period. In India, the even semesters of universities and colleges which usually get operational between January and June, and new sessions in the schools, which start from April have been completely affected. Things might go without the proper teaching and learning capacities, and there is a potential risk of losing the coming semesters in the future. As per the initial evaluation and assessment of the researchers, it is uncertain that when will the normal classroom teaching and learning process be able to resume. This pandemic will surely cause adverse effects on teaching and learning opportunities, as social distancing is essential and mandatory at present. According to the new estimates published by UNESCO, about 1.3 billion students worldwide are unable to go to schools and colleges due to the spread of COVID-19 [2]. In India, schools and colleges were among the first of the several organizations which began to shut down as a precautionary measure to prevent the virus from spreading. Unquestionably, this pandemic has created enormous pressure

K. Kumar
Sikh National College, Guru Nanak Dev University, Qadian, Punjab, India
e-mail: kaushal_kumar302@yahoo.com

B. P. Pande (✉)
Department of Computer Applications, LSM Govt. PG College, Pithoragarh, Uttarakhand, India
e-mail: bp.pande21@gmail.com

on the education system, and nearly 300 million children and 1.4 million schools in the country have been affected. Various studies have been conducted in the past, which support that the closure of educational institutes is a potential intervention to combat a pandemic. Jackson et al. [3] reported in their research that the closure of school and college could be the most successful method to cease the outspread of disease, and it consequently minimized the peak demands on health services. The students, teachers, academic personnel, societies, families, and the country as a whole are required to be saved seriously.

Educational institutions are trying to find a way to resolve this challenging situation and to adopt some multi-pronged strategy to address this crisis in the long term. In the present scenario, various educational units around the world have taken several initiatives to sustain the education system functional. Various educational organizations have integrated the Internet and its technologies to the teaching and learning practices and have started online teaching modules to build a unified teaching and learning system [4]. Online teaching and learning refer to the Internet-based education system, which is nowadays the most prevalent mode of education. Online learning is also known as *e-learning* or *Web-based learning*, and its 24 × 7 access makes it the most popular mode of education at present. Many demerits are also associated with this e-learning mode, like availability and affordability of the Internet and digital gadgets, difficulty to get familiar with it easily, the discomfort of not getting a face-to-face interaction, problems in conducting practical sessions, etc. [5]. However, some people favor the online learning mode as it is easily accessible, the possibility of diversified study material, and the quality of being reachable in remote areas. Some scholars perceived online teaching and learning as a comparatively cheaper mode of education in terms of lower transportation costs and average institution-based learning costs. Before the outbreak of the COVID-19 pandemic, the online learning system was mostly preferred by those students who could not go to schools or colleges because of their busy schedules. Various educational units across the nation agree that online education is critical to their long-term strategy as an alternative to the traditional classroom teaching and learning process. Ministries of education in various countries are also providing remote learning resources for students while schools and colleges are closed. The Indian Ministry of Human Resource Development (MHRD) has also released a list of essential digital learning platforms under the Government of India's initiatives. These platforms cover both school education and higher education in different subject areas and encourage online learning in India. Some of these popular digital learning platforms are discussed in the appendix.

The rest of the present chapter is organized as follows: Sect. 2 presents a brief literature survey and Sect. 3 discusses the features of online teaching and learning processes; in Sect. 4, we present a comparative analysis of digital tools available to aid online teaching and learning process, and Sect. 5 presents a brief survey report, and the final section presents the conclusion of the present work.

2 A Brief Literature Survey

Kim and Bonk [6] presented a survey on the prospects of online teaching in higher education. The authors surveyed college instructors and administrators who had relevant experience and ideas about the factors that could affect the present and future role and scope of the online education system. They reported that the female participants appeared to be more active in the online teaching environment. Moreover, the authors underlined their finding that usage of course management systems (CMSs) would be increased rapidly in the upcoming years, and the tools like video streaming, online testing, and exam, and learning object libraries would become popular eventually. They inferred that the society would enter into a unique and exciting age of online teaching and learning. Sagheb-Tehrani [7] explored the impact of distance learning over online platforms and investigated the advantages and disadvantages of it. They stated that the developments and advances in the IT tools put new challenges in front of the traditional higher education system. This requires advancing the faculties and instructors to teach the courses online with the latest technologies. They commented that the concept of online teaching allowed universities to disseminate their online program and degrees globally. According to the authors [7], in the higher education system, the tendency to register for online courses has been increasing substantially faster than that in the traditional courses. In their meta-analysis and review report, Means et al. [8] studied the available literature of online teaching from 1996 to 2008. Their analysis focused on the following traits of online teaching and learning: the difference between remote and face-to-face environment; outcomes of students' learning; a rigorous research methodology; and calculation of effect size. The authors [8] performed a meta-analysis on the outcomes of their screening and reported that, on average, students who had online teachings performed better than those who received face-to-face instructions. They highlighted their finding that blended teaching and learning, i.e., combination of the elements of the online and face-to-face methods, had the upper hand over teachings conducted entirely in the traditional face-to-face environment. El-Seoud et al. [9] discussed the difficulties in traditional teaching faced by a multitude of universities in Egypt. They argued that technology could help to overcome such obstacles and discussed the interactive features of e-learning. They presented some hypotheses to determine the inclination of students toward the modern e-learning environment and reported that the teachers and instructors should understand the motives of the students when taking online classes. The authors [9] discussed that it is difficult to assess the students' motivation for online teaching and learning system because of the absence of personal contact between the students and instructors. Nguyen [10] examined the effectiveness of online learning in higher education and reported that the supremacy of the traditional classroom teaching appeared to mitigate, and the Internet developed the interest of many educators and researchers in online teaching and learning. The authors concluded that based on the pieces of evidence they found, online teaching and learning processes appeared to be as effective as the traditional teaching and learning process, but the evidence might be conclusive. They commented that online learning had been commenced and its scope and significance in the future would depend on its present treatment. Sun and Chen [5] discussed the theories, practices, and assessments in the realm of the online learning environment. They suggested practical approaches to the development of online courses. They argued that online teaching and learning environment could be more effective with carefully designed course content, interactions among instructors and learners, development of interest for online teaching and learning opportunities, and swift advancements in technologies. The authors [5] highlighted that the concepts and implementations of online education are very likely to continue and grow. Tsai [11] reviewed twelve research works by different authors and presented many approaches, tools, and applications of Web-based learning technologies. The author [11] felt the need to design appropriate and relevant e-learning platforms with the help of contemporary IT tools. The author [11] concluded with the remarks that the ideas he presented from the literature could help educators, teachers, and schools to design their online, blended, or flipped courses more efficiently, and this would eventually improve behaviors, responses, and learning performances of their students. Frazer et al. [12] highlighted the effectiveness of online teaching methods in nursing. They stated that the faculties needed to be competent and skilled in IT tools to influence the online teaching and learning environment. They designed a semi-structured interview for nurse educators from an online university and reported that teaching effectiveness, indicators of quality (like improvement in students' performance, their ability to apply the knowledge, etc.), and students' success were the three key points that reflected from the analysis of data. Roddy et al. [13] presented a review article about the practices employed in online teaching and learning environment. They reported that students and knowledge seekers wish to upgrade their skills, get retrained, and pursue further studies. Therefore, the need for smooth and flexible online pedagogical methods has been increasing. The authors discussed the critical factors for both the facets of the coin: online teaching and online learning. They highlighted the fact that for the successful implementation of online teaching and learning methods, leaning on effective communication, e-content generation, latest technologies, and feedback strategies is essentially required. Rouadi and FaysalAnouti [14] compared the success and failure of online teaching and learning at intermediate and secondary schools in Lebanon during the outbreak of the COVID-19 pandemic. The authors reported that due to the following reasons, most of the respondents considered online learning as a failure: slow speed of the Internet, electricity issues, lack of awareness and motivation among students, and non-availability of more than one gadget at home. However, they also highlighted that the rest of the people in their survey admitted that with good explanation techniques, instructors' ability to teach online, good understanding among teachers and students, and their commitment to participate in e-sessions, online teaching and learning could be more effective and successful.

3 Features of Online Teaching and Learning Process: The Pros and Cons

In the present section, some critical issues related to online teaching and learning processes are being raised. We discuss some issues directly related to the present circumstances under the impact of the COVID-19 pandemic and explore their possible remedies.

3.1 Effectiveness of Online Teaching/Learning as Compared to Classroom Teaching/Learning

Since the COVID-19 outbreak, every nation has been witnessing a distinctive increase in online teaching and learning practices. The deadly pandemic has dramatically changed the flavor of the traditional education system, where teaching and learning are being conducted remotely and on digital platforms. Now, the question arises, whether online teaching and learning practices are as effective as conventional classroom teaching and learning? Many researchers believe that online teaching and learning are not as effective as traditional classroom offerings. Teachers cannot teach discipline, etiquettes, and moral values through online mode to students. Moreover, daily interactions with teachers and classmates improve the perception and experience of students, and they learn how to behave in society [12]. Through online learning, children might not seek opportunities to learn socialization skills which are possible only with classroom teaching. On the other hand, many scholars believe that if students have access to modern gadgets and technologies, online learning can be as effective as classroom learning in several ways. Students can study at their own pace, going back and read, skipping, or accelerating through concepts as they want. Another convenience of online teaching is flexible learning: One can attend online classes or courses in their spare time [15]. A study was conducted by a team of researchers in the *Research Institute of America* which found that online learning has increased student retention rates from 25 to 60% [16]. The *'anyplace-anytime'* characteristic of online learning is useful in crises, for example, man-made disasters, natural catastrophes, and pandemics. Thus, online teaching and learning offer a strong substitute to the traditional classroom teaching and learning at the times of emergency, but the former cannot overtake various dimensions of the latter.

3.2 Infrastructure Requirements for Online Teaching/Learning

According to Schroeder [17], developing the infrastructure to support online classes is similar to building a physical campus that operates with the existing one. The author states that both the teachers and students in online teaching and learning environment have basic needs corresponding to the needs of their physical counterparts in the real campus. These infrastructure requirements should be well addressed for the success of the online teaching and learning project. We present below the basic ingredients of the infrastructure requirements: (a) latest gadgets (computer, laptops, smartphones, tablets, etc.), (b) licensed software and applications (c) high-speed Internet connectivity, and (d) multimedia support (webcam, microphone, etc.). The above-mentioned elements are the essential constituents and are needed as the backbone of the online teaching and learning environment. But, apart from the above list, other factors are equally essential for successful implementation like training of the teachers, students, and staff; support and maintenance of the system; and feedback system. Hussain [18] presented infrastructure requirements for online teaching and learning in terms of hardware, software, and support needs.

3.3 Challenges of Online Teaching/learning and How Do Deal with Them

Online teaching and learning processes are not that simple as they may appear. Many issues can affect the successful manifestation of the online education system in this outbreak of the COVID-19 pandemic. Some vital challenges are discussed below that should be addressed while dealing with teaching and learning practices over the Internet.

3.3.1 Lack of Motivation Among Students

In the physical classroom environment, being attentive and disciplined is the natural phenomenon. It is easy to get distracted when one is trying to learn online lectures from home. Students remain in their comfort zones at their homes, and one can easily be tempted to lose his/her attention and concentration. Moreover, instant expert support may not be available all the time.

3.3.2 Physical and Technical Hurdles

Not every student possesses reliable and robust IT tools to continue his/her online learning smoothly. Students may not have personal gadgets, and they may be dependent on the availability of the devices that belong to their parents or siblings. Internet availability and speed are the major factors which directly affect the remote learning process even if students are very sincere to undertake the online lectures. Students may not be comfortable with the software applications or tools on which their online classes get conducted. Some applications may demand higher hardware require-ments than the devices they have. From the teachers' and institutions' point of view, applications they are using may need a full license to access their complete functionalities.

3.3.3   Isolation

The traditional classroom environment provides an opportunity for the students to be social. They study and learn in groups, they share their understandings about the topics/subjects and other feelings, and there is a sense of healthy competition among pupils. On the contrary, in remote learning, students feel isolated and lonely. This drops their enthusiasm to receive the lessons being taught.

3.3.4   Time-Consuming Process

When teachers are not allowed to stand in class and teach in the usual way, they have to generate the learning resources for their students. Developing e-contents (like presentations, PDFs, videos, animations, etc.) of the syllabi is indeed a challenging and time-consuming task. The verbal lectures that a teacher provides online should be accompanied by written documents so that every student can access and comprehend them. This process gets more complicated if you have to teach a practical subject, where step-by-step instructions, explanations, and demonstrations are needed.

3.3.5   Absence of Common Guidelines or Standard Paradigms

Since the lockdown began in India and different nations, the teaching and learning processes have been kept operational through online medium. However, we may observe the lack of a common framework, model, and guidelines on how to shift from the offline mode to the online mode of teaching and learning processes. Every teacher has been putting his/her best endeavors to carry out the remote teaching process, but the heterogeneity of the approaches can easily be observed. This phenomenon gets more diversified at local level educational institutions. Hardy [19] discussed an exhaustive list of online teaching challenges and suggested feasible solutions. Based on the literature study and remote interviews with teachers and students, the following suggestions can serve as remedies to the aforementioned challenges: (1) The role of parents and family comes into the picture when students are lacking motivation while studying from home; (2) institutions should communicate with the parents to arrange gadgets and proper Internet connection for the students. There should be some finan-cial relaxation in the tuition fee to meet these extra expenses; (3) a separate hotline or grievance cell for the students should be maintained by respective institutions to address the difficulties faced by the students in online learning; (4) To ensure that students must not feel isolated, virtual group activities, tutorial sessions, discussions on virtual boards, and regular check-ins should be maintained by the teachers; (5) There must be strict deadlines associated with each module and assignment submission; (6) teachers should develop e-contents in advance and accompany them with already existing subject-related material (like blogs, e-books, videos, animations, etc.) available online. This may save a lot of precious time for the teachers; (7) the system needs to develop a clear and common guidelines and framework to facilitate online teaching and learning practices homogeneously.

3.4 Skills Required by a Teacher for the Online Teaching Process

In the current scenario of COVID-19, the domain of online pedagogy is continuously expanding, and teaching in online mode is now considered as an essential and integral part of the teaching skills. A major barrier that restricts a teacher from shifting to online teaching mode is their mindset of the traditional classroom model. Online teaching skills have been classified into different hierarchical levels in the literature [20]. The following skills must be possessed by online instructors for the success of the online teaching and learning paradigm: (1) Instructors must have an understanding of the online pedagogical model; (2) instructors should have basic IT skills. This includes computer literacy, familiarity with the operation of software and applications, usage of multimedia devices and corresponding applications; (3) instructors should have the art to convert their traditional lectures into their online counterparts, supported by study material in soft form; (4) they should possess good communication skills; (5) instructors should have strong subject knowledge; (6) they must possess personal characteristics like a good listener, patient, politeness, etc.; (7) instructors should have motivating skills; (8) instructor should have time management skills which are essential in online classroom teaching and learning model.

3.5 Moral Duties of Students and Parents to Support Online Teaching Methodologies

Teaching and learning are a two-way process: Endeavors and hard work are demanded both at the teacher's side and the student's side. Now, in the online teaching and learning model, since the students are at their homes, the role of parents also gets magnified for the successful manifestation of online education. The quest of providing uninterrupted education at the time of the COVID-19 pandemic requires that endeavors and techniques adopted by teachers should significantly be supported by students and their parents. Some ethical notes are presented here which should be followed by students and their families: (1) Students should understand that online lectures and face-to-face lectures may not be equally comparable. Therefore, they should put more effort to try to learn the things by exploring additional resources if needed; (2) students should appreciate the efforts that their teachers put in preparing online lectures and supporting documents in soft form; (3) Student should respond positively by appreciating teacher's job in the online environment, by carrying out given tasks in time, and by submitting assignments within the deadline; (4) parents should play the role of a mediator between teacher and student. They should try to fill the communication gap if any between them; (5) parents should periodically check the progress of the online lectures, percentage of syllabi completion, and progress of their children; (6) parents should motivate their children to support their teachers and their efforts.

3.6   Potential Consequences of Online Education Model on Health

Online teaching and learning are the only possible ways in the present pandemic time, but the longevity of gazing electronic screens and sitting before digital gadgets would lead to many health issues. UNICEF released an official alerting statement that millions of young students are at a higher risk as their screen time has been rapidly increased during the COVID-19 pandemic [21]. Many health experts across the world believe that if online teaching and learning methodologies remain in existence with such a hectic schedule in upcoming months, this will surely result in ill consequences such as headache, weaker eyesight, muscle fatigue, stress, back pain, irregular sleep pattern, schizophrenia, bipolar disorder, etc. A large number of students who are actively participating in online classes experienced noise-induced deafness due to the prolonged usage of earphones. To tackle all the health hazards, it is now essential that administrators of schools and colleges must develop physical and mental health and wellness resources for students and faculty members. The Indian MHRD released a few effective guidelines [22] to cope up with the issues of students' health during online classes, like online classes for pre-primary students should not last more than 30 min; students in grade 1 to 8 should not be required to attend more than two sessions of 30–45 min each; schools are expected to keep four 30–45-min sessions each for students in classes 9–12.

3.7   Scope of Online Teaching/learning in the Post-Pandemic World

Most of the teachers and students have either never practiced online education mode or they have experienced the hybrid mode where online and offline teaching and learning go hand in hand. To encourage complete online teaching and learning, various stakeholders such as governments and private organizations have been trying their best to offer services and training to teachers and students so that they can use online platforms optimally. In India, the central government has taken many initiatives to provide easy access to online learning resources for students and teachers such as PM E-VIDYA and SHAGUN. Globally recognized IT companies have developed easy-to-use virtual online teaching–learning applications so that students can acquire knowledge while staying at home. The scope of online teaching/learning in the post-pandemic world depends entirely on the availability of adequate infrastructure. The reach and impact of online teaching/learning will remain significant after the current pandemic crises only in those institutions which can provide basic infrastructure to their personnel. The past statistics show that online learning and teaching have shown maximum growth and success in tier 1 and tier 2 cities in India as compared to other less developed cities [23]. The craze and scope of online teaching and learning in such areas may continue to expand post-pandemic due to its easy and on-demand access, time–cost feasibility, and abundance of online resources. On the other hand, most of the students come from villages and remote areas, and they face almost unbeatable challenges by not having adequate infrastructure facilities to carry out online learning. There are nearly 638,000 villages in India, where students face many hurdles in attending online classes due to inadequate facilities. To overcome all these challenges and for the digital development of the villages, governments all over the world have been taking many initiatives. Undoubtedly, the COVID-19 pandemic has given an opportunity to academic communities across the world to embrace online teaching and to learn new technological skills. Teachers who are proficient at planning and teaching in classroom teaching are now re-learning the same for online classes. Therefore, the COVID-19 crisis worked as a catalyst for the intensive usage of digital technologies and for promoting e-learning. In the last couple of months, our education system has been going through positive modifications and online learning is now becoming a new paradigm in educational society.

4   Comparative Analysis of Digital Tools Available to Aid Online Teaching and Learning Process

In this era of the digital boom, technology plays a significant role in every dimension of our day-to-day life, including the process of teaching and learning. In the present crisis, the globally affected teaching and learning systems have been witnessing a sort of revolution through the effective use of IT tools. Such tools facilitate real-time communications from one sender to several receivers across remote locations in the form of text messages, voice, video, screen sharing via PPTs, etc. While thousands of applications and tools are available in the market, only a few are popular among educational persons. In this section, some popular digital learning tools are discussed that are assisting teachers and students in the present pandemic crisis and helping them to expand their knowledge and making teaching and learning easy.

4.1 Google Classroom

Google Classroom is a free Web-based application developed by *Google* that assists teachers and students to interact, collaborate, schedule, manage assignments, and it also offers much more functionalities in a single software app. This app provides a very user-friendly interface where a teacher can customize a unique class as per his/her requirements in just a few mouse clicks. The main feature that distinguishes *Google Classroom* from other apps is that it integrates docs, sheets, slides, Gmail, and calendar into a single platform to make communication and collaboration easy.

4.2 Zoom App

Zoom is one of the most popular cloud-based video conferencing application that helps teachers and students to set up a virtual video and audio-conferencing platform. Using the *Zoom* application, a teacher can organize webinars, discussion forums, screen sharing, and other collaborative tasks with students. The network bandwidth consumed by the *Zoom* app is optimized for the best experience and quality service based on the participants' network speed. The reason behind its popularity is its simplicity, lightweight, and user-friendly interface. After the outbreak of the COVID-19 pandemic, the *Zoom* app has touched a new milestone of nearly 300 million active *Zoom* users.

4.3 Webex

Webex is a cloud-based Web application developed by *Cisco*. *Webex* is a highly efficient, secure, scalable, and open global platform for virtual collaboration that integrates audio and video calling, texting, meeting, team collaboration, and offers an excellent experience to its customers. *Webex* has the potential to bring teachers and students together just like a traditional physical classroom. *Cisco* claimed that in the month of April 2020, at the peak of the current crisis, over a half billion people were using *Webex* for virtual communication like business meetings, virtual classrooms, etc.

4.4 Google Meet

Previously named as *Google Hangouts Meet*, it is an audio–video conferencing application provided by *Google* as part of their *G-Suite*. The standard version of *Google Meet* is very popular among teachers and students while the premium version which offers more features is mostly used by larger business enterprises. *Google* started offering *Google Meet's* additional features free of cost in response to the global crises caused by the COVID-19 pandemic for which the standard enterprise account was needed. In the free version of *Google meet*, teachers can host meetings with 250 students at a time and for live streaming; it supports up to 100,000 viewers with the option to record and save meetings in *Google Drive*.

4.5 Microsoft Teams

Microsoft Teams is a collaborative platform by *Microsoft* for Web-based real-time communication, and it integrates workplace chat, video meetings, file storage and sharing (PPT, PDF, CSV, etc.), and application integration. In April 2020, Microsoft declared that the *Microsoft Teams* had reached 75 million users and it recorded 4.1 billion minutes of meetings on a single day. Teams apps have both free and paid premium versions for better service quality and security of data. Its free version offers 2 GB space per user and with no guarantee of the quality of service, while the paid version provides 1 TB and with 99.9% service guaranteed.

For a better understanding of these applications, we have performed a comparative technical analysis over some features which is presented in Table 1.

5 Online Teaching and Learning Practices During COVID-19 Pandemic in India: A Brief Online Survey

A survey was conducted online among the school and college teachers from different states in India with the help of *Google form*. This online survey aimed to find the views and experiences of school and college teachers who have been teaching online since the outbreak of the COVID-19 pandemic. Ten multiple choice questions and two short answer questions were compiled to know and assess the experiences and opinions of teachers who are presently teaching in Indian secondary schools, colleges, and universities. This online survey had been employed to determine teachers' levels of computer literacy, their familiarity with computers and software in general, students' motivation level during online class, the alertness, and inquisitiveness of students in an online class, problems being faced by teachers in online classes, etc.

5.1 Data Sampling

As we all know, the nation's unlock process has been started in phases from June 1, 2020, but schools and colleges have been kept closed in these unlock phases.

Table 1 Comparative technical analysis of some popular online teaching–learning applications

Features	Applications				
	Zoom App	Webex	Google Meet	Google Classroom	Microsoft Teams
Platform supported	Windows, Mac, Android, iOS, Ubuntu	Windows, Mac, Android, iOS, Linux, Chrome OS	Windows, Mac, Android, iOS, Linux, Chrome OS	Windows, Mac, Android, iOS, Linux	Windows, Mac, Linux, iOS
Free option	Yes	Yes	Yes	Yes	Yes
Application size (MB)	115.9	90.3	144.7	198.8	95.9
Monthly fee (paid version)	$14.99 to $19.99 per host	$17.5 to $57.5 per host	$10 to $20 per host	$4 to $22 per host	$2 to $18 per host
Maximum participants	Allow for 100 participants at a time and up to 1000 with pro packages	100 for free version and up to 1000 in premium versions	100 for free version and up to 250 in G-Suite Enterprise Essentials	250 using personal Google account and 1000 using G-Suite with 20 teachers per class	300 desktop or web version and up to 1000 in live streaming
Desktop sharing	Yes	Yes	Yes	Yes	Yes
Group messaging	Yes	Yes	Yes	Yes	Yes
Application sharing	Yes	Yes	Yes	No	Yes
Recording	Yes	Yes	Yes	Yes	Yes
Live streaming	No (only in paid version)	No (only in paid version)	Yes 100 k Viewers (Free till 30th Sep. 2020)	Not supported	No (only in paid version)
End-to-end Encryption	Yes	Yes	No	Yes	Yes

(continued)

Table 1 (continued)

Features	Applications					
	Zoom App	Webex	Google Meet	Google Classroom	Microsoft Teams	
Storage location	Cloud	Local and Cloud	Cloud	Cloud	Cloud	
Minimum hardware requirements	Single Core 1Ghz or Higher, 2 GB RAM	Intel Core2Duo 2.0 GHz or AMD Athlon equivalent and 2 GB RAM	2.2 GHz Intel 2nd-generation processor with 2 GB RAM	1.4 GHz Intel Pentium 4 with 512 MB of RAM	1.6 GHz processor with 2 GB RAM	
Recommended hardware requirements	Dual Core 2Ghz or Higher (i3/i5/i7 or AMD equivalent) with 4 GB RAM	Dual Core 2.5 GHz with 4 GB RAM	Core to Due with 2.6 GHz or i3/i5/i7, with 4 GB RAM	2 GHz Pentium 4 or faster processor with 2 GB RAM	Dual core 2 GHz or Higher (i3/i5/i7 or AMD equivalent) with 4 GB DDR3 RAM	
Bandwidth requirements for group video calling	800 kbps/1.0 Mbps (up/down) for high quality video	0.5 Mbps(up/down) to 3 Mbps for HD quality	1–4 Mbps for up and down connection	512 kbps for audio and 2 Mbps for video communication	30 kbps (P2P audio call) to 2 Mbps (HD group call)	

Compliance with social distancing has always been a mandate too. Therefore, we could conduct the survey in online mode only. The media we utilized to endorse our questionnaire included WhatsApp chat groups, Facebook posts and Messenger chats, LinkedIn posts, ResearchGate posts, and personalized e-mail messages. The targeted population for our survey study was teachers/lecturers who have been teaching through online mode in various schools and higher educational institutions of India. Data were collected in 2 weeks (between July 15 and 30, 2020), and it took approximately 5 min for a participant to complete this survey. The survey contains responses from 750 participants. We are thankful to all the school and college teachers who participated positively in this study with full cooperation and enthusiasm.

5.2 Data Summarization and Analysis

The first ten multiple choice questions and their responses are presented in Table 2.
Now, we summarize the above findings in graphical form as below; see Fig. 1a–h.
The rest of the two survey questions were descriptive. The first is about the difficulties one faces in online teaching/learning, and the second is about the suggestions. We summarize the responses as follows: (1) inadequate resources at students' end; (2) not every student can afford gadgets and Internet bills/recharges; (3) communication problem; (4) no direct control over the class; (5) difficulties in handling practical subjects; (6) lack of motivation and enthusiasm among students; (7) lack of knowledge about IT tools; (8) technical lags during the online sessions; (9) unavailability of library; (10) government/institutions should provide the proper infrastructure; (11) audio/video lectures should be saved on cloud apart from live streaming; (12) training should be provided; (13) feedback and grievance cell should be maintained; (14) weekly motivational sessions should be arranged for both students and teachers; (15) one should constantly upgrade oneself as per the pedagogical and technical requirements.

6 Conclusions

In the present chapter, the authors discussed the substantial growth of online teaching and learning methods during the COVID-19 pandemic. The complete shutting down of schools, colleges, and universities affected the education system thoroughly, and a revolution has come in the education industry. The consequences demanded from teachers, instructors, and students to put more endeavors and adjust themselves to adopt the online teaching and learning practices. The principal hindrances on the way of the online education model are: inadequate infrastructure; poor availability and speed of the Internet; extra financial expenses; lack of proper training, common guidelines, and motivation, etc. One of the atrocious consequences of online teaching and learning practices is the serious adverse effects on health. Online teaching and

Table 2 Questions and responses of the survey

S. No.	Characteristics/Questions	Responses			
1	Gender	Male		Female	
		530 (70.7 %)		220 (29.3%)	
2	Place	Urban	Rural	Semi Urban	
		452 (60.3%)	116 (15.5%)	182 (24.2%)	
3	Discipline	Humanities	Engineering	Languages	Sciences
		212 (28.3%)	150 (20%)	75 (10%)	313 (41.7%)
4	Which app do you use for online teaching?	Zoom App	Google Meet	Cisco Webex	Others
		225 (30%)	247 (33%)	83 (11%)	195 (26%)
5	Do you have sufficient computer knowledge to carry out online teaching?			Yes	No
				621 (82.8%)	129 (17.2%)
6	Are online classes more effective?	Yes, more effective	No, less effective	May be	
		50 (6.7%)	598 (79.7%)	102 (13.6%)	
7	Do students appear motivated in online classes?		Yes	No	
			412 (55%)	338 (45%)	
8	Do students ask queries in online class?		Yes	No	
			437 (58.3%)	313 (41.7%)	
9	Does online teaching take more time than classroom teaching?		Yes	No	
			625 (83.3%)	125 (16.7%)	
10	Would you like to continue online classes after the abolishment of COVID-19 pandemic?		Yes	No	
			350 (46.7%)	400 (53.3%)	

learning in its current form cannot be compared with traditional classroom teaching, but we cannot deny the scope and significance of the former in the post-pandemic world. Governments are also providing several digital platforms across multiple channels to address the needs of online learning resources so that teachers, students, and learners can be benefitted from them. The productive utilization of online teaching–learning methods and the eventual benefits to students rely partly on the extraneous

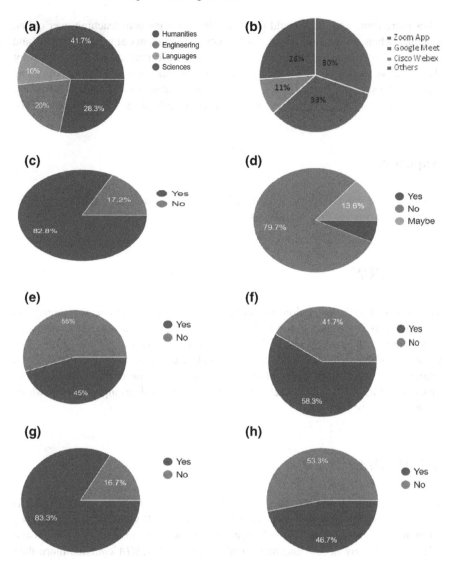

Fig. 1 a Major disciplines, **b** Most popularly used apps, **c** Computer knowledge, **d** Is online teaching more effective? **e** Do students appear motivated? **f** Do students ask queries? **g** Does online teaching take more time? **h** Will you like to continue online classes after the pandemic?

environment, such as availability of appropriate infrastructure, and also to a significant extent, on the attitudes and perceptions of teachers about the role of technology in the modern education system.

In the Indian scenario, our brief survey revealed that most of the teachers are computer literate and the most popular online teaching and learning apps among them are *Zoom* and *Google Meet*. Most of the teachers believe that online teaching takes more time, and they would prefer traditional classroom teaching over online teaching when the current crises finish. Although students appear motivated and attentive in online mode, most of the teachers believe that online teaching is not that effective as it sounds. To expand the ground impact and significance of online teaching we should focus on two things: first, the availability of basic infrastructure and second, proper training to teachers, supporting staff, students, and their parents.

Appendix

Some of these popular digital learning platforms released under the Indian government's initiatives are discussed below:

A.1 SHAGUN

This is related to the education system in schools for more convenient teaching and learning. This is a digital platform through which many e-learning sites have been introduced by the government of India, all states, and union territories (UTs). The main goal of the *SHAGUN* program is to provide teachers and students with a forum where they can connect using Internet technologies for the teaching and learning process. *SHAGUN* program itself contains three other e-learning platforms which are mentioned below:

A.2 DIKSHA

The MHRD introduced the *National Digital Teachers' Infrastructure (DIKSHA)* platform to bring teachers and students of classes I to XII grade into the e-learning environment. This platform provides teaching and learning material to teachers and students with easy access and better understanding. *DIKSHA* contains more than 85,000 e-books prepared by NCERT, CBSE, and states/UTs for classes I to XII, along with a web mobile app. This digital platform is available in multiple languages so that students from various states can access this learning platform. The *DIKSHA* platform can be accessed from this link: https://diksha.gov.in/.

A.3 e-Pathshala

Under the initiative of *Digital India*, the *e-Pathshala* is a collaborative effort of MHRD and NCERT. The *e-Pathshala* platform is enriched with numerous textbooks, audios, videos, and other printable materials for students, teachers, parents, and researchers. This portal is also available in many languages like the other digital learning platforms and can be accessed using this link: https://epathshala.nic.in/.

A.4 National Repository of Open Educational Resources (NROER)

The *NROER* is a project launched by the Ministry of Strategic Human Resource Management, Department of School literacy and education, Government of India. *NROER* is one of the excellent e-learning initiatives with approximately 16,000 registered users across the nation and with more than 15,000 e-learning services. A broad range of video lectures is hosted on the *NROER* database repository which includes experts' lectures from various domains, demonstration of science experiments, etc. NROER repository can be accessed from this link: https://nroer.gov.in/home/repository.

A.5 SWAYAM

SWAYAM, a Hindi abbreviation that stands for *Study Webs of Active-Learning for Young Aspiring Minds* is an Indian *Massive Open Online Course (MOOC)* platform. This digital forum provides study material in the form of video lectures, self-assessment tests, reading material, online discussions, and doubt sessions for students and faculty members. The portal is managed and run by many national coordinators such as *AICTE, NCERT, IGNOU, NPTEL, UGC, NIOS, IIMB*, and *ITTTR*, etc. for delivering and updating reliable and quality contents to the aspirants. This digital portal is very popular across the globe among the learning community which is being used by subscribers from over 60 countries, including India, Canada, UK, USA, UAE, Germany, Australia, Nepal, and Singapore. *SWAYAM* courses can be accessed using this link: https://swayam.gov.in/.

A.6 NPTEL

NPTEL stands for *National Programme on Technology Enhanced Learning*, which is an initiative launched in 2003 by seven IITs (IIT Bombay, Madras, Guwahati, Delhi, Kanpur, Kharagpur, and Roorkee) and the IISc Bangalore to develop study material for engineering and science disciplines. This program is funded by the MHRD to deliver training to teachers on curricula and pedagogy. The primary motivation behind the establishment of this platform was to provide quality and free education online to students seeking to learn from IITs faculty members. The *NPTEL* web portal contains video lectures for undergraduate and postgraduate levels courses in all major branches of engineering and sciences. The online NPTEL repository has more than 2000+ courses available to view and download along with 55,000 h of video transcripts available as PDF. *NPTEL* has been recognized as one of the most accessed online digital libraries of peer-reviewed educational content in the world. The official website of *NPTEL* can be accessed using this link: https://nptel.ac.in/.

References

1. Mackenzie JS, Smith DW (2020) COVID-19: a novel zoonotic disease caused by a coronavirus from China: what we know and what we don't. Microbiol Australia 41(1):45–50
2. Li C, Lalani F (2020) The COVID-19 pandemic has changed education forever. This is how. World Economic Foroum. https://www.weforum.org/agenda/2020/04/coronavirus-education-global-covid19-online-digital-learning/
3. Jackson C, Mangtani P, Hawker J, Olowokure B, Vynnycky E (2014) The effects of school closures on influenza outbreaks and pandemics: systematic review of simulation studies. PLoS ONE 9(5):e97297, 1–10
4. Dhawan S (2020) Online learning: a panacea in the time of COVID-19 crisis. J Educ Technol Syst 49(1):5–22
5. Sun A, Chen X (2016) Online education and its effective practice: a research review. J Inf Technol Educ Res 15:157–190
6. Kim K, Bonk CJ (2006) The future of online teaching and learning in higher education. Educause Q 22–30
7. Sagheb-Tehrani M (2009) The results of online teaching: a case study. Inf Syst Educ J 7(42):1–10
8. Means B, Toyama Y, Murphy R, Bakia M, Jones K (2010) Evaluation of evidence-based practices in online learning: a meta-analysis and review of online learning studies. U.S. Department of Education. https://www2.ed.gov/rschstat/eval/tech/evidence-based-practices/finalreport.pdf
9. El-Seoud MSA, Taj-Eddin IATF, Seddiek N, El-Khouly MM, Nosseir A (2014) E-Learning and students' motivation: a research study on the effect of E-Learning on higher education. Int J Emerg Technol Learn 9(4):20–26
10. Nguyen T (2015) The effectiveness of online learning: beyond no significant difference and future horizons. MERLOT J Online Learn Teaching 11(2):309–319
11. Tsai C (2016) Research papers in online learning performance and behaviour. Int Rev Res Open Distributed Learn 17(1). https://www.irrodl.org/index.php/irrodl/article/view/2441/3588
12. Frazer C, Sullivan DH, Weatherspoon D, Hussey L (2017) Faculty perceptions of online teaching effectiveness and indicators of quality, pp 1–6
13. Roddy C, Amiet DL, Chung J, Holt C, Shaw L, McKenzie S, Garivaldis F, Lodge JM, Mundy ME (2017) Applying best practice online learning, teaching, and support to intensive online environments: an integrative review. Front Educ 2:59. https://doi.org/10.3389/feduc.2017.00059
14. Rouadi NE, FaysalAnouti M (2020) The online learning experiment in the intermediate and secondary schools in Lebanon during the Coronavirus(COVID-19) crisis. Int J Adv Res Sci Eng Technol 7(7):14466–14485
15. Mastel-Smith B, Post J, Lake P (2015) Online teaching: "are you there, and do you care?" J Nurs Educ 54(3):145–151
16. Leeds EM, Campbell S, Baker HM, Ali RM, Brawley D, Crisp JD (2013) The impact of student retention strategies: an empirical study. Int J Manage Educ 7(1/2):22–43

17. Schroeder R (2001) Institutional support infrastructure for online classes. Metropolitan Univ 12(1):35–40
18. Hussain AR (2020) Infrastructure requirements for E-learning implementation and delivery. CommLab India. https://blog.commlabindia.com/elearning-design/infrastructure-for-elearning
19. Hardy L (2017) The A-Z of online teaching challenges. eLearning Industry. https://elearning industry.com/online-teaching-challenges-a-z
20. Jia-Ling L, Atsusi H (2004) Analysis of essential skills and knowledge for teaching online. In: Association for Educational Communications and Technology, 27th, Chicago, IL, pp 534–540
21. UNISEF Press release: Children at increased risk of harm online during global COVID-19 pandemic (2020). https://www.unicef.org/press-releases/children-increased-risk-harm-online-during-global-covid-19-pandemic
22. Department of School Education & Literacy MHRD, GOI: PRAGYATA Guidelines for Digital Education (2020). https://www.mhrd.gov.in/sites/upload_files/mhrd/files/pragyata-gui delines_0.pdf
23. Khaitan A, Shankhwar A, Jeyanth N, Kharbanda M, Dulipala N, Jhunjhunwala S (2017) Online education in India: 2021. A study by KPMG in India and Google (2017). https://assets.kpmg/content/dam/kpmg/in/pdf/2017/05/Online-Education-in-India-2021.pdf

Chapter 15
Robotic Technology for Pandemic Situation

S. Sangeetha and D. Poornima

1 Introduction

The main routes of transmission of coronavirus are respiratory droplets and direct contact. Because of this, anyone who comes in close contact with the individual who is infected is at great risk of getting the infection. When these droplets land on surfaces, they could remain there for a long time, thus making the environment around the infected person a viable transmission source [1]. In the hospitals and quarantine centers where the infected people are admitted, maintenance of sanitation is of prime importance. This work is done by the sanitary persons whose exposure is very high and so are at high risk [1, 2]. Even though these workers are given protective gear and kit, there is always a risk of exposure and therefore a lot of anxiety among all the workers entering into isolation ward where there are infected patients [1, 3]. This is where the usability of a robot comes into the picture. The use of a robot for such infectious disease treatment will be of great help. With this concern in mind, a robot could be designed which is fully automated and gives a good performance [3]. Even if the robot does 10% of the work that humans do, it would also matter as it will reduce a 10% chance of the human being infected. The other desirable features would be ease of operation, financial effectiveness and power requirements. Smart floor cleaning robot, the automatic lavatory cleaning system and robotic nurse are some of the technology-enabled robots that can be employed in the COVID isolation wards to reduce the exposure of the frontline workers like nurses, sanitary workers and even doctors to a great extent. These robots are practically realizable using low-power microcontrollers and line following principle of robots.

S. Sangeetha (✉) · D. Poornima
Department of EEE, Sri Ramakrishna Institute of Technology, Coimbatore, Tamil Nadu, India
e-mail: sangeetha.eee@srit.org

D. Poornima
e-mail: poornima.eee@srit.org

2 Robotic Technologies

Today's generation likes being smart in everything, whether it is their gadgets or workplace or even home. The recent trend in these smart technologies is the adoption of domestic robots. Automation technology has been evolving in recent years and now comes the right time to adopt it practically. The main benefit of automation technology is an easy lifestyle with more free time for people [4]. This free time can be used to do more creative work which is productive for mankind. Automated homes are today's trend, and the first work that everyone wants to be automated is the cleaning of the living place. The same applies to hospitals and caretaking facilities. In this pandemic, it is difficult to employ the sanitary workers to clean the hospital floors and quarantine areas. Robotic hands are preferred in cleaning the floors of such areas so that those workers do not get infected from the patients who are under treatment [2]. There is a demand for automatic vacuum cleaners as they are convenient than manual vacuum cleaners. Many automated vacuum cleaners are there in the market but most of them clean only dry floors. Wet mopping is still not common. The main components of an automatic vacuum cleaner are Arduino, Arduino shield, real-time clock, LDR sensor, ultrasonic sensor, infrared (IR) sensor and motor shield.

For an automatic cleaning robot, the movement around the house or office or the caretaking facility is very important. It has to clean the whole place with minimum human assistance. For doing this, the robot should have the following specifications:

- It should be able to avoid obstacles.
- It should be able to identify between the floor and carpet.
- It should be able to monitor the fan motor.
- It should be able to do light sensing.
- It should be able to keep track of the real clock time.
- It should be able to switch ON and OFF automatically.

These features will help to achieve the desirable behaviors expected from an automatic floor cleaner robot.

3 Automatic Vacuum Cleaner Robots

Automatic vacuum cleaners are based on a set of data input from the sensors mounted on it which tells the cleaner about the condition of the floor around it. The sensors can be sonars, digital compass or touch sensors. The sensors sense the data from its surroundings and send it to the main processor. The program inside the processor analyzes the data from the sensors and decides the direction of the movement of the cleaning robot. The movement is achieved by sending signals to the appropriate motor drives [5].

3.1   Components of the Cleaning Robot System

The main components of the cleaning robot system are as follows:

- Arduino Mega 2560 microcontroller
- Motor driver
- DC motor
- Bluetooth
- IR sensor
- LDR sensor
- Ultrasonic sensor
- Real-time clock
- 20 × 4 LCD.

3.1.1   Arduino Mega 2560 Microcontroller

The Arduino microcontroller has an ATmega1280 processor embedded in it. It consists of analog inputs, digital I/O pins, crystal oscillator of 16 MHz, ICSP header, UARTs, power jack with USB connection and reset button. The USB cable can be used to connect the microcontroller to a computer. It is powered either with a 5 V battery or an AC-to-DC adapter. Two voltage levels of 3.3 and 5 V are provided in the controller board which gives the flexibility to use the required voltage needed for the particular application. There are four hardware serial ports (USART) which helps in establishing a high-speed connection. This controller is aimed at applications with complicated circuits and requires much memory space to store many instructions. It has many numbers of digital and analog pins for input and output which facilitates employing it in complex circuits [6].

Powering the Arduino board can be done in three ways. A simple USB cable can be used from a device like a laptop or mobile or we can use the V_{in} pin of the board from a power supply, using power jack and battery. Arduino IDE is a software used for programming the controller board. This software is user-friendly and commonly used to code all Arduino family boards. The software code written in Arduino IDE is called sketch. Sketch is burned in the software first and then transferred to the physical board through USB cable. A built-in boot loader is present in the Arduino board so an external burner cannot be used to burn the code into the board. Another good feature of Arduino is its ability to multitask, whereas its software does not support multitasking. So operating systems like Free RTOS and RTX can be used to incorporate multitasking. This gives the user an added flexibility of building their own program using the ISP connector.

Table 1 Motor outputs for different input conditions

Direction	Motor 1		Motor 2	
	Input 1	Input 2	Input 3	Input 4
Forward	High	Low	High	Low
Reverse	Low	High	Low	High
Left	High	Low	Low	High
Right	Low	High	High	Low

3.1.2 Motor Driver

The commonly used motor driving IC is L293D chip, a dual H-bridge motor driver IC that has the ability to drive two motors simultaneously. It has a 16-pin chip and is configured to generate bidirectional currents in the range of 600-mA and voltage range of 4.5–36 V. The drivers are enabled when its associated enable inputs are made high. The outputs of the drivers are in phase with the inputs and are active. The drivers get disabled with low input, and they enter a state of high impedance. The solenoid and motor in any application are controlled by H reversible drive with proper input data [6] (Table 1).

3.1.3 DC Motor

In automation applications, mechanical movements are practically implemented with electric motors. A motor is given electrical energy as the input, and the mechanical energy is obtained as the output. Everyday devices like automobiles, food blenders, vacuum cleaner, etc., run with the help of motors. A DC motor works on DC supply, and the salient feature is its controllability of speed over a wide range, by changing either the supply voltage or the current in the field windings [6]. Figure 1 shows the motor and the IC connection. Generally, we prefer DC motor due to its good performance, ease of speed control, less weight and comfortable controller design. The fact that it can also be battery operated adds to its advantage.

3.1.4 Bluetooth

Bluetooth device is used for communication between the robot and the control device. The control device can be a cell phone or a laptop. Figure 2 shows the Bluetooth unit. The control device transmits the control signal which is received by the Bluetooth device attached to the robot. The robot can also transmit data, and so it is a two-way communication. The structure of Bluetooth is good enough for creating personal area networks and is made for low-power equipment such as mobiles and laptops. Bluetooth protocol makes use of the device's MAC address for communication between the two devices.

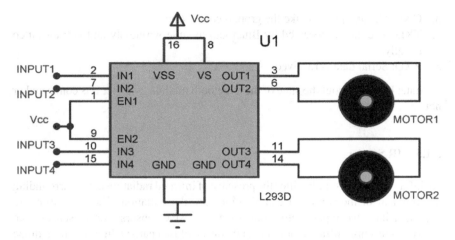

Fig. 1 DC motor and drive connection

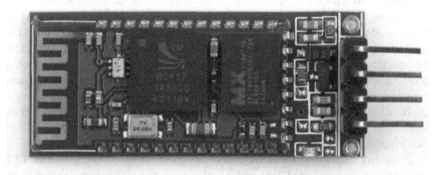

Fig. 2 Bluetooth module

Bluetooth will work up to a distance of 100 m but this range depends upon atmosphere, geographic conditions and the transmitter and receiver. Frequency-hopping spread spectrum (FHSS) method is utilized to send data through the atmosphere. Bluetooth has serial modules which permit the serial-enabled devices to interconnect with each other. The following are six pins in the Bluetooth module.

1. Key/EN: When this key is enabled, the module is set to be in command mode or else it is always set in data mode. The two modes of operation are as follows:

   - Data mode: In this mode, there is an interchange of data between the devices.
   - Command mode: In this mode, AT commands are utilized to change the setting of the module.

2. V_{CC}: A regulated input supply of 5 V or 3.3 V DC supply can be given to this.

3. GND: Ground pin to make the ground connection.
4. TXD: The data is received by Bluetooth module wirelessly and is transmitted serially.
5. RXD: Serial data is received.

State: Informs about the state of the Bluetooth module, whether it is connected or not.

3.1.5   IR Sensor

An infrared (IR) sensor identifies the presence of infrared radiation in the surrounding environment of the sensor. It can also measure the radiation. The IR sensors are classified into two types: active sensors and passive sensors. Active sensors can transmit and sense infrared radiation and consist of two parts: a light-emitting diode (LED) and a receiver [7]. When an object blocks the path of light between the transmitting LED and the receiver, the infrared light from the LED gets reflected by the object. This reflected light is sensed by the receiver, and the difference in the time of traveling of the infrared light is the parameter that helps the receiver to detect the presence of an object. Active IR sensors can be used as proximity sensors and find application in robots as obstacle detection systems. Passive infrared (PIR) sensors are the ones that cannot emit radiation but can detect it. They are widely used for motion detection applications like home security systems. Any object which emits infrared radiation enters the range of the passive sensor, and it detects the object. PIR sensors use the difference in IR levels between the object and the surroundings to detect the presence of a moving object. The sensor sends a signal to the microcontroller which then triggers an alarm. Figure 3 shows the IR sensor.

The sensor used in the vacuum cleaner consists of two eyes. One eye is the LED emitter which emits infrared light, and the other eye is the detector which receives the reflected infrared light. This detection is converted into the distance, and then the data is sent to Arduino for further processing and decision making. Three wires coming from the sensors are connected to 5 V, ground and analog input pin of Arduino, respectively.

Fig. 3 IR proximity module

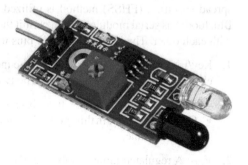

3.1.6 LDR Sensor

The light-dependent resistor (LDR) is a light intensity sensor in which the resistance decreases with an increase in intensity of light. The principle underlying its working is photoconductivity. The light-dependent resistor makes use of a semiconductor material having high resistance [7]. Visible light, when incident on such a semiconductor device, transfers some of the energy of its photons to the valence electrons in the outermost shell. The valence electrons thus get some additional energy and jump from the valence band of the atom to its conduction band. Electron and hole pairs are produced due to the electron jump. This movement of charge carriers improves the conductivity of the device, reducing its resistivity.

Figure 4 shows the structure of an LDR. The cadmium sulfide (CdS) curved line is the film which goes through the sides. Metal films are placed on the top and bottom and are connected to the terminals. The design is done to be able to give the maximum possible area of contact between the two metal films. The whole setup is encased in resin or clear plastic case. This provides the LDR with free access to external light. Cadmium sulfide, the main element of LDR, is a photoconductor and holds very few electrons when no light falls on it. It is designed to attain a large resistance when kept in dark. The resistance is usually in the range of megaohms. When the LDR is illuminated, many free electrons are produced as per the principle explained above, and this increases the conductivity of the material. The energy absorbed by the electrons will increase as the frequency of the incident light increases. Once the frequency exceeds a limit, the electrons will have enough energy to jump from the valence band to the conduction band. The electrons present in the conduction band are free and are capable of conducting electricity. This is the reason behind the dramatic decrease in the resistance of the LDR which will be less than one-kilo ohm.

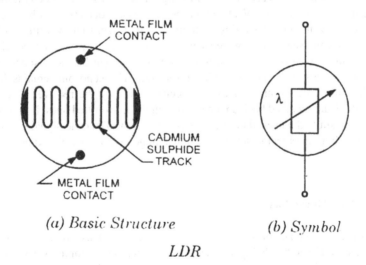

(a) Basic Structure   *(b) Symbol*

LDR

Fig. 4 LDR sensor

Fig. 5 Ultrasonic module

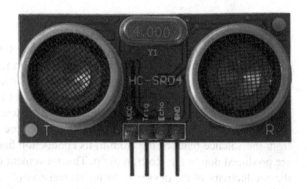

3.1.7 Ultrasonic Sensor

An ultrasonic sensor is a range finder as depicted in Fig. 5. It has a very high performance rating and uses the ultrasonic sound reflection principle. It is compact and is available in a wide range of sizes from 2 cm to 4 m. This ultrasonic range finder is very suitable for all robotic applications and applications where precise ranging data is required. This is a very user-friendly sensor and can be directly connected to the digital input–output lines of the microcontroller [8]. The distance is calculated by measuring the time taken for a sound signal to travel from one point to another. This is done by the use of a simple formula as below.

$$D = (E * V/2) \text{ or}$$

where D = distance, E = echo pulse width high time, V = sound velocity (340 m/s).

The module works on 5 V DC input and accurately detects any obstacle up to a distance of 4 m and gives a direct output signal. To start the working cycle, the pin "Trig" on the sensor is powered with a 10 μs input. This commences the first cycle of range conversion, and the transmitter sends eight bursts of sound waves. This also triggers the echo pin which goes high. The echo pin remains in high until the transmitted sound waves are received back by the receiver. The sound waves which are received back are checked with the transmitted ones. If they are the same as transmitted waves, then the echo pin goes low. The echo signal will go low automatically if no object is detected within a range of 5 m after checking for 30 ms [5].

3.1.8 Real-Time Clock

A real-time clock (RTC) makes a note of the current time. This term usually points at the clocks used in embedded systems, servers and personal computers but nowadays they are embedded in all electronic devices which need to keep track of the accurate time. It is available as an integrated chip. Time tracking can also be done without using RTC, but RTC has some advantages:

- Consumes less power which becomes very crucial when supplied from alternate power sources.
- Time-critical tasks may be well managed by making the main system free during that time.
- Accuracy is better than other methods.

3.1.9 20 × 4 LCD

A liquid crystal display (LCD) can do visual or video display, and it utilizes liquid crystals. Liquid crystals cannot radiate light directly but have light modulating properties. The LCDs are usually referred by the number of rows and number of characters in that row. 20 × 4 denotes that the LCD has four rows, and each row can display a maximum of 20 characters. This means totally eighty characters can be displayed as a message at a given time. Figure 6 illustrates the pin configuration of the LCD and its connection to the Arduino.

The app to control the operation of the cleaner can be developed by any one of the application software. The abovementioned components which are used in the design of a user-friendly robotic vacuum cleaner can operate in both autonomous and manual mode as per our requirements.

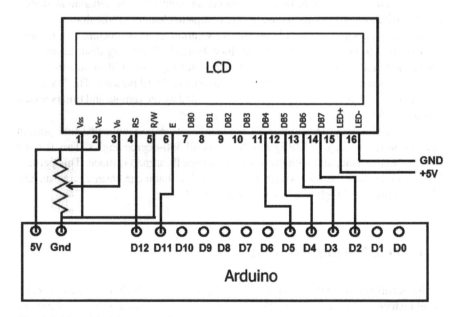

Fig. 6 LCD and Arduino connection

4 Smart Wet Cleaning Robots

Floor cleaning is the frequent task in both clinics and quarantine centers to free the surface from the virus that reaches it during the sneezing or coughing of infected patients [1]. Presently, it is carried out by manual work risking the health of the worker. But this can be overcome by robot technology. The designed floor cleaner robot is programmed to work in two modes: manual or automatic as per the requirement [9]. This robot can facilitate both sweeping and mopping, and the communication between the remote control and the robot is possible for a distance of 50 m. They communicate wirelessly using RF modules. Water is sprayed automatically using a pump, and it avoids the collision with obstacles. Both these functions are made possible with IR sensors. Water pumping, cleaning and wheel movement are done by separate motors. Separate dual relay circuits are used for the motors pumping the water and the cleaners [5].

In the automatic mode, the machine controls all the operations by itself and moves to a different lane in case of difficulty in detection [9]. A keypad is provided for the user to make the robot perform the desired task in the manual mode so that the power requirement can be minimized. There are separate switches to control different operations like basement cleaning, water flow control, to and fro movement and 360° rotation [5]. This device also facilitates both rotational as well as horizontal movement for wet floor cleaning. Switch belonging to water control can be pressed ON to sprinkle water over the surface area of a sheet. Along with water, any disinfectant can be added. To and fro vertical movements are controlled by separate switches, and the switch for 360 rotation ensures the complete cleaning of the floor.

The robot also uses sodium hypochlorite solution as a disinfectant to eliminate any COVID-19 microorganisms on the floor. Instead of spraying disinfectant, UV sterilization that uses short-wavelength ultraviolet rays that kill or inactivate the microorganism can be used in hospitals treating COVID-19 patients. The UV tower is portable in design, battery operated and controlled by the remote and timers which effectively sterilize public places wherever required.

Recent technology development has given rise to robots with real-time terrain recognition technology (RT2RT) which covers all 360-degree angles. This is done six times in a second, and with this data a real-time floor map is made. This permits the devices to clean the floor within a short period so that it can cover a large surface with less power and high efficient performance [9].

5 Robotic Nursing Assistant

Health departments of all countries are working round-the-clock to trace contact and travel history of the infected people, beef up the infrastructure for medical care of the patients and ensure social distancing to contain the spread of the coronavirus pandemic. The greatest risks during the outbreak of any contagious disease are the ones associated with the health workers and attenders of the patients [2]. The health workers are very prone to infections due to contacts with patients, handling the materials used for and by the infected patients, safe removing of protective equipment, etc. This brings an opportunity where the implementation of remote-controlled robots can be shown to be useful. They can be used for doing nursing duties in infected clinical areas which helps in reducing the exposure of nurses and caretakers to disease infections and other biohazards. The implementation of robotic nurses in health care has several benefits. It can help the hospital or nursing home reduce wastage, improved patient care and save costs in the long run. This also results in better management of the facility as every move is tracked and recorded [4].

Robotics in health care is presently entering an establishment stage where they can be trusted to be used for risky jobs. They have been implemented in such a successful manner that they are famous for their assistance to the healthcare industry [2]. Some of the famous robots in usage in the healthcare industry are described below.

5.1 Dinsow

Robot Dinsow is used by some of the Asian country hospitals for giving care to the patients, to video monitor elderly patients and to help in video chatting with their relatives. The patient's activities are also monitored, and the caregivers are alerted via phone [10]. Dinsow also alerts the patient about the timing of exercise and medication. The lighter side of it includes entertaining the patients by offering karaoke and games that help in improving their mental health which is also important for isolated patients [11].

5.2 Paro

Paro is a seal-like robot employed in hospitals and other caretaking institutions. It helps in building up communication between patients and their caregivers [10]. It imitates the voice of a baby harp seal for relaxing the patients. In addition to this, Paro adjusts with the patient's behavior via its five sensors: sound, temperature, light, posture and tactile [12]. In a nutshell, this robot helps in reducing patient stress, improving relaxation, motivation and improving their social relations with caregivers and other patients [4].

5.3 Pepper

Pepper is a humanoid robot that has been put into practical use in the reception area of two hospitals in Belgium. It greets the people coming in, checks their temperature and guides them to the concerned department [11]. The most important features of Pepper are that it can identify 20 languages, identify gender and emotions of joy, sadness, anger and surprise. It can also identify non-verbal gestures like frowns, smiles, head tilts and changes in vocal tones [10].

Pepper has high-resolution cameras and a 3D camera for its vision. It captures images through this camera and processes them using the image recognition software that is embedded in it. The robot is very mobile which is powered by twenty engines and three multi-directional wheels. Pepper moves at 3 km/h speed, navigated using the six laser sensors, two ultrasound transmitters and three obstacle detectors in its legs. It can detect obstacles within a 3 m range and steer its course accordingly.

In China, when COVID-19 caused sudden havoc, the flow of patients into the hospitals was way more than the medical staff could handle. So to accommodate and give medical care to more patients, Wuhan Hong Shan Stadium was converted into a smart field hospital fully assisted by robots. A total of 14 robots were brought out on the field from Cloud Minds. The main works of these robots were cleaning and disinfecting the surfaces and utensils used by the patients, measuring their temperatures, giving them food and medicine, entertaining and comforting them with various activities.

In Italy, during the peak COVID times, robot named Tommy was deployed to reduce the direct interaction time between the patients and the medical team. Tommy was equipped with a monitor and a keypad that was used for visual and acoustic communication between the patient and medical staff both at different locations. Tommy could also measure blood pressure and oxygen saturation of the patients, the two critical parameters when COVID is concerned. Robots are increasingly and efficiently able to run initial tests, complete preprogrammed routine tasks and help doctors with remote a diagnosis, which helps in reducing the spread of infections [10].

5.4 Trina

TRINA—Tele-robotic Intelligent Nursing Assistant is a robot which is designed with the basic features required for the machine that replaces a man, like human-safe, versatile, used by unskilled, easy to assemble and relatively less expensive [13]. It can do duty manipulation tasks which are light and medium range such as serving food, giving medication and even pushing carts. The nursing assistant robot is expected to perform all the unexpected duties and contingencies that arise while taking care of a patient. It must also work according to the judgment of medical experts [12]. TRINA has been designed with high degrees of freedom and is expected to function over a range of activities requiring varying strength and precision. It does coarse manipulation tasks like pushing and lifting to fine manipulation tasks like clicking on screen that too with the same accuracy but with varying strength. The robot has a height of 1.7 m and weights 140 kg approximately. Important features of TRINA are as follows:

- Free movements in a hospital wards and room.
- Ability to perform light and medium-duty tasks.
- Safe in close proximity and human touch tasks.
- Facilitates audio and video communication between a caretaker and patient.
- Continues in operation round the clock.

The major components of TRINA system are.
(1) Mobile manipulator.
(2) Operator console.
(3) Software meant for the control operation and user interface.

5.4.1 Mobile Manipulator

The robot uses a dual-armed humanoid torso, a unidirectional mobile base and three-fingered grippers on both the hand for manipulation and indoor navigation purpose. The components like mike, speakers and screen are available in the body to allow audio and visual communication among robot operators, patients and rest of the healthcare employees in the hospital premises [13]. An additional feature of this product is its ability to provide visual feedback. The length of the power chord is 30 feet that provides enough motion range to move around the isolation wards where the COVID patients are admitted and quarantined.

The safety of the patients is the major issue about which there has to be a major concern while designing the device. But there is always a trade-off. Here the trade-off is the precision loss and the robot hands having big fingertips. Precise-positioning unit (PPU) is mounted on the forearm of the robot for simple tasks such as button pressing with a positioning accuracy of millimeter level [12, 14]. TRINA also has rich sensory feedback with ultrasonic range finders to discover people around it. A collision during the motion is detected using joint torque sensors.

The visual sense of the robot is enriched with 180° camera placed on the head, a Microsoft Kinect 2 fixed to the chest and a couple of Intel Real Sense F200 3D cameras that are connected to the wrist to facilitate the enhanced visual feedback [13].

5.4.2 Operator Console

The operator console is the remote place from which robot can be controlled with the help of different input devices. The controlling devices are normal mouse, 3D mouse, keyboard and kinesthetic robot miniatures. The control and user interface permits the control of the robot by the operator using both direct teleoperations and semiautonomous assistance. There is also provision for users to teleoperate various parts separately such as gripper, arm and base using joint or Cartesian position control to change from preprogrammed poses [13, 14]. It also has autonomous assistance functionality for many shared control modes like hand movements, bimanual coordination control and stop a collision. The operator's GUI collects data from all the cameras fixed in the body of robots about its status.

5.4.3 Software

The input signals from sensors and devices are communicated to the console, which can send back the control signal to the robot through system state service. The controller has a dispatcher which constantly monitors the performance of the robot on posted tasks and sends commands to the motion server by the task-specific controller. Visual sensory feedback, such as videos of the connected cameras and 3D display of the cognitive map, is sent to the console with the help of robot operating system (ROS) [13].

To make the system simpler, an assistance module is provided for the operator. The module does all the tedious and repetitive tasks with a high level of precision [14]. At present, only a few functions are available that are highlighted in yellow color in Fig. 7. Existing software can be used for low-level assistance for enforcing actuator limits, Cartesian end-effector control and collision avoidance.

The development is in progress where higher-level assistance will be designed in the future. This will include lowering the learning curve, improving ergonomics and better performance [15]. Future robots will be provided with human guidance in click form and automatic mobile base navigation (Fig. 8).

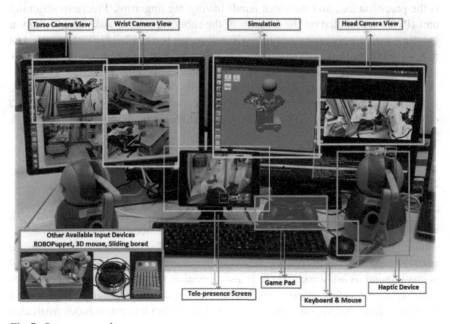

Fig. 7 Operator console

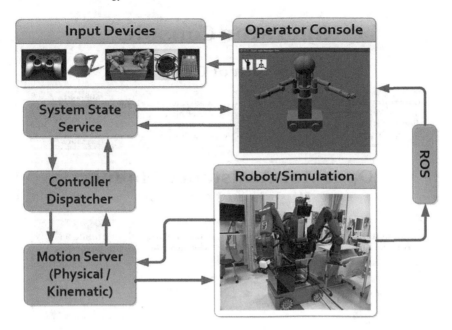

Fig. 8 TRINA software architecture

Future plans include two main features grasping in human-guided or point and click the form and mobile base navigation. Direct teleoperation and supervisory control interpolation can be done with an adjustable autonomy interface in which the users will have the choice to select the assistance level [15] (Fig. 9).

TRINA has been tested and is found to be very effective in manipulation tasks, like moving carts, carrying food tray and shifting the medical accessories. Still, there are issues and challenges in some teleoperated tasks performed by the robots, whereas it is simple for humans [15, 16]. The arm of the robot is similar to a human arm, but there are two problems One is its elbow points rest in "up" rather than "down" during its rest configuration, i.e., it could not reach the human elbow down postures. The second one is that wrist flexion creates a big movement at the gripper. Similarly, the rotatory movement of the palm or opening of the fingers results in a big movement of the wrist and elbow. The grippers are designed to be compliant and are underactuated, with only one motor per phalanx. This supports power grasp and pinch modes and leads to accuracy and dexterity better than a human hand [13, 16].

TRINA, the advanced technological robot, is found to be very effective at gross tasks and less effective at finer tasks that are common in clinical care. To make it do minute tasks, care has to be taken in strength, safety, control and hardware precision. This can be done by improving operator transparency and semiautonomous control [15, 16].

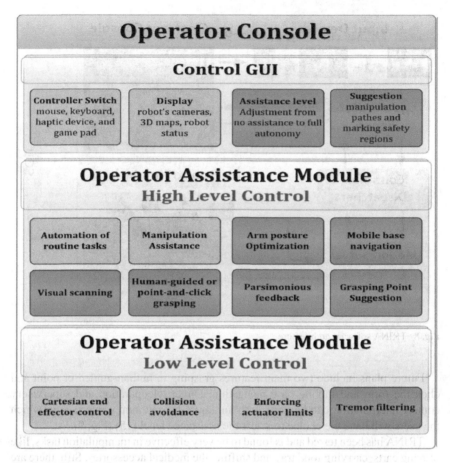

Fig. 9 Architecture of operator console

6 Hospi Robot

The Matsushita's robot is used for the blood sample courier system. It consists of a group of autonomous mobile robots controlled and operated by the main computer [17]. The robotic system is designed to collect blood samples and deliver in the required location where testing can be done using automatic analyzers and collect back the tested samples. The robot can also be employed for other transportation tasks within the hospitals and the laboratories. The main computer which acts as a server assigns various tasks to individual robots and tracks its activities. It has a laser scanner to detect obstacles while moving around to accomplish its assigned duty [18]. The group control system that monitors robot activities, solves failure situations and also controls the robot's battery level. Each autonomous unit is equipped with a positioning mechanism that ensures high precision in pickup and delivery of blood samples and other things [12].

7 Helpmate Robot

HelpMate is a new robotic technology developed by Evans that can be used in a hospital to carry things from one place to another to help patients and assist nurses and others in their work [17, 18]. The operators place the materials in the spaces provided on the robot's body as shelves and then select one or more destination in the map built on robot's graphical user interface (GUI). After getting instructed, it follows the built mission plan and starts to reach its destination on a preplanned path. While moving if it finds an obstacle, the robot tries to go around, and if not possible then it waits till obstacles are removed. When goods carried are received by the person in the selected location, they need to confirm the same, which can be monitored from remote and to maintain dispatch database.

8 Automated Guided Vehicle

TransCar AGV is an Automated guided vehicle (Fig. 10) developed by the Swisslog company for carts transportation. They are flat robots that can move under the cart with the ability to lift and deliver the same to the desired location expected by the particular application [18]. To employ this automated vehicle in the hospital, its environment should support the spaces with minimal obstacles and so has to get altered accordingly. The advantage of this robot is that it can carry most of the cart types on its body. It requires wide trailers that are high enough so that these robots could go under them. But we need not replace already existing carts with the new one which suits for the automated vehicle. Already existed systems could be adapted by automatically guided vehicles to fulfill its purpose which makes ease of its role in hospital application with less operation cost and increased efficiency.

Fig. 10 Swisslog AGV

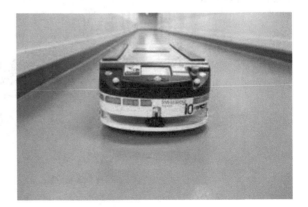

9   Delivery Robots

The collection of swab samples for testing is the first essential step to find the infected person for treatment of contagious diseases. They need to be isolated from the remaining population to prevent the spreading of the disease. CCS robots can render their service for an efficient specimen delivery system. It is built with features that facilitate them to navigate without artificial landmarks. While establishing the robot in a particular environment, it builds a map, and the same can be used for planning and execution of the mission [18]. The delivery request is sent to the interface of the robot body with its necessary information of destination after placing the items on the robot. After completing the task, the robot returns to its own station with appropriate acknowledgment.

10   Delivery Drone Robot

In this contagiousness period, it is wise to minimize human-to-human contact since the main issue in COVID-19 is its speed of transmission from one to another. Nowadays, people prefer online shopping but then delivery of the purchases involves human interaction. Robots can be the solution to this problem also. Special type of robots can be designed for the purpose of delivering the household items to their destination homes in case of online purchasing and also for those who were advised to be in-home quarantine. The same method can be implemented for home delivery of the drugs and food delivery service. It can also be employed to supply food for quarantined individuals who reside in a hotel when they migrate from other countries and states (Fig. 11).

Fig. 11 Delivery drone robot

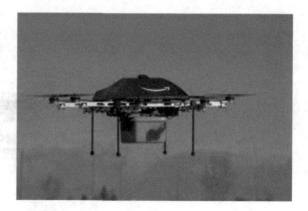

Fig. 12 Sanitizing drone robot

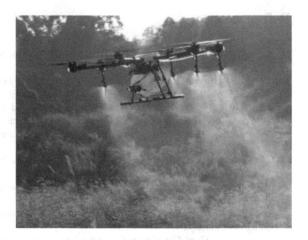

11 Sanitizing Drone Robot

Sanitizing is the common measure taken by the government in common places where there is a possibility of spreading the virus. It is a challenging task for officials to make arrangements to sanitize every street as it involves huge human force. In such a situation, drones can be employed for this purpose as we use drones in agriculture for seeding and applying fertilizers in the fields. This drone robotic technology also reduces the risk of sanitary workers whose role is vital in this pandemic situation. As per the plan, drones will be used to spray disinfectants, to sanitize the roads, metros and hospitals across the state (Fig. 12).

12 Conclusion

In this chapter, the applications of the robotic technology in the form of automatic floor cleaners, automatic lavatory cleaners and robotic nurses have been discussed. Robotic blood sample courier system, automated guided vehicle, delivery robots, delivery drone robot and sanitizing drone robot were also introduced. These robots can be used in this pandemic situation to avoid physical contact with the patients by the frontline workers like doctors, nurses, sanitary workers, delivery personal, etc., who are prone to get an infection due to their continuous exposure to infected personal. Although robot's performance is not compared with humans due to lack of emotional intelligence, this technology can be a good solution for these outbreaks of contagious diseases.

References

1. Lupia T, Scabini S, Pinna SM, Perri GD, Rosa FG, Corcione S (2020) 2019-novel coronavirus outbreak: a new challenge. J Glo Antimicr Resi 21:22–27
2. Robots, Intelligent Medical Care Respond to Coronavirus Outbreak. https://www.chinadaily.com.cn/a/202002/02/WS5e366cb4a3101282172742b8.html
3. Paparizos C, Tsafas N, Birbas M (2020) A Zynq-based robotic system for treatment of contagious diseases in hospital isolated environment. J Tech 8:0–17
4. Pervez A, Ryu J (2008) Safe physical human-robot interaction-past, present and future. J Mech Sci Tech 22:469–483
5. Liu K, Wang C (2013) A technical analysis of autonomous floor cleaning robots based on US granted patents. Eur Intel J Sci Tech 2:1–6
6. Stevens Institute of Technology. https://web.stevens.edu/ses/me/fileadmin/me/senior_design/2007/group01/DesignFinal.pdf
7. Roomba Robotic Vacuum Cleaners. https://www.irobot.com/For-the-Home/Vacuum-Cleaning/Roomba.aspx
8. Autonomous Floor Cleaning Robot. https://eprints2.utem.edu.my/4710/1/Design_And_Implementation_Of_Vacuum_Robot_-_24_pages.pdf
9. Gawande AC, Telrandhe S, Satone A, Kade P (2018) Design and fabrication of advanced mechanism for indian toilet dome cleaning with multi Washer's assembly. Intl J Res Adv Tech 6:259–262
10. Park H, Hong H, Kwon H, Chung M (2001) A nursing robot system for the elderly and the disabled. Intl J Hum Frie Welf Rob Syst 2:11–16
11. Fong SJ, Dey N, Chaki J (2020) AI-enabled technologies that fight the coronavirus outbreak, artificial intelligence for coronavirus outbreak. Springer Briefs in Computational Intelligence Book Series, pp 23–25
12. Sampsel D, Vermeersch P, Doarn CR (2014) Utility and effectiveness of a remote telepresence robotic system in nursing education in a simulated care environment. J Telemed e-Health 20:1015–1020
13. Li Z, Moran P, Dong Q, Shaw RJ, Hauser K (2017) Development of a tele-nursing mobile manipulator for remote care-giving in quarantine areas. In: IEEE international conference on robotics and automation, pp 3581–3586
14. Heavey BM, Stelly EM. Telenursing RoboPuppet. https://digitalcommons.wpi.edu/mqp-all/2209
15. Quigley M, Conley K, Gerkey B, Faust J, Foote T, Leibs J, Wheeler R, Ng AY (2009) ROS: an open-source robot operating system. In: ICRA workshop on open source software, vol 3. Kobe, pp 1–5
16. Pineaua J, Montemerloa M, Pollack M, Roy N, Thrun S (2003) Towards robotic assistants in nursing homes: challenges and results. Robot Autonomous Syst 42:271–281
17. Works ME. Automatic robotic blood sample courier system. https://www.mew.co.jp/e/corp/news/2006/0610-01
18. Qureshi MS, Singh P, Swarnkar P, Goud H (2020) Robotics solutions to combat novel Corona virus disease-2019 (COVID-19). Elsevier, SSRN

Chapter 16
Face Mask Detection Using AI

Saini Pooja and Saini Preeti

1 Introduction

World Health Organization (WHO) has professed the Covid-19 (severe acute respiratory syndrome coronavirus 2, SARS-CoV-2) as public health emergency of international concern. As per WHO report, in the last week of December 2019, for the very first time, the information about the detected cases of pneumonia of unidentified etiology (unknown cause) in Wuhan Metropolis, Hubei State, China, had submitted to the WHO China Country Office. In addition, on January 3, 2020, the national authorities in China reported that there are total of forty-four cases with pneumonia of unknown etiology. Eleven cases out of total forty-four are severely ill, while the remaining 33 patients are in steady condition. As per media reports, on January 1, 2020, the concerned market in Wuhan had been shut down for ecological cleanliness and disinfection. The clinical signs noted were mostly temperature, having some of cases getting difficulty in deep breathing. Until that time, there was zero case had been reported with this new disease anywhere else aside from Wuhan. Even prior to the announcement of coronavirus as a worldwide outbreak, as per sources, there was 7711 infected people and 170 reported deaths in China.

S. Pooja (✉)
Department of Computer Science and Engineering, Ambala College of Engineering and Applied Research, Ambala, Haryana, India
e-mail: spst.08@gmail.com

S. Preeti
Chitkara University, Rajpura, Punjab, India

On January 30, 2020, WHO Director-General, Dr. Tedros Adhanom Ghebreyesus declared "the novel coronavirus outbreak as global pandemic". As per WHO situation report-190, on July 28, 2020, there was over 16 341 919 confirmed Covid-19 cases and more than 650 803 deaths. Covid disease has spread speedily across the globe and has become a cause many issues related to health and fitness, economical, the environmental and societal to overall population.

Infected person's respiratory droplets (coughing, sneezing) and physical contact are the two major sources of transmission of the Covid-19 virus. One recent report presented that "we spray thousands of droplets invisible to the naked eye into the air just by saying the words stay healthy". At present, more than 20 vaccines are in developing and trial phase around the world. Rather than, just waiting for vaccines, presently, there are certain things that every human being can practice to guard themselves and their loved ones. WHO suggests that individuals ought to put on face masks to prevent the danger associated with Covid virus and also maintain the interpersonal distance of a minimum of 2 m to avoid person-to-person virus transmission. Face mask could help to reduce the Covid virus which spread into the community and potentially causes more infections. Masks have become vital to stay safe in the fight against Covid-19.

To get back to our workplaces and performing our day-to-day duties safely, new demand has emerged in the market, and that is face mask detection. It is one such technology capable of detecting a face with a mask or without mask. From a security perspective, detecting and identifying those who wear masks could be a necessity, but in the epidemic, alerting authorities of someone not wearing a mask is most critical for safety reasons. Hence, the face mask detection system has become the crucial need to have safe society.

1.1 Application Areas of Face Mask Detection System

Following are the areas where face mask detection system can be implemented.

- **Public Transport**

At airports, railway stations, buses, etc., to detect passengers without masks on public transport. Face mask detector can send the information to the concerned authorities, if a passenger is found to be without a face mask.

- **Healthcare Organizations**

With face mask detection system in hospitals/healthcare organizations, the isolated people, who are required to wear face mask, can be easily identified whether they are doing so or not.

- **Workplaces**

Authorities can take appropriate actions and warn employees to follow instructions to wear a mask and to maintain safety standards at work.

- **Surveillance Systems**

Face mask detection system can be integrated with existing surveillance setup to enforce the compulsory wearing of face masks in public places.

Thus, face mask detection system has become the need of the time to safe our society from the invisible demon. Thankfully, the advanced technology, namely artificial intelligence, has provided us helping hand to design and implement such systems efficiently and effectively. In next section, we will briefly explain the artificial intelligence terminology.

2 Artificial Intelligence (AI)—The Right Way Solution

Intelligence is "the capacity to learn and solve problems". Professor John McCarthy defined, "Artificial intelligence is the science and engineering of making intelligent machines, especially intelligent computer programs". AI enables the machine to mimic like human behavior. For example, a machine can identify a face in an image, recognize human speech, play game, automated fraud detect fraud automatically, read checks automatically, verify signature, etc. AI makes possible for machine to learn from experience. Based on new inputs, the machine updates their response, thereby performing tasks just like human. By processing a large volume of data and identifying patterns in them, AI can make a machine to perform specific tasks just like human. Nowadays, in day-to-day life, it has spread and found its applications in each field such as health care, agriculture, media, data security, transportation, finance, e-commerce and many more.

AI is an umbrella that covers other subareas, namely, machine learning and deep learning. Figure 1 shows the relationship between artificial intelligence and its subsets.

Machine learning enables the system to handle a particular job through data-driven decisions. The programs and algorithms have developed such that they can learn and enhance with time whenever subjected to new information.

Deep learning field is a subset of machine learning that is stimulated by the human mind cells, called neurons. Collections of neurons are known as artificial neural network. For learning, model considers all the data between these neurons and regulates them as per the pattern of data. For large data, more neurons added. It automatically features learning at multiple levels of abstraction. Irrespective of any specific algorithm, the model allows the system to learn multifaceted function mapping. For example, recognize the square from other shapes; recognize the specific object in an image or in a video.

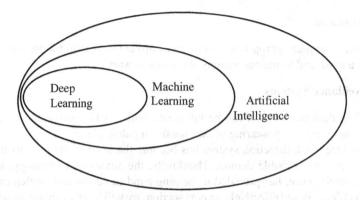

Fig. 1 Relationship between artificial intelligence and its subsets

In next section, we will provide a brief introduction of deep learning and the basic architecture of convolutional neural networks (CNN).

3 Deep Learning

Deep learning is a subclass of machine learning that learns via unstructured information, like images, video, sound or text, which processed through sophisticated algorithms to train a new multilevel neural network. It is a new "superpower" that allows to build such AI systems that were not even imaginable a few years ago. Just like a human brain, in deep learning, an artificial neural network is the brain to learn and allows the machine to evaluate the information in almost the same manner human beings carry out. A number of applications of computer vision techniques, which are now parts of our everyday lives, are feasible only with the use of deep learning. These include image classification, object detection, photo stylization or machine vision in self-driving cars. Deep learning is the most advanced technology available today. Following are major reasons why researchers prefer deep learning over traditional machine learning.

- **Raw Data Training**

Deep learning is the first and only AI method capable of training directly on raw data. It therefore achieves better resilience and can be trained for extreme scenario. Unlike traditional machine learning which trained only on handcraft features.

- **Independent of Human Intervention**

Deep learning models are capable to extract directly the data representation without the human intervention. Based on the data, patterns and their relationship generated.

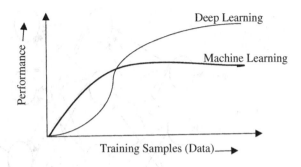

Fig. 2 Learning capacity of deep learning vs traditional machine learning

- **Analyze Different Data Types**

Deep learning can analyze any type of data. Deep learning is best to apply on unstructured data like images, video, sound or text.

- **Nonlinear Correlations**

Highest detection rate and lowest false positives can be achieved with deep learning. In complex patterns, deep learning can analyze multiple levels of nonlinear correlations.

- **Unbounded Training Samples**

The training dataset constantly grows which improves the learning continually. In traditional machine learning, the learning curve will always ultimately reach saturation, but deep learning can scale to hundreds of millions of training samples. Figure 2 shows the learning capacity of deep learning versus traditional machine learning.

By applying a large volume of labeled data and neural network architectures, deep learning models can be properly trained. They are capable to learn features directly from the raw input only, independent of human intervention. The most popular deep neural networks architecture is convolutional neural networks (CNN) [1–3]. A CNN uses 2D convolutional layers and combines the learned features with input data. To process the 2D data, such as images, the CNN architecture is well suited. Figure 3 shows a typical fully connected convolution neural network. Layers often learn in an unsupervised mode and discover general features of the input space. First layer learns the first-order features like color and edges. The second layer learns higher-order features liks boundaries. The third layer learns about textures, etc. The network can have tens or hundreds of hidden layers. More the layers implies more complex architecture but more deeply the features can be extracted. Then, the final layer features are fed into a supervised layer to complete the task, such as regression or classification. To train deep learning models, a number of deep learning libraries have developed which deliver numerous help and support for video or graphic recognition. Tensorflow, Pytorch, Caffe, MxNet, CNTK, Keras, etc., are the libraries which are used to build deep learning models.

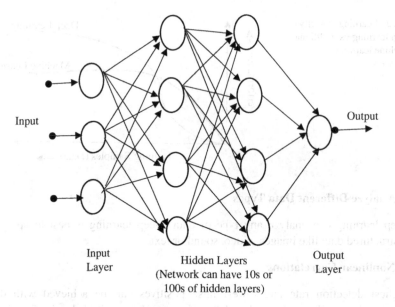

Fig. 3 Typical fully connected convolution neural network

4   Deep Learning in Face Mask Detection

It will be challenging to recognize faces with masks on any monitoring systems, while maintaining touch less access control in buildings. Conventional facial recognition technology becomes ineffective, in many cases, on masked face. Advanced face recognition approaches are designed which incorporate AI-enabled pattern recognition systems that uses a large dataset. This dataset consists of a large number of face samples for both classes wearing a mask and not wearing a mask. These systems extract facial features and classify them in different categories. Besides, system can also identify people without masks by generating an alarm or a notification to notify security or officials. Once the dataset is available, normally, face mask detection system processes in two phases.

Phase 1—Build and train the learning model.

Phase 2—Deploy mask detector over images or live videos.

Figure 4 shows the two phases of face mask detection system. Image preprocessing steps such as to resize the input image, color filtering over the channels, scaling or normalizing images, cropping the image and subdividing them into sub arrays are applied to all the raw input images to have augmented data, which could be fed to a neural network machine learning model.

Then, in first phase, build a model and train the system with mask and without mask images with an appropriate algorithm. Once the models are trained, then in second phase, load the face mask detector, perform face detection, and then, classify each face. Once an image has uploaded, the classification happens automatically.

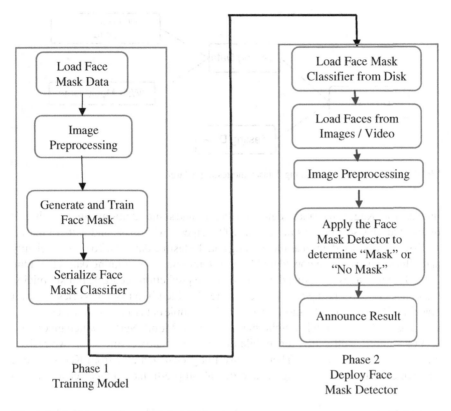

Fig. 4 Basic phases of face mask detection system

5 Face Mask Detection—A Simple Implementation Using OpenCV

In this section, we will learn the basic steps to implement a face mask detection system. For implementation, we subdivide our task into a set of three sub tasks as follow.

Task 1: Data collection and preprocessing.
Task 2: Building and training the learning model.
Task 3: Deploying the deep learning model with OpenCV.

5.1 Task 1: Data Collection and Preprocessing

The system uses a large volume of data set consisting of face images that have labeled and used for the training of our model. We have used the dataset, which comprises

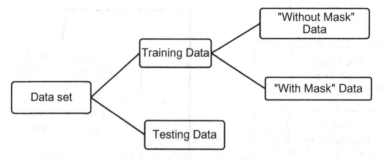

Fig. 5 Categorized data as training dataset and testing dataset

images from Kaggle face mask detection data set and some additional images (clicked by us). Our dataset contains more than 900 images—with mask and without mask.

Now, we divided dataset as the training and the testing datasets. To train efficiently and effectively, we have considered 80% of total images as training dataset and the 20% of total images as testing data set to test the prediction accuracy. For simplicity, the images in our training data collection are classified into two categories as "with mask" and "without mask" shown in Fig. 5. The sample data from our dataset is shown as in Fig. 6. We used a lightweight image classifier, MobileNetV2, which gives high accuracy and is well suited for mobile devices. In preprocessing steps, we resized image to 224 × 224 pixels. Then, we use ImageDataGenrator from Keras to have augmented data in the training set and download pre-trained ImageNet weights to

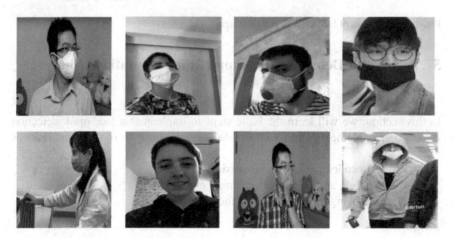

Fig. 6 Sample data from our dataset

make the algorithm's prediction efficiency accurate. Following code segment shows what the necessary libraries are and how to import them.

```
import tensorflow as tf
import os
import datetime
from keras.preprocessing.image import
ImageDataGenerator
from tensorflow.keras.models import Sequential
from tensorflow.keras.layers import
GlobalAveragePooling2D, Activation, Dropout, Dense,
Flatten
from tensorflow.keras.optimizers import Adam
from keras import layers
import numpy as np
from keras.preprocessing import image
from tensorflow.keras.applications import
MobileNetV2
import cv2
```

Once the needed libraries are imported, now it is time to preprocess our input images. Image preprocessing includes steps such as to resize the input image, color filtering over the channels, scaling or normalizing images, cropping the image and subdividing them into sub arrays are applied to all the raw input images to have augmented data, which could be fed to a neural network machine learning model. In following code snippet, we used the ImageDataGenrator to have augmented data for training.

```
trainGen = ImageDataGenerator(rescale=1./255,
shear_range=0.2,horizontal_flip=True, zoom_range=0.2)

testGen = ImageDataGenerator(rescale=1./255)

train_data = trainGen.flow_from_directory (
dir_for_train_data, target_size=(224, 224),classes=
['with_mask','without_mask'], class_mode =
'categorical',    batch_size=batch_size, shuffle=True)

test_data = testGen.flow_from_directory (
dir_for_test_data, target_size=(224,224),
classes=['with_mask','without_mask'], class_mode =
'categorical', batch_size=batch_size)
```

At this stage, our input data is ready with us. Let us move onto next step, i.e., to build and train our model.

5.2 Task 2: Building and Training the Learning Model

To build and train our model, we have used class GlobalAveragePooling2D to have global average pooling operation for spatial data, "relu" as activation function and "softmax" final layer activation. To train our model, we used Adam optimizing algorithm, with initialized parameters as number of epochs = 10 and batch size = 32.

```
model.compile(optimizer=Adam(lr=0.00001), loss =
'categorical_crossentropy',metrics=['accuracy'])
model.fit(train_data, epochs=epochs)
```

Now, save the model on disk. Once the model has trained with the training data set and the pre-trained weights given, we predicted and check the accuracy of the model on the test dataset using following code snippet.

```
process_img = image.load_img(path, target_size =
(224,224))
process_img = image.img_to_array(process_img)
img = np.expand_dims(process_img,axis=0)
result = model.predict_classes(img)
```

Once we are satisfied with the validation accuracy of model, we can now move to our next and final step, i.e., to deploy our model in real life.

5.3 Task 3: Deploying the Deep Learning Model with OpenCV

Now, we will deploy our trained model with OpenCV to detect who is "with mask" or who is "without mask". OpenCV can be used to deploy deep learning models from various frameworks such as Tensorflow, Caffe, Darknet and Torch. To deploy our model, we will consider a real-time image, which is not a part of our dataset; neither from training data nor from test data. We will apply our model on this image using following code snippet. Here, "haarcascade_frontalface_default.xml" will help to classify the face region in the image. Figure 7 shows the prediction and accuracy of our model on given test data and the real-time image.

```
result = {0:'With Mask',1:'PLEASE wear Mask'}
def prepImg(pth):
 return
cv2.resize(pth,(224,224)).reshape(1,224,224,3)/255.0
classifier=cv2.CascadeClassifier(cv2.data.haarcascades
+ 'haarcascade_frontalface_default.xml')
path = r'G:\Deeplearning\deploy12.jpg'
img = cv2.imread(path)

faces = classifier.detectMultiScale(cv2.cvtColor (
img,cv2.COLOR_BGR2GRAY),1.1,2)
for (x1,y1,x2,y2) in faces:
 img1=cv2.rectangle(img,(x1,y1),(x1+x2,y1+y2),color,2)
pred = model.predict(prepImg(img))
pred = np.argmax(pred)
img = cv2.resize(img, (224, 224), interpolation=
cv2.INTER_LINEAR)
imgx=cv2.putText(img,
resMap[pred],(30,200),cv2.FONT_HERSHEY_SIMPLEX,0.5,(25
5,255,0),2)
plt.imshow(imgx)
```

Thus, our face mask detection system can automatically and efficiently detect whether or not people wear mask in public place. In this section, we have focused on the simple implementation of face mask detection system for understanding purpose

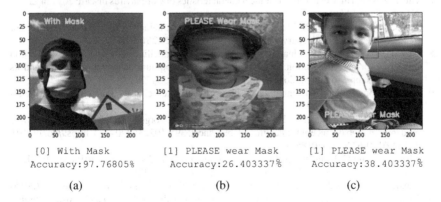

[0] With Mask   [1] PLEASE wear Mask   [1] PLEASE wear Mask
Accuracy:97.76805%   Accuracy:26.403337%   Accuracy:38.403337%

       (a)   (b)   (c)

Fig. 7 Trained model outputs: **a, b** show prediction and accuracy on test sample images. **c** shows prediction and accuracy on real-time image

only. Reader may modify this implementation to deploy the trained model on the live videos by mean of camera feeds.

6 BibTeX

```
@misc{make ml,
    title = {Mask Dataset},
    url = {https://makeml.app/datasets/mask},
    journal = {Make ML}}.
```

Acknowledgements We would like to express our sincere gratitude to all those who have willingly helped us out with their abilities.

References

1. Masita L, Hasan KAN, Satyakama P (2018) Pedestrian identification by mean of R-CNN object detector. In: IEEE Latin American conference on computational intelligence. https://doi.org/10.1109/LA-CCI.2018.8625210
2. Ren S, He K, Girshick R, Sun J (2015) Faster R-CNN: towards real-time object detection with area proposal networks. In: Proceedings of Advance Neural Inf. Processing Systems, pp 91–99
3. Liu H, Chen Z, Li Z, Hu W (2018) An powerful method of pedestrian detection based on YOLOv2. Math Eng. https://doi.org/10.1155/2018/3518959
4. World Health Organization. https://www.who.int/dg/speeches/detail/who-director-general-s-statement-on-ihr-emergency-committee-on-novel-coronavirus-(2019-ncov)
5. Chawla S, Mittal M, Chawla M, Goyal LM (2020) Corona Virus—SARS-CoV-2: an insight to another way of natural disaster. EAI Endorsed Trans Pervasive Health Technol 6(22)
6. Guan W, Ni Z, Hu Y et al (2020) Clinical characteristics of Coronavirus disease 2019 in China. New England J Med
7. Liu L, Ouyang W, Wang X, Fieguth P, Chen J, Liu X, Pietikäinen M (2020) Deep learning for generic object detection: a survey. Int J Comput Vis 128(2):261–318
8. Mohamed SS, Tahir NM, Adnan R (2010) Background modelling and background subtraction efficiency for object detection. In: 6th International colloquium on signal processing and its applications, pp 1–6. https://doi.org/10.1109/CSPA.2010.5545291.
9. Singh S. Cousins of artificial intelligence. https://towardsdatascience.com/cousins-of-artificial-intelligence-dda4edc27b55
10. Wang Chen S, Horby Peter W, Hayden Frederick G, Gao George F (2020) A novel coronavirus epidemic of global concern for health. It's the Lancet. 395(10223):470–473. https://doi.org/10.1016/S0140-6736(20)30185-9
11. Chen S, Zhang C, Dong M, Le JRM (2017) Using ranking CNN for age estimates. In: IEEE Conference on Computer Vision and Pattern Recognition (CVPR)
12. Najafabadi MM, Villanustre F, Khoshgoftaar TM, Seliya N, Wald R, Muharemagic E (2015) Deep learning applications and challenges in big data analytics. J Big Data 2, Article number 1
13. Wu W, Qian C, Yang S, Wang Q, Cai Y, Zhou Q (2018) Look at boundary : a boundary—aware face alignment algorithm. In: 2018 IEEE conference on Computer Vision and Pattern Recognition (CVPR)

14. Krizhevsky A, Sutskever I, Hinton G (2012) ImageNet classification with deep convolutional neural networks. In: Neural Information Processing Systems (NIPS), pp 1097–1105
15. Liu W, Anguelov D, Erhan D, Szegedy C, Reed S, Fu C-Y, Berg AC (2016) SSD single shot multibox detector. In: European conference on computer vision. Springer, Heidelberg, pp 21–37
16. Ren S, He K, Girshick R, Sun J (2015) Faster r-CNN: towards real-time object detection with region proposal networks. In: Advances in neural information processing systems, pp 91–99
17. Deng J, Guo J, Zhou Y, Yu J, Kotsia I, Zafeiriou S (2019) Retinaface: single-stage dense face localisation in the wild. arXiv preprint arXiv:1905.00641
18. Zou Z, Shi Z, Guo Y, Ye J (2019) Object detection in 20 years: a survey. arXiv preprint arXiv: 1905.05055
19. Piccardi M (2004) Background subtraction techniques: a analysis. In: IEEE international conference on systems, man and cybernetics, vol 4 (2004), pp 3099–3104. https://doi.org/10.1109/ICSMC.2004.1400815
20. Sreenu G, Saleem Durai MA (2019) Intelligent video surveillance: a review through deep learning techniques for crowd analysis. J Big Data 6, Article number: 48
21. Java Virtual Machine (JVM). Difference JDK, JRE & JVM—Core Java, https://beginnersbook.com/2013/05/jvm/
22. Farfade S, Saberian M, Li L (2015) Multi-view face recognition using deep convolutional neural networks. In: ACM ICMR, pp 643–650
23. Emami S, Suciu VP (2012) Facial recognition using OpenCV. J Mobile Embedded Distributed Syst IV(1): 38–43
24. Lin T-Y, Dollár P, Girshick R, He K, Hariharan B, Belongie S (2017) Type pyramid networks for object detection. In: IEEE conference proceedings on computer vision and pattern recognition, pp 2117–2125
25. Matrajt L, Leung T (2020) Evaluating the efficacy of social distancing strategies to postpone or flatten the curve of coronavirus disease. Emerg Infect Dis Man
26. Sandler M, Howard A, Zhu M, Zhmoginov A, Chen L-C (2018) Mobilenetv2: inverted residues and linear bottlenecks. In: IEEE conference on computer vision and pattern recognition, pp 4510–4520
27. Fu C, Liu W, Ranga A, Tyagi A, Berg A (2017) DSSD: deconvolutional single shot detector model. arXiv preprint arXiv:1701.06659
28. Dalal N, Triggs B (2005) Histograms of oriented gradients for human detection. In: 2005 IEEE computer society conference on computer vision and pattern recognition (CVPR'05), vol 1. IEEE, pp 886–893
29. Girshick R (2015) Fast R-CNN. In: Proceedings of IEEE international confrence computer vision, pp 1440–1448
30. Zhu X, Ramanan D (2012) Face detection, pose estimation, and landmark position in wild. In: IEEE CVPR, pp 2879–2886
31. Howard A, Zhu M, Chen B, Kalenichenko D, Wang W, Weyand T, Andreetto M, Adam H (2017) MobileNets : effective convolutional neural networks for mobile vision applications
32. Zhu X (2020) Semi-supervised study of learning literature survey. Computer Science, University Of Wisconsin-Madison 2(3):4. Int J Res Appl Sci Eng Technol 8(VII)
33. Oro D, Fernández C, Saeta JR, Martorell X, Hernando J (2011) Real-time GPU-based face detection in HD video streams. IEEE Int Conf Comp Vis
34. Glass RJ, Glass LM, Beyeler WE, Min HJ (2006) Targeted social distancing architecture for pandemic influenza. Emerg Infectious Dis 12:1671–1681
35. Ge S, Li J, Ye Q, Luo Z (2017) Detection of masked faces in the wild with LLE-CNNs. In: IEEE Conference on Computer Vision and Pattern Recognition (CVPR), Honolulu, HI, pp 426–434

Chapter 17
Machine Learning Tools to Predict the Impact of Quarantine

Amandeep Kaur, Neerja Mittal, Praveen Kumar Khosla, and Mamta Mittal

1 Introduction

The outbreak of COVID-19 (coronavirus disease) has put the world of Industry 4.0 into quarantine mode. It has been declared by World Health Organization (WHO) on January 30, 2020, that this outbreak is a Public Health Emergency of International Concern (PHEIC) and on March 11, 2020, this disease was recognized as a pandemic which is taking a bad shape globally [1, 2]. Ever since, the infections caused by this disease are rising in numbers due to the non-availability of vaccine. As of August 30, 2020, the global coronavirus cases have exceeded 25 million [3]. Since there is no vaccine available for this disease, quarantine-based control [4] becomes the only possible method which could assist in breaking the chain of the virus. However, the impact of these quarantine measures needs to be studied in order to impose state-wide plans for disease mitigation and control. This may also facilitate the governments to devise effective quarantine measures in order to mitigate the effects of COVID-19. The region-wise situation has been shown from Figs. 1, 2 and 3.

A. Kaur (✉)
Computer Science and Engineering, Punjab Engineering College (Deemed to be University),
Chandigarh, India
e-mail: amandeepkaur@pec.edu.in

N. Mittal
Computational Instrumentation, CSIR-CSIO, Chandigarh, India
e-mail: neerjamittal_2k1@yahoo.com

P. K. Khosla
Centre for Development of Advanced Computing (C-DAC), Ministry of Electronics & IT, Mohali,
Punjab, India
e-mail: pkk7@yahoo.com

M. Mittal
G.B Pant Government Engineering College, Delhi, India
e-mail: mittalmamta79@gmail.com

P. K. Khosla et al. (eds.), *Predictive and Preventive Measures for Covid-19 Pandemic*,
Algorithms for Intelligent Systems, https://doi.org/10.1007/978-981-33-4236-1_17

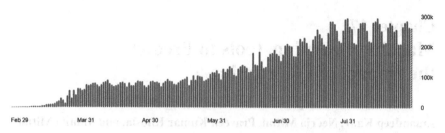

Fig. 1 Global situation as of August 31, 2020: 25,118,689 confirmed cases

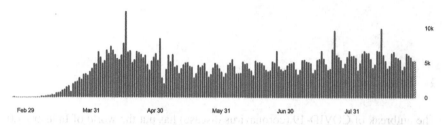

Fig. 2 Number of deaths globally as of August 31, 2020: 844,312

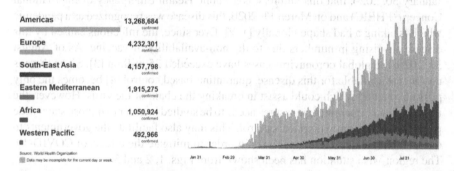

Fig. 3 Region-wise situation of COVID-19 confirmed cases

During the Spanish flu pandemic of 1918, the medical and technological advances were not like the present times. But nowadays, there is advanced technology available which is augmented with buzzwords like artificial intelligence, machine learning, Internet of things, cloud computing, etc. Machine learning is an application area of artificial intelligence that provides for the development of various computer programs which access and learn from data. Such programs are structured around machine learning models, which are applicable on a variety of data and their tuning. This chapter explores various machine learning models and techniques, which have been used to develop tools that quantify the effects of quarantine as a measure of control in several parts of the world. In order to predict the impact of quarantine and estimate the spread of the disease, various research investigations have been presented in this chapter.

2 Machine Learning Models to Quantify Quarantine Impact

The researchers have developed a neural network-based machine learning model which can be used to quantify the impact of quarantine-based COVID-19 mitigation and control measures [5]. It has been observed that the number of cases rises exponentially in case the quarantine protocol is not imposed in a particular region, as shown in Fig. 4. The countries which have deployed quarantine-based mitigation models are doing better off in terms of rise in the number of infections. This quantification of the impact of quarantine could help the people understand why it is so important not to relax the quarantine norms and lift the lockdowns. In order to quantify the impact of quarantine, publicly available data has been used, and mixed first-principles epidemiological equations have been applied. Data-driven neural network model forms the basis of these quantifications [6].

The major reason behind low rise in number of cases because of quarantine is the break in COVID-19 infection chain. The highly infectious virus, which travels from human to human in different ways, makes it necessary to break the chain of physical communication between the people by imposing social distancing, quarantine and lockdown guidelines.

The effective use of machine learning models has proven to be quite beneficial for various countries. Already established corona mitigation models by countries, which have been successful in controlling the disease, could be considered as case studies by other countries which are lacking behind. However, there are certain risks and challenges such as non-availability of authentic datasets and the de-falsification of the data obtained from random sources. Even a minor update in the pattern of the data can bring a large amount of change in the predictions of the model. Therefore,

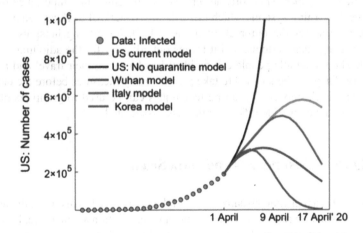

Fig. 4 Rise in number of cases with respect to quarantine models. *Source* https://news.mit.edu/2020/new-model-quantifies-impact-quarantine-measures-covid-19-spread-0416

it is very important to build standard publicly available datasets which can be trusted to carry out research activities. Interactive GUI tools based on these models could be built to represent various results as an extension to the model-based research. Following are some of the important research studies in this direction.

- Research has been conducted to find out whether or not mass quarantine and isolation effective measures to control the spread of COVID-19 by considering the case of Wuhan, China [7]. To answer this question, epidemiological model-driven approach augmented by machine learning has been used to build models to identify its effectiveness as a social tool. As per the results obtained from this study, quarantine and isolation for a defined period of time prove to be efficient methods for mitigation of the disease. The neural network-based models are being used as quarantine control models to check global COVID-19 spread [8].
- SIRNet [9] is a hybrid machine learning model which integrates itself with epidemiological models to forecast the COVID-19 spread. The knowledge of this spread can help in developing quarantine and isolation strategies in the worst hit areas. It also takes into consideration the parameters of social distancing and brings out facts which could help in keeping the disease at bay [10–13].
- In order to minimize the human contact especially to protect frontline corona warriors in hospitals and other medical facilities, artificial intelligence-powered robots are being deployed to deliver food and medicine to infected people, thereby strengthening the quarantine measures. Robots can act as an intermediary and protect people from potential threats by coming in contact with other people during the pandemic. Even the diagnosis and treatment can be done by using robots. A list of such robots has been provided in Table 1.

- Bluedot is an outbreak risk software which was among the first in the world to identify the risk of COVID-19 in Hubei and also published the first COVID-19 scientific paper. This software brings into limelight the importance of early outbreak warning systems which prove highly beneficial to check readiness and preparedness for the outbreak of diseases [14]. Identifying hotspots becomes easier using such systems, and it brings out advisory for the adjoining areas as well. The vulnerable people can be identified based on their travel and medical history. They can be advised to take precautionary measures before the outbreak hits with high impact. Clustering techniques can be used to group people who have high fever and identify potential risks associated.

3 Big Data Dashboards and Data Science

A dashboard is a real-time visualization portal which is used to display authentic and reliable information related to the topic under consideration at one place. In order to make the users aware about the number of COVID-19 infections happening locally as well as globally, dashboards are being used by different countries including various agencies and organizations such as World Health Organization. These dashboards

Table 1 List of robots with their functions related to COVID-19

Sr. No	Robot Name/Country	Functionality
1	Zafi and Zafi Medic/India	Deliver food and medicine to COVID-19 patients under quarantine
2	KARMI-bot/India	Similar to Zafi and Zafi Medic but has added functionality of disinfecting the floors with ultraviolet radiation
3	Sona 2.5/India	Deliver food and medicine
4	Minus Corona UV Bot/India	Sterilization of hospital wards, ICUs using ultraviolet radiation
5	Pepper/Japan	Enforcing social distancing and greeting COVID-19 patients
6	iMap 9/India	Floor cleaning using sodium hypochlorite solution
7	Humanoid/ELF	Record and transmit isolation ward activities and helps nurses and doctors contact with patients remotely
8	Tommy the robot nurse/Italy	Nursing purposes
9	Spot/USA	To interview patients
10	Violet/Ireland	Ultraviolet light robot that can kill virus, bacteria and germs
11	Little Peanut/China	Deliver food to quarantined people
12	Video-conferencing bots by ZoraBots/Belgium	Help the contact between elderly and their loved ones
13	UV light robots by Netcare/South Africa	To sanitize hospitals
14	Robots deployed in supermarkets/Germany	To advise about panic buying and crowd gatherings

provide necessary information about total number of infected cases, recovered cases, number of deaths, number of active cases, etc. The information may be visualized by plotting in the form of different types of graphs which makes the analysis of the disease-related trends possible so that government can make informed decisions to implement lockdowns and social distancing in the most affected areas.

Ever since coronavirus has taken the shape of a pandemic, heaps of data are being generated worldwide which can be termed as big COVID-19 data. The surveillance, tracking and continuous monitoring of exposed people as well as those who violate the social distancing and quarantine norms are being done using various Internet of things-based approaches. To analyze such huge amount of accumulated data, various emerging big data tools and techniques could be practiced.

Thermal scanners are being used to detect body temperatures all over the places [15]. Alert systems are in practice to inform people about the potential threats that may be around them. Smart ID cards are being issued in order to check the health status of the employees in various organizations. Security cameras are being used to track the movements of citizens [16]. Various smartphone apps are providing information to the users.

Big data dashboards are being developed by various government as well as non-governmental agencies to provide interactive information interfaces to the people across the globe. This information is quite important for one to ensure self-control and safety measures in case their neighborhood lies in a quarantine zone. People can also upload information regarding those who violate the norms in order to ensure the safety of everyone around them. These dashboards bring about a sense of responsibility among the citizens so as to become self-aware and self-dependent to take the necessary precautions without any enforcement at the state level. Table 2 displays a list of dashboards developed during COVID-19 crisis.

Considering the case study of Taiwan, it was initially assumed that it will be one of the worst hit states as it is in close vicinity of China as per geographic location. But the preparedness of the state was so effective that COVID-19 disease was in their control rather than them being controlled by the disease. Integration of the national health insurance database and immigration and customs database were done in order to generate real-time alerts. QR code scanning systems were used along with online reporting of travel and health symptoms. This information could be further used to keep a track of the health status of the recent travelers. All these effective mitigation strategies helped Taiwan to counter the attack of the virus with strong capability. Therefore, technology-based strategies have proven to be vital in fighting the coronavirus disease, and these could become a basis for handling any future crisis that entails.

The impact of quarantine and isolation measures on world economy is observed to be quite dramatic. Almost every industry had to transform their businesses drastically in order to keep up during the pandemic. Small businesses have been affected the most since these have not been able to shift their work using technological platforms like big firms have, due to lack of infrastructure and resources. Data science has played an important role in data-driven decision making. With the exploding number of data sources, descriptive and data analysis techniques are being widely used instead of predictive and automated machine learning-based techniques.

4   Crowd Counting Algorithms

Crowd counting is a technique of counting the number of objects in a given region. The most common algorithm takes as input the images of the given region and provides a count of the objects under consideration. There are numerous crowd counting algorithms which have been developed based on different notions. Real-time crowd counting finds its application in traffic control systems at streets by using live CCTV data feed as input source. Crowd counting may also be applicable in imposing quarantine and social distancing norms by taking into consideration various kinds of inputs. Various standard crowd counting methods have been listed in Table 3.

Table 2 List of dashboards which display COVID-19-related information

Sr. No	Dashboard name	Details
1	John Hopkins University Dashboard	Provides real-time updates of coronavirus disease
2	WHO COVID-19 Dashboard	Provides visualization features to understand pandemic details
3	The University of Washington Dashboard	Provides an overview of COVID-19 infections worldwide
4	SharedGeo	Uses data analytics to track COVID-19
5	South China Morning Post Dashboard	Provides details about the virus outbreak
6	CDC Dashboard	Evaluates the pandemic over infection dates and racial groups
7	COVID tracking project	Provides details about positive and negative cases along with deaths
8	Epidemic Calculator	Collects region-wise data and provides information about disease outlook
9	ECDC Dashboard	Provides efficient visualization maps for distribution of COVID-19
10	University of Virgina COVID-19 Dashboard	Provides visualization maps with real-time updates on COVID-19 outbreak
11	91-DIVOC	Normalizes country and state-wise data to provide virus tracking information
12	Carnegie Melon Dashboard	Provides simulation of coronavirus patterns
13	Stanford COVID-19 Dashboard	Provides data on location and cumulative deaths
14	COVID Trends	Performs graphical analysis on total and new coronavirus cases
15	COVID19-SEIR	Transmission and death rates could be used to assess the coronavirus situation in a given region
16	Rt Covid-19 Dashboard	Monitors the rate of spread in a given population
17	IHME COVID-19 Dashboard	Focuses on curve flattening by simulating the variables
18	Worldometer	Provides information about aggregate number of virus cases
19	COVID ACT Now Dashboard	Explains growth curve of COVID-19
20	COVID-19 Measures Oxford	Provides visualizations to show government data on COVID-19
21	Microsoft Bing COVID-19 Tracker	Provides a web portal to track coronavirus cases worldwide
22	HealthMap	Provides disease monitoring and real time surveillance for health threats

Table 3 Crowd counting methods

Method	Description
Detection-based methods	Using a window-like detector to find the count
Regression-based methods	Ability to extract low-level features also
Density estimation-based methods	Learning a linear mapping between the extracted features and density maps
Convolutional neural network(CNN)-based methods	Take entire image as input and generate count. CSRNet architecture based on deep learning is widely used

CNN-based crowd counting algorithms could be highly beneficial to assist in maintaining social distancing at public places. A template of an algorithm has been shown in Fig. 5. Let n be the number of permissible number of people in an area and d be the permissible distance between them. Then, a basic algorithm can be designed as shown to build a social distancing mechanism.

There are numerous techniques of crowd counting such as counting by detection, counting by regression, counting by density estimation, counting by clustering and counting using convolutional neural networks (CNNs). CSRNet is a popular architecture which uses deep CNN to capture high-level features and generate efficient density maps [17].

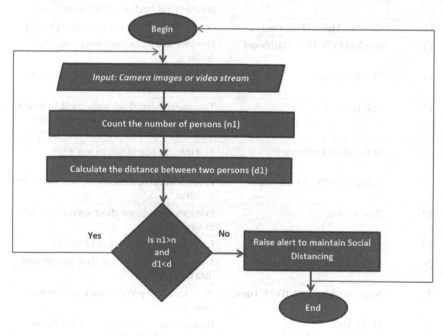

Fig. 5 Algorithm for social distancing using crowd counting

Crowd counting algorithms along with facial feature recognition software can also be used in order to find out number of unmasked people out of a population in an area and accordingly raise alarms. Nowadays, data would normally contain sparse crowds due to lockdowns and the fear of the disease; algorithms may be devised and modified according to the need of the hour.

5 Quarantine Impact on Mental Health

The quarantine and social distancing norms imposed during COVID-19 pandemic have led to numerous psychological and mental disorders. As per a case study on Italian population, participants were divided into various groups depending upon how exposed they were to the virus. Assessment was done using surveys and questionnaire, and it was concluded that the quarantine may have detrimental effect on mental health. Therefore, preventive measures need to be taken in order to address these issues. To deal with mental health issues, artificial intelligence chatbots prove to be an effective measure as these do not involve any intervention by people. The stereotypes associated with mental health are deep rooted in the minds of people, which may be addressed by building AI chatbots [18]. According to various studies [17], there are about 41 unique chatbots in practice to assist in mental health issues, most of them being in the USA. These chatbots can be used for training, therapy and screening. Siri and Cortana are the voice assistants which are used by millions of people worldwide. Following are some of the examples of mental health chatbots [19, 20].

5.1 Woebot

This chatbot monitors the moods of the people and provides thoughts and emotions sharing platform. It is built on the model of cognitive behavioral therapy (CBT). Natural language processing is at the core of these chatbots. It becomes quite comfortable for the mentally upset people to share their thoughts and feelings with the bots as there is no risk of being judged or misinterpreted.

5.2 Moodkit and Moodnotes

Moodkit is developed by mobile application development company named Thriveport to deliver a kit to the users which can help alleviate mental illness issues. The kit consists of a number of applications to address various issues. Moodnotes takes as input the mood of the user and provides a rating and description on the mood.

5.3 Pacifia

This application deals with anxiety issues by providing tools for meditation, relaxation and health tracking. There are audio exercises for breathing and muscle relaxation. Health tracker monitors anxiety issues related to sleeplessness, caffeine, alcohol intake, etc.

5.4 Wysa

It is an emotionally intelligent conversational entity which may help users control their emotions and thoughts by using various applications and tools.

5.5 Joy App

This app is founded by Danny Freed for a friend who suffered from depression. This app measures physical activity, movement and moods of the people.

These applications may be modified to include the more tools and techniques to address mental health issues caused due to quarantine and isolation imposed during the pandemic for the safety of the people.

6 AI/ML/DL Algorithms

Various artificial intelligence, machine learning and deep learning algorithms are being used by the researchers all over the world to perform various kinds of investigations related to COVID-19 pandemic. The relation between various kinds of techniques has been shown in Fig. 6. The research studies are being conducted using various publically available datasets as listed in Table 4.

Various techniques of machine learning such as decision trees, association rules, data mining, predictive analytics, reinforcement learning and big data visualizations are being used to identify patterns in data and yield new information [27, 28].

CT scan images can be processed using deep learning to automatically detect the presence of the disease so that the monitoring of the patient could be effective. A sample machine learning model has been shown in Fig. 7. Such techniques of automatic detection may prove beneficial by providing faster results, so that the strict quarantine norms could be applied on the basis of the rise in the number of cases in a particular area.

The impact of imposing quarantine norms and their effectiveness can also be measured by comparing with the rise in the number of cases over a period of time

Fig. 6 Relation between various techniques

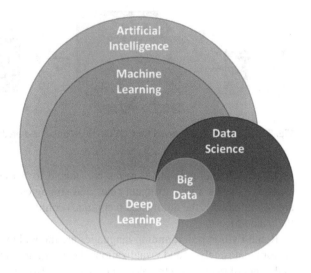

Table 4 Various COVID-19 datasets

Sr. No	Dataset Name and Access Information	Description
1	COVID-19 Open Research Dataset Challenge (CORD-19) [21] https://www.kaggle.com/allen-institute-for-ai/CORD-19-research-challenge	An AI challenge with AI2, CZI, MSR, Georgetown, NIH & The White House
2	Novel Corona Virus 2019 Dataset [22] https://www.kaggle.com/sudalairajku mar/novel-corona-virus-2019-dataset	Provides day level information on COVID-19 affected cases
3	COVID-19 in India [23] https://www.kaggle.com/sudalairajku mar/covid19-in-india	Dataset on Novel Corona Virus Disease 2019 in India
4	CORONAVIRUS (COVID-19) TWEETS DATASET [24] https://ieee-dataport.org/open-access/cor onavirus-covid-19-tweets-dataset	It contains IDs and sentiment scores of the tweets related to the COVID-19 pandemic
5	Novel Coronavirus (COVID-19) Cases Data [25] https://data.humdata.org/dataset/novel-coronavirus-2019-ncov-cases	Novel Corona Virus (COVID-19) epidemiological data since January 22, 2020
6	COVID-19 Coronavirus data [26] https://data.europa.eu/euodp/en/data/dat aset/covid-19-coronavirus-data	This dataset contains the latest available information on COVID-19 including a daily situation update, the epidemiological curve and the global geographical distribution (EU/EEA and the UK, worldwide)

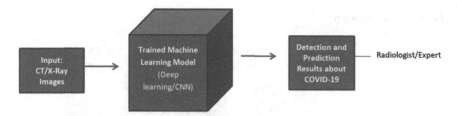

Fig. 7 Machine learning model for COVID-19 detection and prediction

in an area. If the quarantine norms are unable to witness a steady decline in the number of cases, more stringent rules and strategies could be developed for those areas. In this way, the automated techniques could assist in mitigating the effects of the pandemic.

R and Python programming languages are the widely used languages in order to perform data analysis and visualizations. Due to quarantine, there have been changes in the diet of people and the physical activity is also low. Therefore, a rise in the risk of cardiovascular diseases has been observed [26]. Such issues need to be taken into consideration while developing quarantine norms.

7 E-Quarantine Systems

E-Quarantine [29] systems refer to smart health monitoring systems for people who have been quarantined at remote places, rather than being available in the hospital itself. It has been difficult to accommodate people in large numbers in the hospitals, and the risk of infection is more if people with mild symptoms are also quarantined at the hospitals. Therefore, such people can be remotely monitored to check their health status with respect to the disease.

This system involves the use of sensors to monitor various body parameters rather than exposing the health staff to the virus carriers. These parameters include measuring the patient's body temperature, respiration rate, pulse rate, blood pressure and time. Routine monitoring can be carried out, and medication can be suggested on the basis of the health condition. The data collected from various sensors is combined using data fusion technology and then alerts may be sent to hospitals or emergency services. The risk levels of the patients can be traced.

8 Risk Assessment of Easing the Quarantine and Social Distancing Norms

Since almost all commercial activities, schools, universities and industries are shut in the wake of the pandemic, it is necessary to identify the risks associated with easing the quarantine and social distancing norms. This risk assessment may help in effective decision making whether or not to ease the norms. Machine learning algorithms can be used to assist in this risk assessment by analyzing the available public data. In case there is a rise in the number of cases in a particular region, the ease in social distancing norms should be revised and stringent measures should be taken.

The identification of high-risk patients in an area also provides necessary information to health systems to scale up and expand their services on demand. Machine learning-enabled chatbots have the capability to automatically screen people for COVID-19 symptoms [30]. Risk assessment also provides timely information to manage agricultural sector as well by introducing crop monitoring systems based on artificial intelligence.

9   Alert Generation Systems

When people are enforced to stay in quarantine due to travel history to infected regions or contact tracing with infected people, there is a necessary requirement of continuous monitoring to check whether they are following the government imposed quarantine period or not. This needs to be ensured so that others can be safeguarded [31]. Therefore, there are several alert generation systems being implemented as follows:

- Several COVID quarantine alert generation systems have been implemented by various government agencies to track the movement of people during quarantine period.
- GPS-enabled monitoring apps, drone camera systems, CCTV surveillance, facial recognition and wrist bands are some of the systems which help in generating alerts in case of any violations [32].
- In China, a color-coded health rating system had been deployed which monitored millions of people in various cities. It assigned green, yellow or red color on the basis of travel and medical history of the people. At various public spaces, the color codes and the temperature of the person were checked to allow entry. Only those who were assigned green color codes were allowed to move in public spaces [33].
- Drones having facial recognition capability were used to give warnings to people to not to move out of their homes [34].

Therefore, the use of alert generation systems has proven effective in controlling the spread of coronavirus.

10 Conclusions and Discussions

Due to the lack of availability of vaccine of coronavirus disease, quarantine, social distancing and isolation are the only measures which could help control its infectious spread. Quarantine and isolation are suggested in case a person comes into direct contact with a potential victim of the virus or has infected himself.

Social distancing is however a means to be followed by all individuals to safeguard themselves. The quarantine norms may be relaxed in the areas where the infection cases are not severe. However, continuous risk assessment of the effects of relaxations in quarantine norms needs to be done. This is where technology comes into picture.

Artificial intelligence and machine learning tools and techniques help in measuring the impact of quarantine in various areas and provide recommendations for decision making. In this chapter, following points have been addressed.

- Machine learning models can be implemented on publicly available data in order to detect and predict the disease in various regions of the world. The quarantine impact can be analyzed by comparing the number of cases in different regions.
- The data that is being generated with respect to the COVID-19 pandemic from different sources and having different volume and variety may be termed as big data. To view the analysis of such data, big data visualization tools can be used.
- Data science is an important technology to address various challenges during the pandemic as it is a science that revolves around the study of data. The huge amount of data related to COVID-19 has huge potential to provide predictions and insights into the disease and its patterns. These patterns may be useful to impose required norms in the said regions.
- Machine learning-based crowd counting algorithms can be deployed to check for social distancing violations at public places. The simultaneous location-based tracking can be done for those who violate the social distancing norms.
- Mental health, stigma and psychological imbalances are some of the major issues associated with the quarantined people. These may be analyzed with the help of conversational entities called chatbots. There are numerous chatbots which are freely as well as commercially available for this purpose.
- E-quarantine systems are a new paradigm in the age of coronavirus disease. Since the number of cases is rising, the limited resources at hospitals have witnessed huge challenges of accommodating infected people. To address this issue, people are quarantined away from hospitals. To monitor them, e-quarantine systems could be highly beneficial.
- Risk assessment of ease and relaxations in the quarantine norms should be done on a regular basis, since most of the people are now exhausted with the lockdowns, so they are moving out despite huge risk. People should be made aware of why such risks need to be avoided.
- There are some famous chatbots which can help to curb COVID-19 induced mental anxiety such as PinkyMind, YourDost, VentAllOut, IWill, Wysa and MFine [2].

- The survival rates of the infected people can also be predicted with the help of medical AI. This also involves many machine learning techniques. The survival rate is also an important parameter in planning the mitigation of the disease.
- Early warning systems using wearable devices may be used to ensure preparedness.

Therefore, the planning and response in COVID-19 pandemic can be assisted with the help of digital technologies especially artificial intelligence and machine learning. Governments have been working hard to develop strategies of quarantine and phased lockdowns. The streets of the world are now reopening amidst the strong waves of the virus to handle the declining economy. This brings out the most challenging phase of the pandemic, where the cases are rising exponentially but still the life has to go on.

The quarantine and social distancing norms play an important role here, which need to be addressed with careful considerations. Machine learning tools may be effectively used to address all these challenges and help in solving the major issues during the worldwide crisis. Various open-source softwares such as Python, R and DialogFlow can be exploited in order to develop more tools. The challenges posed by existing techniques, the accuracy and privacy concerns should be taken into consideration while devising new tools in accordance with the sustainability with the environment which should be the most important parameter.

References

1. WHO (2020) WHO Director-General's opening remarks at the media briefing on COVID-19. Available (Online). https://www.who.int/dg/speeches/detail/who-director-general-s-opening-remarks-at-the-media-briefing-on-covid-19---8-june-2020
2. Ai T, Yang Z, Hou H, Zhan C, Chen C, Lv W et al (2020) Correlation of chest CT and RT-PCR testing in Coronavirus Disease 2019 (COVID-19) in China: a report of 1014 cases. Radiology, p. 200642
3. WHO Situation Reports. https://www.who.int/emergencies/diseases/novelcoronavirus-2019/situation-reports
4. Mahalle PN, Sable NP, Mahalle NP, Shinde GR (2020) Predictive analytics of COVID-19 using information, communication and technologies
5. Gallagher MB. Model quantifies the impact of quarantine measures on Covid-19's spread. Available (Online). https://news.mit.edu/2020/new-model-quantifies-impact-quarantine-measures-covid-19-spread-0416
6. Dandekar R, Barbastathis G (2020) Quantifying the effect of quarantine control in Covid-19 infectious spread using machine learning. medRxiv
7. Dandekar R, Barbastathis G (2020) Neural Network aided quarantine control model estimation of COVID spread in Wuhan, China. arXiv preprint arXiv:2003.09403
8. Dandekar R, Barbastathis G (2020) Neural network aided quarantine control model estimation of global Covid-19 spread. arXiv preprint arXiv:2004.02752
9. Soures N, Chambers D, Carmichael Z, Daram A, Shah DP, Clark K, Kudithipudi D (2020) SIRNet: understanding social distancing measures with hybrid neural network model for COVID-19 infectious spread. arXiv preprint arXiv:2004.10376
10. Machine Learning predicts the impact of quarantine. Available (Online). https://www.upgrad.com/blog/machine-learning-predicts-the-impact-of-quarantine/

11. Machine Learning tools predict impact of quarantine on COVID-19. Available (Online). https://healthitanalytics.com/news/machine-learning-tools-predict-impact-of-quarantine-on-covid-19

12. Big Data dashboard tracks COVID-19 cases and response in Indiana. Available (Online). https://healthitanalytics.com/news/big-data-dashboard-tracks-covid-19-cases-and-response-in-indiana

13. New MIT machine learning model shows relaxing quarantine rules will spike COVID19 cases. Available (Online). https://techcrunch.com/2020/04/16/new-mit-machine-learning-model-shows-relaxing-quarantine-rules-will-spike-covid-19-cases/

14. It's a Record-Breaking Crowd! A Must-Read Tutorial to Build your First Crowd Counting Model using Deep Learning. Available (Online). https://www.analyticsvidhya.com/blog/2019/02/building-crowd-counting-model-python/

15. Data Science, Quarantined. Available (Online). https://sloanreview.mit.edu/article/data-science-quarantined/

16. Abd-alrazaq AA, Alajlani M, Alalwan AA, Bewick BM, Gardner P, Househ M (2019) An overview of the features of chatbots in mental health: a scoping review. Int J Med Informatics 132:103978

17. Giallonardo V, Sampogna G, Del Vecchio V, Luciano M, Albert U, Carmassi C, Pompili M (2020) The impact of quarantine and physical distancing following COVID-19 on mental health: study protocol of a multicentric Italian population trial. Front Psychiatry 11

18. Top 6 chatbots helping to curb Covid-19 induced mental anxiety. Available (Online). https://www.analyticsinsight.net/top-6-chatbots-helping-curb-covid-19-induced-mental-anxiety/

19. Lovejoy CA (2019) Technology and mental health: the role of artificial intelligence. Eur Psychiatry 55:1–3

20. Moore JR, Caudill R (2019) The bot will see you now: a history and review of interactive computerized mental health programs. Psychiatric Clinics 42(4):627–634

21. COVID-19 Open Research Dataset Challenge (CORD-19). Available (Online). https://www.kaggle.com/allen-institute-for-ai/CORD-19-research-challenge

22. Novel Corona Virus 2019 Dataset. Available (Online). https://www.kaggle.com/sudalairajkumar/novel-corona-virus-2019-dataset

23. COVID-19 in India. Available (Online). https://www.kaggle.com/sudalairajkumar/covid19-in-india

24. CORONAVIRUS (COVID-19) TWEETS DATASET. Available (Online). https://ieee-dataport.org/open-access/coronavirus-covid-19-tweets-dataset

25. Novel Coronavirus (COVID-19) Cases Data. Available (Online). https://data.humdata.org/dataset/novel-coronavirus-2019-ncov-cases

26. COVID-19 Coronavirus data. Available (Online). https://data.europa.eu/euodp/en/data/dataset/covid-19-coronavirus-data

27. Jesus AD. Chatbots for mental health and therapy—comparing 5 current apps and use cases. Available (Online).:https://emerj.com/ai-application-comparisons/chatbots-mental-health-therapy-comparing-5-current-apps-use-cases/

28. Wang S, Kang B, Ma J, Zeng X, Xiao M, Guo J, …, Xu B (2020) A deep learning algorithm using CT images to screen for Corona Virus Disease (COVID-19). MedRxiv

29. El-Din DM, Hassanein AE, Hassanien EE, Hussein WM (2020) E-Quarantine: a smart health system for monitoring coronavirus patients for remotely quarantine. arXiv preprint arXiv:2005.04187

30. Mattioli AV, Sciomer S, Cocchi C, Maffei S, Gallina S (2020) Quarantine during COVID-19 outbreak: changes in diet and physical activity increase the risk of cardiovascular disease. In: Nutrition metabolism and cardiovascular diseases

31. Machine Learning Models Estimate Seasonal Impact of COVID-19. Available (Online). https://healthitanalytics.com/news/machine-learning-models-estimate-seasonal-impact-of-covid-19

32. Wearable provides COVID-19 early warning system. Available (Online). https://www.eenewsembedded.com/news/wearable-provides-covid-19-early-warning-system

33. Yan L, Zhang HT, Xiao Y, Wang M, Sun C, Liang J, …, Tang X (2020) Prediction of survival for severe Covid-19 patients with three clinical features: development of a machine learning-based prognostic model with clinical data in Wuhan. medRxiv
34. Medical AI can now predict survival rates—but it's not ready to unleash on patients. Available (Online). https://theconversation.com/medical-ai-can-now-predict-survival-rates-but-its-not-ready-to-unleash-on-patients-127039
35. Chawla S, Mittal M, Chawla M, Goyal LM (2020) Corona Virus-SARS-CoV-2: an insight to another way of natural disaster. EAI Endorsed Trans Pervasive Health Technol, May 2020

Author Index